# *Comparative Neurobiology*

Peter J. Mill

Senior Lecturer in Pure and Applied Zoology,
University of Leeds

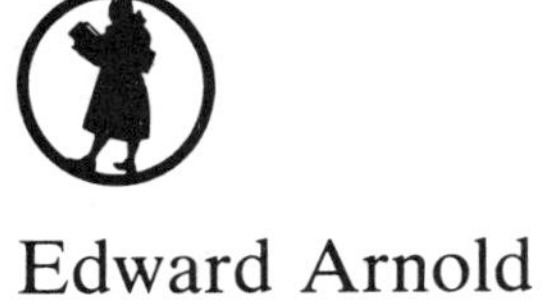

Edward Arnold

First published 1982
by Edward Arnold (Publishers) Limited
41 Bedford Square, London WC1B 3DQ



**British Library Cataloguing in Publication Data**

Mill, Peter J.
Comparative neurobiology. – (Contemporary biology)
1. Neurobiology
I. Title II. Series
591.1′88 QP355.Z

ISBN 0-7131-2810-0



Text set in 10/11pt Linotron 202 Times, printed and bound in Great Britain at The Pitman Press, Bath

# *Preface*

The primary aim of this book is to serve as an introductory neurobiology text for undergraduates. As far as possible the approach is comparative, with examples chosen from both invertebrate and vertebrate work, since I feel that this will help to give the reader a greater feeling for, and depth of understanding of, neurobiology. The first chapter deals with the structure of nerve and muscle. Nerve and muscle cells share the ability not only to maintain a large potential difference across their surface membranes (Chapter 2), but also to restore this potential difference after a change in its level has been effected by an event external to the cell, such as an environmental stimulus or activity in another nerve cell. Information passes from one cell to the next via narrow discontinuities, called synapses, which in most cases only conduct the information in one direction. Two types of potential change occur, graded potentials and action potentials. Graded potentials are not propagated and are hence decremental and serve for integration at a local level, while action potentials have an 'all-or-none' property and are propagated and hence are used to code information for transport over long distances. The concept of excitability and the basic differences between the two types of potential change are dealt with in Chapter 3. Chapter 4 is concerned with the graded potentials, which occur both in sensory cells, as a result of the transduction of external stimuli, and post-synaptically in nerve and muscle cells. Chapter 5 considers synaptic transmission in more detail, while Chapter 6 deals with the action potential and Chapter 7 with muscle physiology. The next two chapters are concerned with the structure and physiology of the various types of sense organs, Chapter 8 dealing with mechanoreceptors, Chapter 9 with photoreceptors, chemoreceptors, thermoreceptors and electroreceptors. Central nervous systems and the integration of sensory information are dealt with in Chapter 10, while the last chapter considers the neural control of behaviour, a rapidly expanding area of neurobiology. The figures have been carefully selected to supplement the text and to cover a wide range of literature. Further references, in the form of reviews, edited volumes and books are given at the end of the book. These methods of referencing should provide the reader with sufficient sources to enable him or her to follow up any area of neurobiology, and have the merit that the flow of the text is not interrupted by innumerable literature references.

I should like to thank Professor E. J. W. Barrington, F.R.S., who suggested to me that I should write this book, and who has since offered encouragement and much useful advice, and the staff of Edward Arnold for their help, particularly during the editorial stages. I should also like to thank my wife for her continued support and understanding throughout the preparation and writing of this book.

University of Leeds, P.J.M.
1982.

# Contents

# 1

# *The Structure of Nerve and Muscle*

## NEURONS (NERVE CELLS)

Neurons which conduct information towards the central nervous system are classically called ***sensory*** or ***afferent neurons***; those which conduct information out from the central nervous system are called ***motor*** or ***efferent neurons***; while those which are contained completely within the central nervous system and whose function it is to distribute and integrate information within the latter are termed ***interneurons*** or, in vertebrates, ***internuncial neurons***. Implicit in this definition of interneurons is that they both receive information from, and transmit it to, other neurons. However, there are some neurons which do not fall neatly into one of the above three categories. These are the so-called dual-function neurons which have an output both on to other neurons and on to an effector organ such as a muscle. An example of this type of neuron is the Right Pedal Giant (RPG) of molluscs. Many mammalian motor neurons could also be ascribed to this category as they synapse with interneurons (the Renshaw cells) as well as with muscle fibres (see p. 204). In this case, however, the Renshaw cell is a controlling device for the same motor neuron which synapses with it and is thus functionally an integral part of the motor output.

All neurons have certain features in common, but there is no such thing as a typical neuron—Fig. 1.1 shows just a few of the many different forms which they take. There is always a cell body (***soma***) and, in many cases, a division of the peripheral processes into one or more which receive information (***dendrites***), and one which conducts information towards the next cell (***axon***).

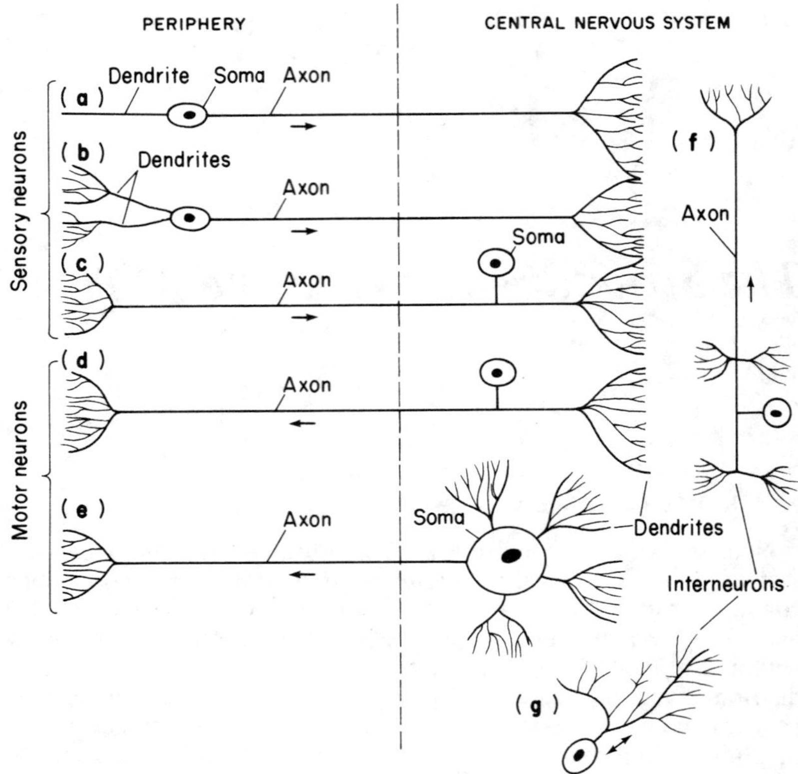


**Fig. 1.1** Diagrammatic representation of a selection of neuron types. (**a**) Arthropod bipolar sensory neuron; (**b**) arthropod multipolar sensory neuron; (**c**) vertebrate sensory neuron; (**d**) arthropod motor neuron; (**e**) mammalian motor neuron; (**f**) arthropod intersegmental interneuron; (**g**) amacrine cell (local interneuron). Arrows indicate the direction of information flow.

Arthropod sensory neurons (Fig. 1.1a,b) nearly always have their cell body in the periphery and, in addition to a long axon, have either one dendrite (bipolar cells; Fig. 1.1a) or several dendrites (multipolar cells; Fig. 1.1b). The dendrite of a bipolar cell may be unbranched, as in some stretch receptors (p. 129) and in chordotonal organs (p. 140), or branched as in the majority of stretch receptors (p. 129). The dendrites of multipolar cells are typically branched. In contrast to these neurons the cell body of the vertebrate sensory neuron (Fig. 1.1c) lies in a ganglion adjacent to the nerve cord and is connected to its axon by a short process, an arrangement termed pseudo-unupolar. The relationship between the soma and its processes in the arthropod motor neuron (Fig. 1.1d) is similar to that in the vertebrate sensory neuron, while the mammalian motor neuron (Fig. 1.1e) has several branched dendrites arising directly from its soma and is thus a multipolar neuron. The axon of all these cells is branched at one end and the terminations of the branches are often dilated into 'axon terminals'. Interneurons may also have a long axon (Fig. 1.1f).

If can be seen from the above examples that there is a functional paradox in the use of the term 'axon'. In the arthropod sensory neuron information in the form of action potentials (see Chapter 7) is transmitted along the axon away from the cell body, whereas in the vertebrate sensory neuron the axon transmits information towards the cell body over much of its length. Thus the term axon is applied to any long nerve cell process which is unbranched except at its end(s). However, it also applies to the long processes of interneurons which, in many instances, have side branches (Fig. 1.1f).

There are many interneurons in which an axon, as defined above, is not present. One example is the amacrine cell (microneuron), which has a single, branched process (Fig. 1.1g), some branches of which receive information whilst others distribute it; although it cannot be ruled out that some branches may do both. The branches are all of limited extent and, in arthropods for example, remain within the confines of the ganglion which contains the cell body.

When fixed and stained in what is currently the conventional manner for examination in the transmission electron microscope (i.e. fixation in glutaraldehyde with post-fixation in osmium, followed by staining the sections with lead citrate and uranyl acetate), sections of a neuron reveal the following structure.

The cell is surrounded by a membrane consisting of a light zone bordered by two electron dense zones, each zone being about 2.5 nm wide. It is not obviously different from other plasma membranes and, like them, is called a unit membrane. The appearance of this membrane has been explained as a double layer of phospholipid molecules sandwiched between two layers of protein molecules (Fig. 1.2). The phospholipid molecules each have a centrally directed hydrophobic (water-repellent) non-polar region and an outwardly directed hydrophilic (water-attracting) polar region; the protein molecules are attached to the latter. Ion channels (pores) in the membrane may well be lined with protein, and the passage of ions through them (pp. 33, 77) may be regulated by their diameter and/or by the charge on their walls.

The nucleus of a neuron often has a prominent nucleolus (or nucleoli). Rough endoplasmic reticulum is fairly abundant in the soma region and smooth endoplasmic reticulum associated with vesicles (Golgi body) is often in evidence. Where the rough endoplasmic reticulum is juxtaposed to the Golgi body there tends to be a heavy concentration of ribosomes. This corresponds to the Nissl substance of light microscopy. Neurotubules (microtubules) occur in

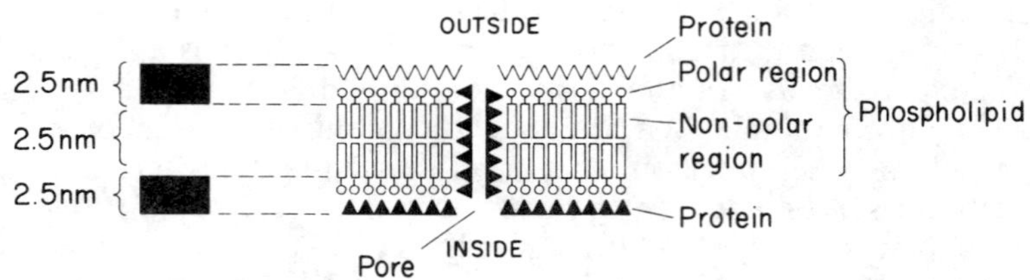


**Fig. 1.2** Hypothetical structure of the unit membrane of a neuron. Its appearance in the electron microscope after osmium treatment is indicated on the left hand side. (After Usherwood, P.N.R. (1973). *Nervous Systems.* Studies in Biology, no. 36. Edward Arnold, London.)

both soma and axon, particularly the latter, where they are longitudinally oriented. With appropriate fixation techniques they have also been observed in the axon terminals. Details of the regions associated with connections between neurons or between neurons and muscles (synapses) will be deferred until the structure of muscles has been dealt with (see p. 22).

## SHEATH CELLS

Associated with neurons are other cells which ensheath them. Within the central nervous system the ensheathing cells are called ***glial cells*** in invertebrates and ***oligodendrocytes*** in vertebrates; in the periphery they are usually referred to simply as ***sheath cells*** in invertebrates and ***Schwann cells*** in vertebrates. In receptors, other names are often used for sheath cells which have a particular functional or structural relationship with the receptor ending. Examples are the tormogen and trichogen cells of insect hairs (p. 117), and the enveloping, scolopale and canal cells of crustacean chordotonal organs (p. 143).

The sheath cells are generally small in volume in comparison with the neurons, although in the central nervous system they often have many ramifying processes. Several cells are required to ensheath a long axon, although at any one point along its length there is generally only a single sheath cell. Several small diameter axons may share a common sheath cell (Fig. 1.3a), but large diameter axons generally have their own (Fig. 1.3b). The juxtaposition of the sheath cell against itself is called the ***mesaxon***. The most complex arrangement seen in invertebrates is when the sheath cell is wrapped several times around an axon (Fig. 1.3c), but in many vertebrate peripheral

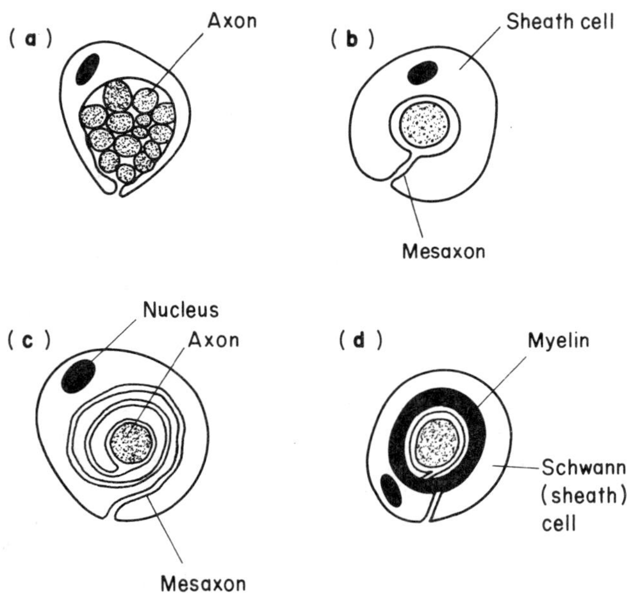


**Fig. 1.3** Diagrams illustrating the types of axon sheath cells. (**a**) A group of several small axons surrounded by a single sheath cell; (**b**) an axon with a single sheath cell and a simple mesaxon; (**c**) an axon surrounded by a sheath cell which is wrapped several times around the axon; (**d**) an axon with a myelin sheath.

axons the enveloping layers of the Schwann cells become closely apposed to each other and fuse to form a myelin sheath (Fig. 1.3d). Such axons are said to be ***myelinated*** or ***medullated***. Since a number of Schwann cells are required to ensheath a whole vertebrate axon, discontinuities occur in the myelin sheath where adjacent Schwann cells meet. These discontinuities are called ***nodes of Ranvier***.

## MUSCLE CELLS

Muscles consist of a number of cells or ***muscle fibres*** which may or may not have a striated appearance. In striated muscles the striations either run at right angles to the longitudinal axis of the muscle fibres (***cross-striated muscle***), or are oriented at an oblique angle (***obliquely striated muscle***). Non-striated muscle is generally called ***smooth muscle***.

All muscle fibres contain protein filaments concerned with the contractile mechanism, as well as sarcoplasmic (endoplasmic) reticulum and mitochondria (sarcosomes). They may possess a single nucleus or be multinucleate.

**Cross-striated muscle**

All arthropod muscles and vertebrate skeletal and cardiac muscles are cross-striated. Each muscle fibre contains two types of longitudinally oriented protein filaments, generally referred to as ***actin*** and ***myosin***, but often called thin and thick filaments respectively. These filaments are organized to varying extents in different muscles into groups called ***myofibrils***. Within each myofibril, and to some extent between adjacent myofibrils, the actin and myosin filaments are each closely aligned. It is primarily this alignment which gives cross-striated muscle its characteristic appearance (Fig. 1.4a–c).

Under the light microscope the individual myofilaments are not visible, but the striations resulting from their alignments can be seen clearly. Thus zones of high birefringency (Anisotropic- or A-bands) alternate with zones of lower birefringency (Isotropic- or I-bands) along the length of the muscle fibre. Under the electron microscope the same basic appearance is seen, with the A-bands darker (i.e. more electron-dense) than the I-bands (Fig. 1.4a–c). Each I-band is bisected, at right angles to the fibre, by a dark narrow line, the Z-line; while the centre of the A-band is generally observed to have a lighter region (the H-zone). The H-zone often has a dark central M-line bounded on either side by a very narrow light zone; this is especially noticeable in vertebrate muscles.

The region between two successive Z-lines is called a ***sarcomere***. Its length varies in different muscles (also in the same muscle, depending on the degree of contraction; see Chapter 7). In relaxed vertebrate skeletal muscle the sarcomere is about 2.5 $\mu$m long. In insect flight and cardiac muscle it is of similar length (2–4 $\mu$m), but is longer in

---

**Fig. 1.4** Cross-striated muscle. (**a**), (**b**) Electron micrographs of longitudinal sections of frog skeletal muscle; (**c**) electron micrograph of longitudinal section of aphid flight muscle. (**d**) Diagram of a longitudinal section through a sarcomere to show the principal regions and to illustrate the relationship between the filaments and these regions. A, A-band; H, H-zone; I, I-band; M, M-line; m, mitochondrion; sr, sarcoplasmic reticulum: t. T-system tubule: Z. Z-line. ((**a**). (**b**) From Franzini-Armstrong, C. (1970). *Journal of Cell Biology*, **47**, 488–99; (**c**) from Smith, D. S. (1965). *Journal of Cell Biology*, **27**, 379–93.)

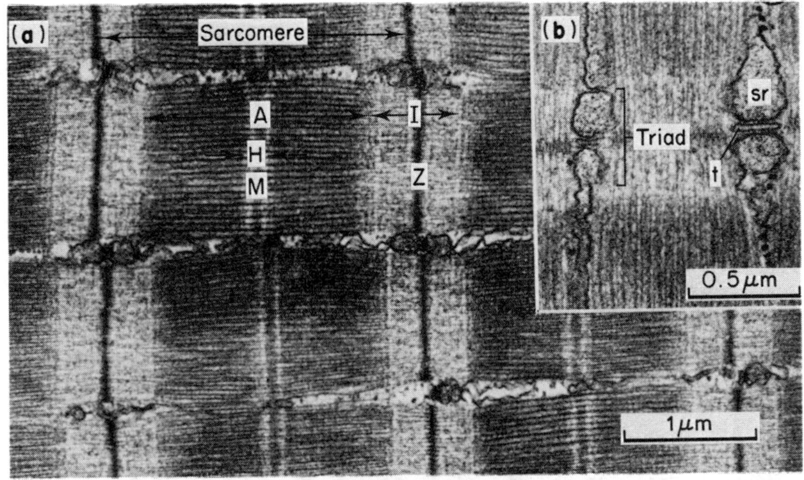

(a)
Sarcomere
A
I
H
M
Z
1 μm
(b)
Triad
sr
t
0.5 μm


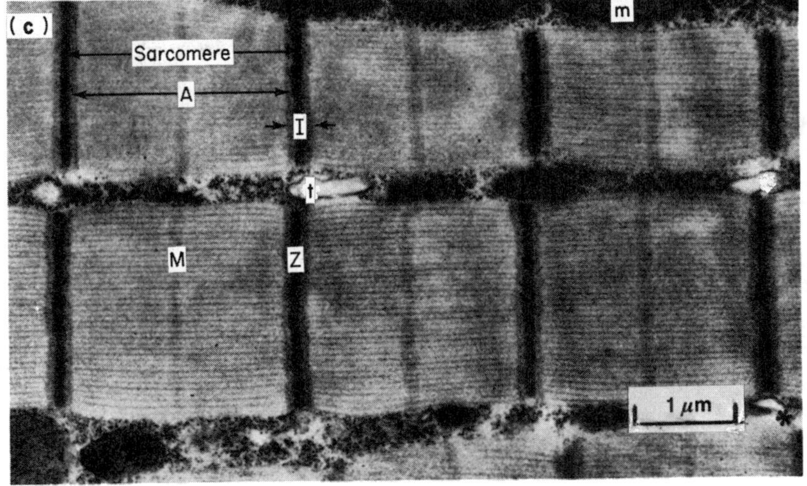

(c)
m
Sarcomere
A
I
t
M
Z
1 μm


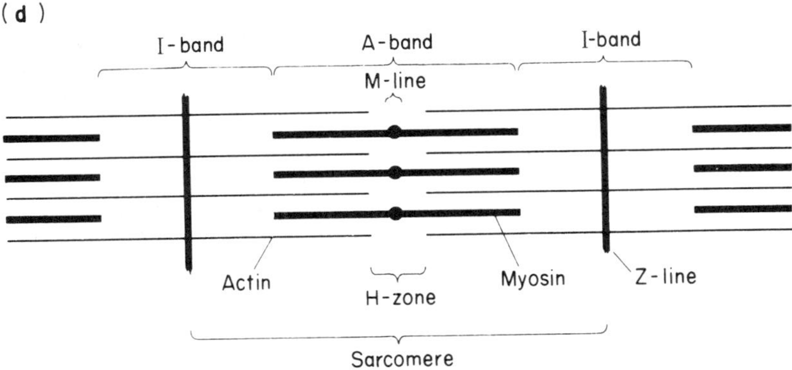

(d)
I-band
A-band
I-band
M-line
Actin
H-zone
Myosin
Z-line
Sarcomere

other insect skeletal (3–7 $\mu$m) and visceral and alary (7–8 $\mu$m) muscles.

Examination with the electron microscope has revealed the detailed structure responsible for the cross-striations. The actin and myosin filaments are arranged in overlapping bands. Thus the I-band contains only actin filaments, attached at one end to the Z-line, while the A-band contains myosin and the ends of the actin filaments (Fig. 1.4d). In relaxed muscle the actin filaments do not reach to the centre of the A-band and this central zone, where the myosin filaments are not overlapped by actin filaments, is the H-zone. The M-line results from a thickening of the myosin filaments in their central region.

In transverse sections, the actin and myosin filaments are seen to be arranged in a regular matrix within each fibril (Figs 1.5, 1.6).

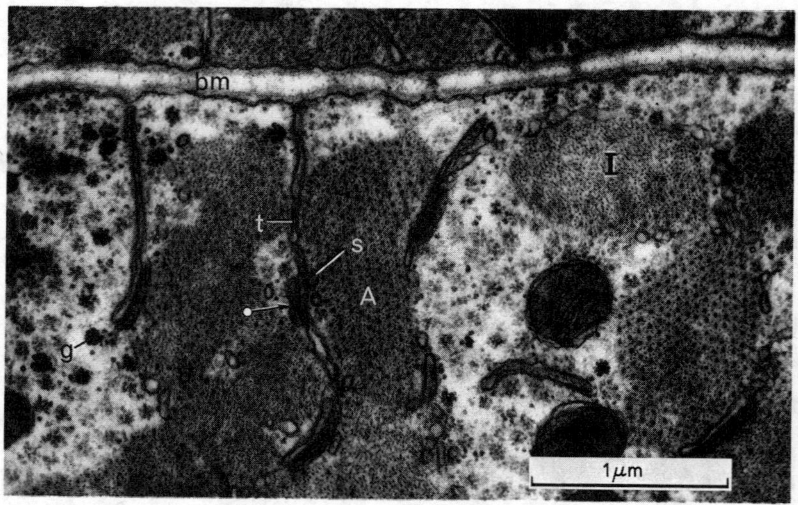


**Fig. 1.5** Cross-striated muscle. An electron micrograph of a transverse section through a skeletal muscle of a dragonfly larva. Due to the slight stagger of adjacent sarcomeres in this muscle, sections through A- and I-bands can be seen. bm, basement membrane; g, glycogen; s, sarcoplasmic reticulum; t, T-system tubule; ○→, dyad. (From Mill, P. J. and Lowe, D. A. (1971). *Journal of Insect Physiology*, **17**, 1947–60.)

Figure 1.6 shows the patterns in various muscles in the region where the actin and myosin filaments overlap (i.e. in the A-band outside the H-zone). Obviously, sections through the I-band and the H-zone will show only actin and myosin filaments respectively (Fig. 1.5), but their matrices remain as in the zone where they overlap. In vertebrate skeletal muscle and insect fibrillar flight muscle, each myosin fila-

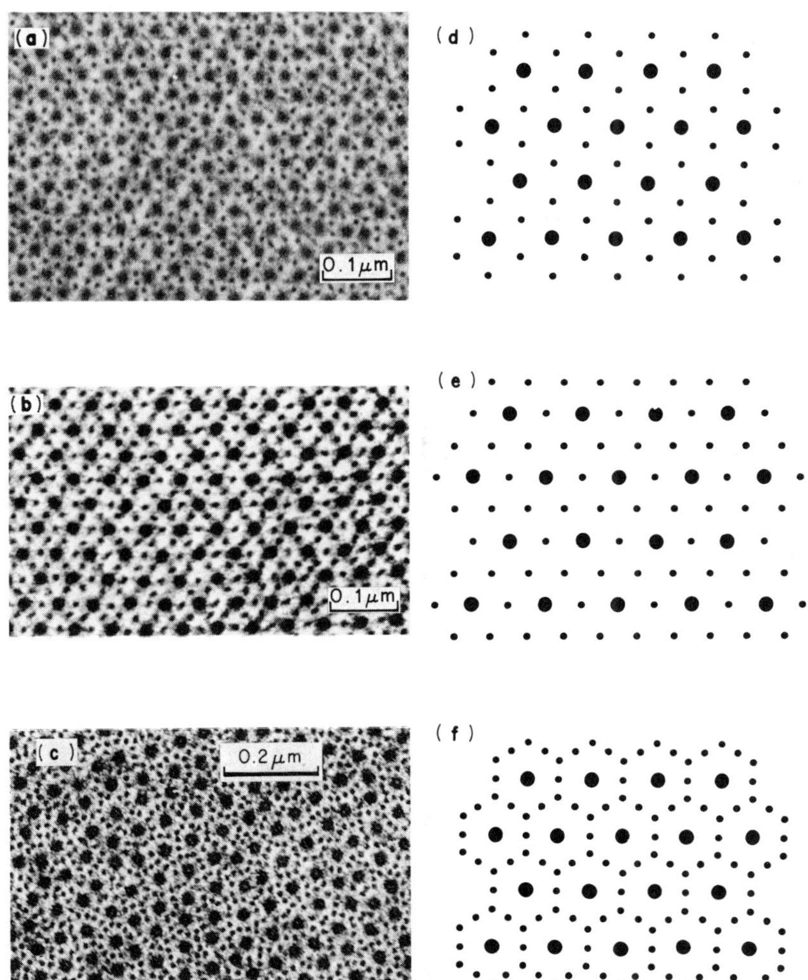


**Fig. 1.6** Cross-striated muscle. Electron micrographs and corresponding diagrams of transverse sections through the overlapping zone of the actin and myosin filaments in various muscles to illustrate the arrays. (**a**), (**d**) Vertebrate (rat) skeletal muscle; (**b**), (**e**) insect (giant water bug) fibrillar flight muscle; (**c**), (**f**) insect (dragonfly larva) skeletal muscle. ((**a**) Photograph by D. Ashworth, Astbury Department of Biophysics, University of Leeds; (**b**) from Ashhurst, D. E. (1967). *Journal of Cell Science*, **2,** 435–44; (**c**) from Mill, P. J. and Lowe, D. A. (1971). *Journal of Insect Physiology*, **17,** 1947–60; (**d**) after Huxley, A. F. (1957). *Progress in Biophysics*, **7,** 255–318; (**e**), (**f**) after Toselli, P. A. and Pepe, F. A. (1968). *Journal of Cell Biology*, **37,** 445–61.)

ment is surrounded by six actin filaments, although there is a different arrangement in the two groups. Thus, in vertebrate muscle, adjacent myosin filaments share two actin filaments (Fig. 1.6a,d), producing an overall actin:myosin ratio of 2:1, whereas in insect fibrillar flight muscle adjacent myosin filaments share only one actin filament (Fig. 1.6b,e), with a consequent actin:myosin ratio of 3:1. In most other insect muscles there is a circle of 10–12 actin filaments surrounding each myosin filament (Fig. 1.6c,f).

The myosin filaments possess side branches (Fig. 1.7) which may be joined to the actin filaments where they overlap, thus forming

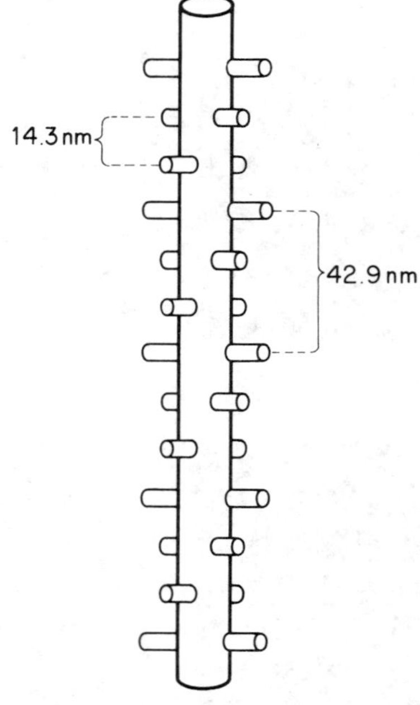


**Fig. 1.7** Diagram of a myosin filament to show the arrangement of the side branches on the backbone of the filament (see text for details). (Redrawn from Huxley, H. E. and Brown, W. (1967). *Journal of Molecular Biology*, **30**, 383–434.)

cross-bridges. These side branches do not occur in the central region of the myosin filaments, and this is thought to be the explanation for the light zone bordering the M-line in the centre of the A-band. There is evidence that the myosin projections occur in opposing pairs, with adjacent pairs lying 14.3 nm apart along the backbone of the myosin filament and rotated by 120° with respect to each other.

The absence of projections in the central region can be explained if the myosin molecules form a myosin filament in the manner shown in Fig. 1.8. The projections are not envisaged as being rigid, as is shown for convenience in Figs 1.7 and 1.8.

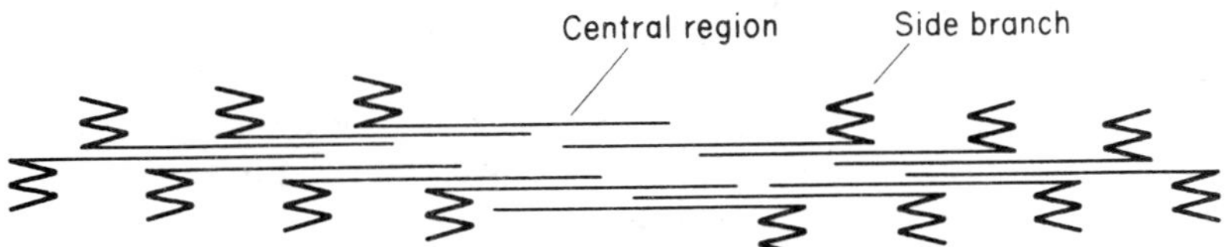


**Fig. 1.8** Diagram showing a possible arrangement of the myosin molecules to form a myosin filament. (Redrawn from Huxley, H. E. (1963). *Journal of Molecular Biology*, **7**, 281–308.)

Thus, each myosin molecule consists of two parts, ***light meromyosin*** forming the backbone of the filament, and ***heavy meromyosin*** forming the side branches (Fig. 1.9). The heavy meromyosin is further separable into a rod-like portion ($S_2$) and a globular portion ($S_1$). The latter is an ATPase, possessing an ATP-binding site as well as an

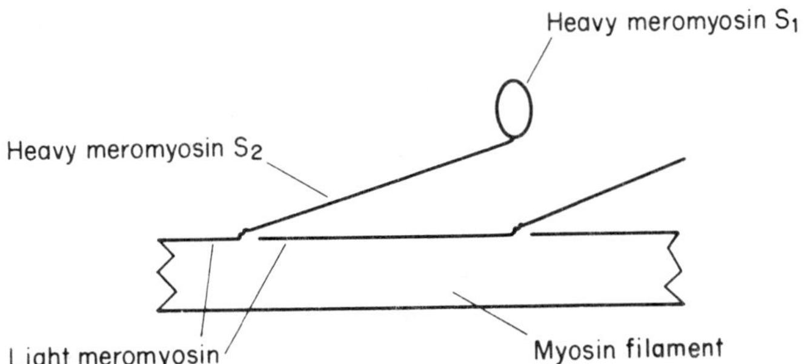


**Fig. 1.9** Diagram illustrating the possible relationship between the light and heavy meromyosin parts of the myosin molecule. The light meromyosin forms the backbone of the myosin filament; the heavy meromyosin the side branch. Heavy meromyosin is divisible into rod-like ($S_2$) and globular ($S_1$) portions. (Redrawn from Huxley, H. E. (1969). *Science*, **164**, 1356–66.)

actin-binding site. In addition, the myosin molecule has a calcium-binding site. It has been suggested that flexible linkages occur in the myosin molecule between the light and heavy meromyosin parts and between the rod-like and globular portions of the heavy meromyosin (Fig. 1.9). The former linkage enables cross-bridges to be established between the myosin and actin filaments at varying distances apart;

the latter allows rotation between the globular component of the heavy meromyosin and the actin filament. These are important elements in the theoretical explanation of the contraction mechanism (see Chapter 7). In some insect flight muscles the myosin filaments also contain some paramyosin.

The actin filaments consist of two chains of actin monomers arranged in a double helix, and are presumed to have active sites at which the myosin projections attach to form the cross-bridges. A tropomyosin molecule lies between the two actin chains, and a third protein, troponin, is attached to the tropomyosin. There is one tropomyosin and one troponin molecule for each seven actin molecules (Fig. 1.10). The troponin molecule consists of three globular

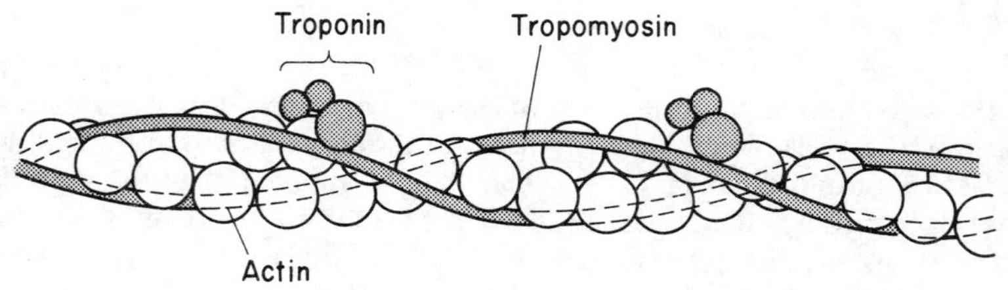


**Fig. 1.10** Diagram illustrating the components of an actin filament. There is a double helical array of G-actin molecules. The tropomyosin molecules are rod-shaped and bonded end to end to form two continuous strands which lie along the sides of the grooves formed by the arrangement of the actin core. Each tropomyosin molecule contacts seven actin molecules and has one troponin complex molecule bonded to it about one third of the way along its length. (After Cohen, C. (1975). *Scientific American*, **233** (No. 5), 36–45 and Squire, J. M. (1975). *Annual Review of Biophysics and Bioengineering*, **4**, 137–63.)

subunits, troponin T, troponin C and troponin I. The T subunit bonds the molecule to the tropomyosin, while the I subunit bonds it to the actin. The C subunit bonds to the T and I subunits (but not directly to the actin or tropomyosin molecules) and also bonds calcium ions.

The actin filaments do not run straight through the Z-line, but are interconnected with the actin filaments of the adjacent sarcomere by short Z filaments.

Mitochondria are generally in evidence in muscle cells and, in the radial flight muscles of dragonflies for example, may occupy a considerable proportion of the cell. Glycogen deposits are also often present in large amounts between the fibrils.

There are two tubular systems—the sarcoplasmic reticulum and the T-system. The sarcoplasmic reticulum corresponds to the endoplasmic reticulum of other cells and is organized with respect to the fibrils in muscle cells. The degree to which it is developed varies considerably in different muscles. In vertebrate and many insect skeletal muscles it is well-developed (Fig. 1.11) and forms a fenestrated envelope around each myofibril. Sarcoplasmic reticulum is also well-developed in the radial and close-packed fibrillar flight muscles of insects. In some crustacean limb muscles it is rather more restricted and consists of collars in the A- and I-band regions, while in some insect muscles it is still less well-developed. In the true fibrillar flight muscles of dipterans, coleopterans and hymenopterans, which are asynchronous (p. 15), the sarcoplasmic reticulum is reduced to isolated vesicles.

The T-system was so named because it is transversely oriented in the muscles in which it was first described (fish skeletal muscle) and, indeed, this is the case in most muscles. It consists of inpushings of the surface membrane of the muscle fibre, of which it is thus a continuation. The system is normally well-developed, although it never reaches the complexity of the sarcoplasmic reticulum (Fig. 1.11).

At certain sites the two tubular systems become closely apposed and septate junctions form between them. In fish and frog skeletal muscle the T-tubules are associated with a pair of sarcoplasmic reticulum tubules in the region of the Z-lines to form triads (Fig. 1.11a, b). In other vertebrates (reptiles, birds and mammals) the triads occur at the A–I-band boundaries (of relaxed muscle). In insects, triads are rarely seen; more usually the T-system tubules are associated with only a single element of the sarcoplasmic reticulum, the resulting structure being termed a dyad. As with the triads of higher vertebrates, dyads are normally found at the A–I-band boundaries of relaxed muscle (Fig. 1.11c).

In some arthropod skeletal muscles there is evidence for a longitudinal component of the T-system. In some cases it is possible that there are two functionally distinct components of the T-system. One consists of the A-tubules, associated with the sarcoplasmic reticulum (forming dyads) and involved with the excitation–contraction coupling process (p. 110). The other consists of the Z-tubules, bearing dilations associated with the Z-material via desmosomes, and possibly having a mechanical role.

*Fast and slow muscles*

Cross-striated muscle fibres can be broadly divided into ***fast (twitch) fibres*** and ***slow (tonic) fibres*** (see p. 106). In crustaceans, fish, amphibians and birds both types are common, but in mammals slow fibres appear to be restricted to the extraocular muscles. In many

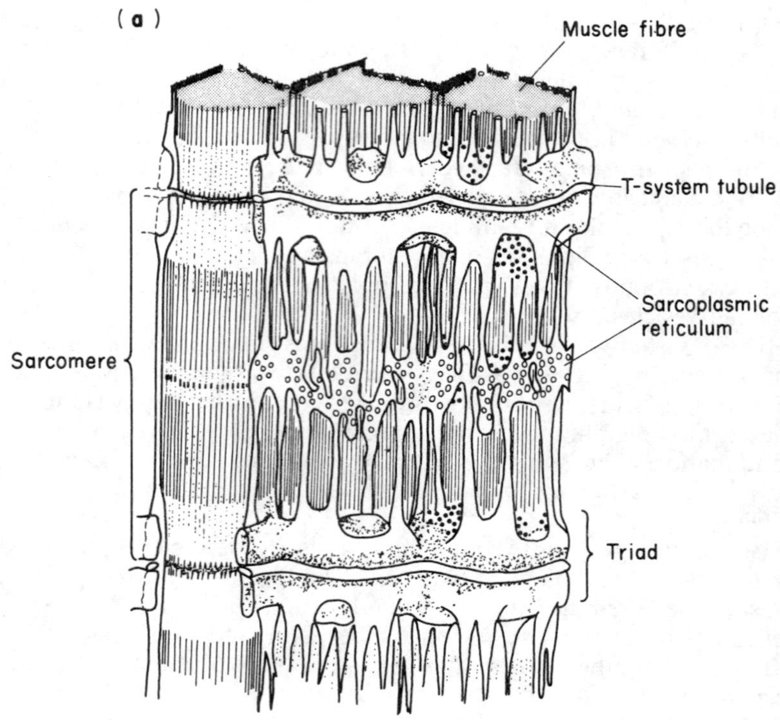


**Fig. 1.11** (**a**) The arrangement of the sarcoplasmic reticulum and the T-system in a frog sartorius muscle fibre. (**b**) Electron micrograph of a longitudinal section of frog skeletal muscle (fast fibre); (**c**) electron micrograph of longitudinal section of dragonfly fibrillar flight muscle. m, mitochondrion; sr, sarcoplasmic reticulum; t, T-system tubule; Z, Z-line. ((**a**) Redrawn from Peachey, L. D. (1965). *Journal of Cell Biology*, **25,** 209–32; (**b**) from Page, S. G. (1965). *Journal of Cell Biology*, **26,** 477–97; (**c**) from Smith, D. S. (1966). *Journal of Cell Biology*, **28,** 109–26.)

cases fast fibres are characterized by complete separation of the fibrils (which produces a punctate appearance in transverse section), abundant sarcoplasmic reticulum and a regular T-system; in vertebrates, the postsynaptic membrane (sarcolemma) is highly folded (see Fig. 1.17). In contrast, the slow fibres are of smaller diameter, the fibrils tend to merge together to give a rather diffuse appearance in transverse section, the sarcoplasmic reticulum is not well-developed and the T-system is irregular or aberrant. Furthermore, in the slow fibres of vertebrates the postsynaptic membrane is not folded; while in arthropods the Z-line is generally wavy and the sarcomere length is relatively long.

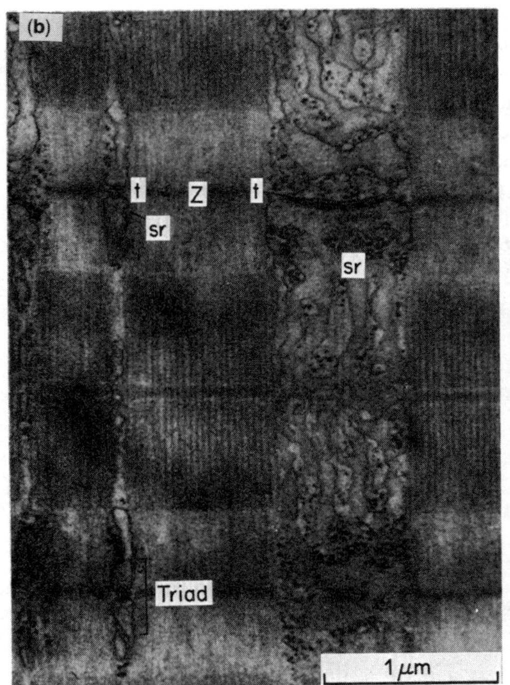


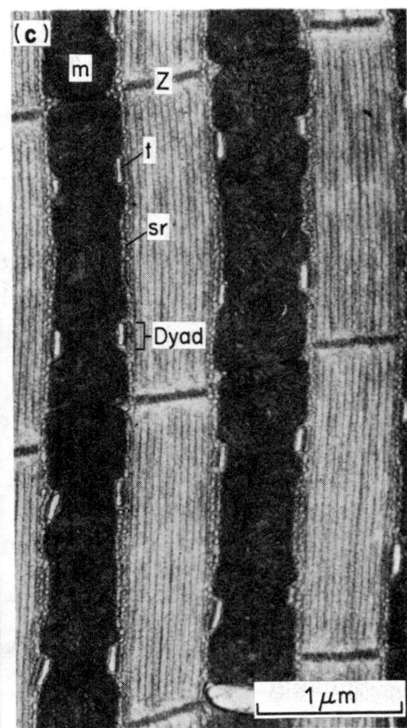


In some crustacean muscles, fibres occur with different sarcomere lengths. Those with short sarcomeres are fast fibres, those with long sarcomeres are slow fibres, while those with intermediate sarcomere lengths exhibit intermediate properties. In other crustacean muscles the fast and slow fibres are not differentiated in this manner; presumably the differences are more at the biochemical level. Some insect muscles contain both long and short sarcomere length fibres but, in the majority, the structural differences between fast and slow fibres are slight. The sarcoplasmic reticulum and the T-system tend to be better developed in fast muscles. However, the fast flight muscles of dipterans present something of a paradox in that their sarcoplasmic reticulum is reduced to small vesicles. This is a rather unusual type of muscle, termed asynchronous because the mechanical oscillations (contractions and relaxations) are not linked, as in most muscles, in a 1:1 manner with the motor input. There is also evidence that in insect muscles the number of actin filaments surrounding each myosin filament is inversely related to the maximum contraction rate of the muscle fibre.

In mammalian skeletal muscle there is a range in the structure and physiology of the fast (twitch) fibres. Thus, A type fibres have a high capacity to utilize glycogen, a low oxidative metabolism and a low myoglobin content; C type fibres have a low capacity to utilize glycogen, a very high oxidative metabolism and a high myoglobin content. The B type fibres are intermediate with respect to glycogen metabolism and myoglobin content but have a high oxidative metabolism. Commensurate with their capacity for oxidative metabolism, the mitochondrial content of the fibres increases from type A through type C. The 'white' muscles of mammals contain a mixture of all three of these fibre types, while the 'red' muscles contain only types B and C. In consequence, although both the white and the red muscles are twitch type muscles, the former are often referred to as 'fast' muscles, the latter as 'slow' muscles. The terms 'fast twitch' and 'slow twitch' respectively will be used in this book in order to avoid confusion.

**Vertebrate cardiac muscle**

Vertebrate cardiac muscle is comprised of two main types of cell: the Purkinje fibres, which are modified for the rapid conduction of the heart contraction, and the contractile cells. While the latter are undoubtedly cross-striated, their structure differs from that of other vertebrate cross-striated muscles in that the individual fibres do not run the full length of the muscle, are not precisely aligned (in terms of their cross-striations) with one another, and are joined to each other by intercalated discs (Fig. 1.12). Part of each disc contains a region where the membranes of the two adjacent cells are closely apposed to form a tight junction or nexus, which functions as an electrical synapse (see Chapter 5). Cardiac muscle also differs from skeletal muscle in that it is innervated by the autonomic nervous system (p. 226).

**Obliquely striated muscle**

Obliquely striated muscle is found in many of the soft-bodied invertebrate phyla. In annelids and nematodes all of the muscles are of this type; in molluscs it is of more limited occurrence.

Obliquely striated muscle, like cross-striated, consists of sarcomeres which contain both thin and thick myofilaments. The thin filaments are composed of actin but the thick ones are composed of paramyosin instead of myosin, and are consequently thicker than the corresponding filaments in cross-striated muscle. The actin filaments are attached to Z-material at one end and interdigitate with the paramyosin filaments at the other, thus producing the same sarcomere arrangement of an A-band flanked by two half I-bands.

However, in cross-striated muscle the Z-material is arranged in discs or plates and hence there is a three dimensional array of actin

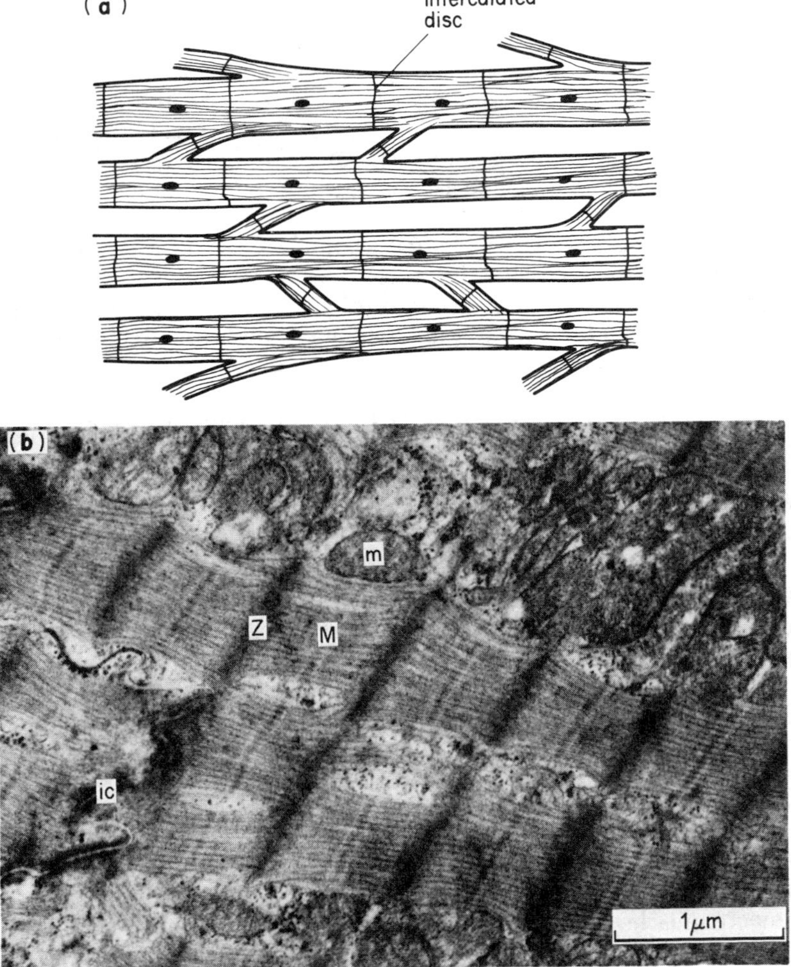


**Fig. 1.12** Cardiac muscle. (**a**) Diagram illustrating the organization of cardiac muscle fibres; (**b**) electron micrograph of a longitudinal section of muscle fibres from the heart of a rat. ic, intercalated disc (those shown do not include a nexus); m, mitochondrion; M, M-line; Z, Z-line. ((**b**) Photograph by D. Ashworth, Astbury Department of Biophysics, University of Leeds.)

filaments arising from each Z-disc. Furthermore, the Z-discs are aligned at right angles to the fibre axis and the bands in adjacent fibrils are aligned more or less with each other. In contrast, the Z-material in obliquely striated muscle is arranged in narrow rods (small dense bodies in the pelecypodan mollusc *Crassostrea*) so that the actin filaments arise from them in a more or less sheet-like array (Fig. 1.13). The Z-rods are arranged in parallel rows which lie obliquely with respect to the long axis of the muscle fibre. In the earthworm, *Lumbricus*, the angle of these rows to the long axis is about 5° in relaxed muscle and is greater in contracted muscle. (In Fig. 1.13 this angle has been exaggerated for clarity.) The arrangement of Z-rods and A- and I-bands produces the obliquely striated appearance of this muscle.

In transverse sections the A- and I-bands are cut through alternately and there is no plane in which the transverse appearance of cross-striated muscle will be seen (Figs 1.13, 1.14a). In cross-striated muscle a longitudinal section in any plane shows the sarcomeres and their composite bands (see Fig. 1.4), but in obliquely striated muscle there is only a single plane (*yz* in Fig. 1.13) which will give this picture. Longitudinal sections will usually have an appearance approaching that of the *xz* plane (Figs 1.13, 1.14b).

In nematode muscle there are two tubular systems, as in cross-striated muscle: a sarcoplasmic reticulum, consisting of flattened vesicles, and a transversely-oriented T-system. The two systems come into contact with one another at dyads. In annelid body wall muscle and in the obliquely striated translucent part of the oyster adductor muscle only the sarcoplasmic reticulum is present. This consists of peripheral vesicles and, in annelids, tubular projections from them which run parallel to, and alternate with, the Z-rods (Figs 1.13, 1.14). The peripheral vesicles are connected to the surface membrane of the fibre by septate junctions which appear to be structurally the same as dyads. Hence inpushing of the surface membrane to produce a T-system has not occurred in the obliquely striated muscles of these two phyla.

**Smooth muscle**

The visceral muscles of vertebrates lack any banding pattern and are hence called smooth muscles. With conventional fixation techniques only actin filaments are seen under the electron microscope, but there is very good biochemical and X-ray evidence for the presence of myosin, which is very labile in this type of muscle. X-ray diffraction pictures have also indicated the presence of myosin bridges. The

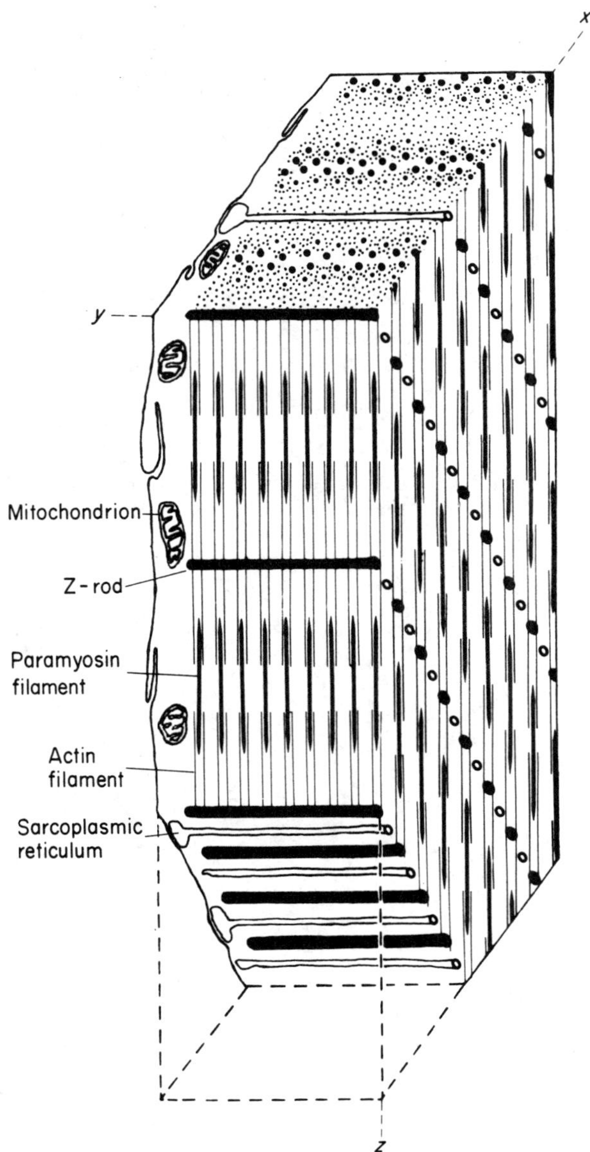


**Fig. 1.13** Diagram illustrating the structure of an obliquely striated earthworm muscle fibre. *x, y,* and *z* are the three perpendicular axes. The angle of the striations is the *xz* plane has been exaggerated for clarity. (From Mill, P. J. and Knapp, M. F. (1970). *Journal of Cell Science*, **7**, 233–61.)

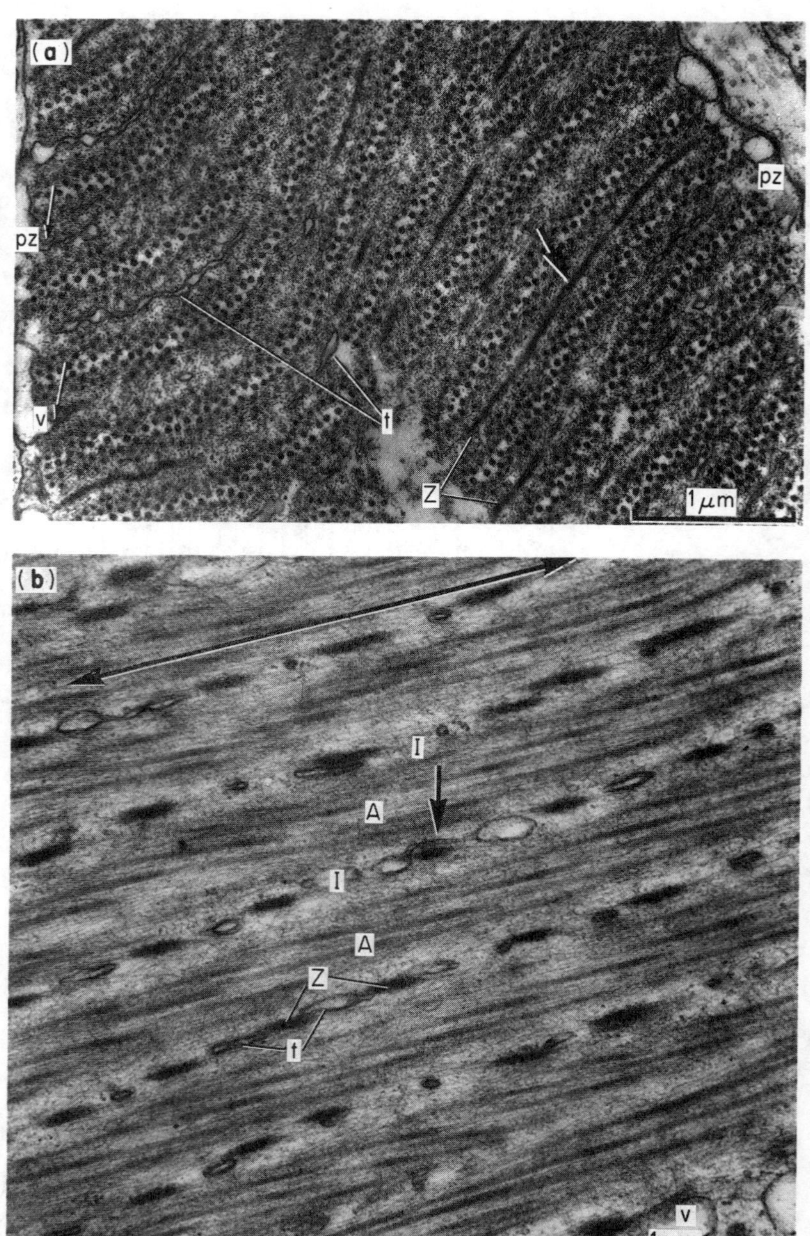
(a)
pz
pz
v
t
Z
1 μm
(b)
I
A
I
A
Z
t
v
1 μm

sarcoplasmic reticulum is poorly developed and is primarily located close to the periphery of the fibre.

The individual muscle cells are interconnected by two types of junction: ***attachment plaques*** and ***tight junctions*** (nexuses). At attachment plaques the adjacent cell membranes have electron dense material on their inner surfaces and there may also be some electron dense material in the gap, whereas at tight junctions the two cell membranes are very closely apposed. The latter are thought to be sites of electrical coupling between the cells, i.e. electrical synapses (see Chapter 5).

## NEUROMUSCULAR INNERVATION

Vertebrate skeletal muscle is typically innervated by a large number of motor neurons, each of which synapses with one or more muscle fibres; although any one muscle fibre is only innervated by a single axon (Fig. 1.15a). There is usually only a single synapse (motor end-plate) on each fast muscle fibre (or sometimes a small group of synapses), but several synaptic contacts are made with each slow muscle fibre (***multiterminal innervation***). All of the motor axons are excitatory.

In contrast, arthropod muscles are innervated by a very small number of motor neurons, often as few as one or two. All of the muscle fibres (i.e. both fast and slow) receive multiterminal innervation and may be innervated by several or even all of the motor axons innervating the muscle (***polyneuronal innervation***) (Fig. 1.15b). Furthermore, the motor axons can be categorized into excitors and inhibitors. In many muscles, the fast and slow fibres are innervated by fast and slow motor excitor axons respectively, while muscle fibres with intermediate characteristics are innervated by both. In other cases the excitors are not divided functionally and the fast and slow effects are then dependent entirely on the membrane properties of

**Fig. 1.14** Obliquely striated muscle. Electron micrographs of earthworm body wall muscle. (**a**) Transverse section (*xy* plane in Fig. 1.13). The A-band strips contain thick and thin myofilaments; the I-band strips contain only thin myofilaments. The transverse tubules of the sarcoplasmic reticulum are connected to the peripheral vesicles (small arrows). The large arrow indicates a Z-rod extending from the periphery to the centre of the fibre. (**b**) Longitudinal section (*xy* plane in Fig. 1.13). ⟷ indicates the longitudinal axis of the fibre. Note that the myofilaments lie approximately parallel to this axis but that the rows of Z-rods and transverse tubules are at a slight angle to it. A, A-band; I, I-band; pz, peripheral zone of sarcoplasm; t, tubule of the sarcoplasmic reticulum; v, peripheral vesicle of the sarcoplasmic reticulum; Z, Z-rod; ↓, connection between two tubules. (From Mill, P. J. and Knapp, M. F. (1970). *Journal of Cell Science*, **7**, 233–61.)

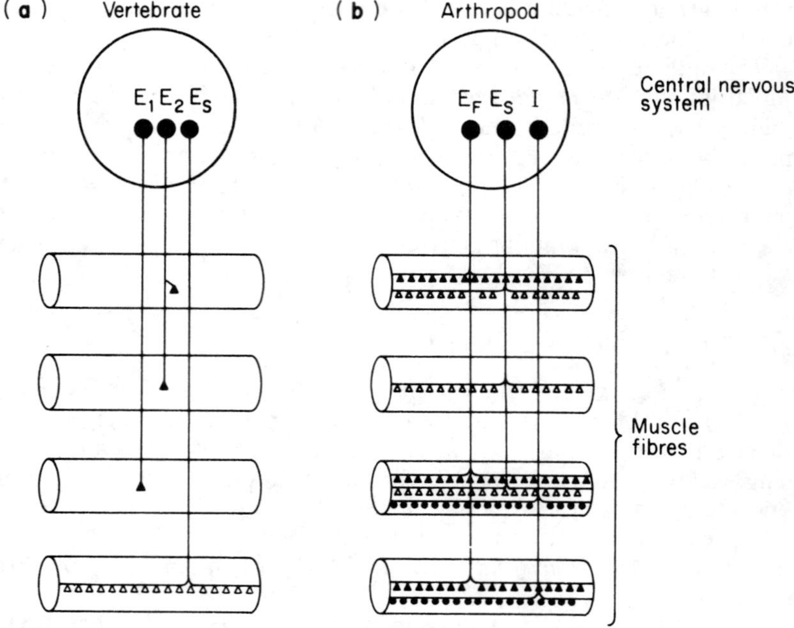


**Fig. 1.15** Diagram illustrating the pattern of muscle innervation in (**a**) a vertebrate and (**b**) an arthropod. $E_1$, $E_2$, $E_F$, fast excitatory neurons; $E_S$, slow excitatory neurons; I, inhibitory neuron. (After Usherwood, P. N. R. (1973). *Simple Nervous Systems*. Studies in Biology, no. 36. Edward Arnold, London.)

the fast and slow muscle fibres. The inhibitor motor axons may synapse directly with the muscle fibres, with the presynaptic terminals of the excitors, or with both.

In vertebrates and arthropods the motor axons synapse directly with the main body of the muscle (except as noted above for the inhibitors), but in annelids it is not unusual for synaptic contact to be made with a muscle tail which is devoid of contractile material. In nematodes the muscle tails extend to the central nervous sytem and it is here that the neuromuscular contacts are made.

## SYNAPSES

Two main types of information-transmitting junction occur between excitable cells—electrically-transmitting synapses (ephapses, tight junctions, gap junctions, nexi) and chemically-transmitting synapses. Electrical synapses are restricted to interneuronal and intermuscular connections. Chemical synapses are found between receptor cells and neurons and at interneuronal and neuromuscular connections.

*Electrical synapses*

Electrical synapses between neurons have been described in annelids, molluscs, crustaceans and lower vertebrates. At all such synapses the gap between adjacent cells (***synaptic cleft***) is either very small (i.e. less than 10 nm) and filled with electron dense material, or the outer layer of each of the two juxtaposed cell membranes is fused. Small vesicles (***synaptic vesicles***) are often present in the region of the junction, sometimes in only one cell (the presynaptic cell, see p. 24), sometimes in both cells. Electrical synapses also occur between the muscle fibres of vertebrate smooth muscle.

*Chemical synapses*

In chemically-transmitting synapses the synaptic cleft is relatively wide, usually in the range 15–30 nm. However there are some instances, such as the neuromuscular synapses on *Tenebrio* flight muscle, where it is less than 15 nm; and others, such as the neuromuscular synapses on vertebrate skeletal muscle, where it is 50–60 nm. Both normal and wide neuromuscular junctions occur on some muscles (e.g. mouse visceral muscle, the intrafusal muscle fibres of frog, the abdominal skeletal muscles of the blowfly larva, and earthworm body wall muscle). The narrower clefts of chemical synapses can be distinguished from those of electrical synapses by the absence of electron-dense material from the cleft of the former, although such material does occur in the wider chemical synaptic clefts.

The form which synapses take shows some variation. Most receptor-neuronal and neuro-neuronal synapses are a simple juxtaposition of the two cells, often with dilation of the presynaptic element. Sometimes these synapses can be categorized further as axo-dendritic, axo-somatic or axo-axonal. Axo-axonal synapses are often serial synapses, with the postsynaptic axon making almost immediate presynaptic contact with another cell (nerve or muscle) (Fig. 1.16a). There are also a number of examples of cells making synaptic contact with each other in adjacent areas of membrane, with one of the synapses being excitatory and the other inhibitory. These are called reciprocal synapses and are probably involved in feedback pathways (Fig. 1.16b).

Many neuromuscular synapses are also fairly simple, but in vertebrate fast skeletal muscles the presynaptic ending is partially sub-

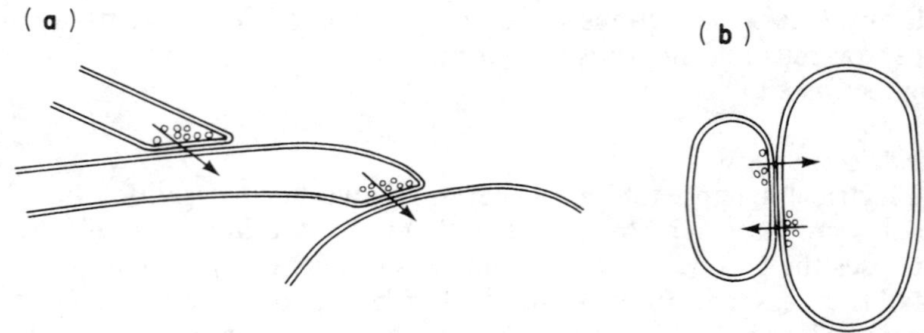


**Fig. 1.16** Diagrams to show the arrangement of (**a**) serial synapses and (**b**) reciprocal synapses. The arrows indicate the direction of transmission.

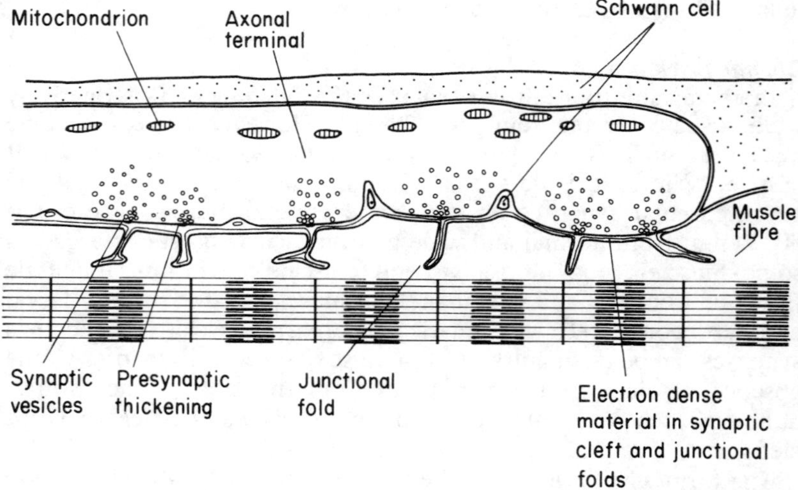


**Fig. 1.17** Diagram to show the structure of a motor end-plate of frog skeletal muscle. (Based on McMahan, U. J., Spitzer, N. C. and Peper, K. (1972). *Proceedings of the Royal Society of London, B*, **181**, 424–30.)

divided into a large number of synaptic areas and there is extensive folding of the postsynaptic (muscle) membrane. This synaptic region is called an ***end-plate*** (Fig. 1.17).

**The presynaptic cell**

At the majority of synapses, vesicles of 30–60 nm diameter are found in the presynaptic cell close to the synaptic region (Fig. 1.18). These synaptic vesicles contain the neurotransmitter substance, which is instrumental in transferring information across the synapse.

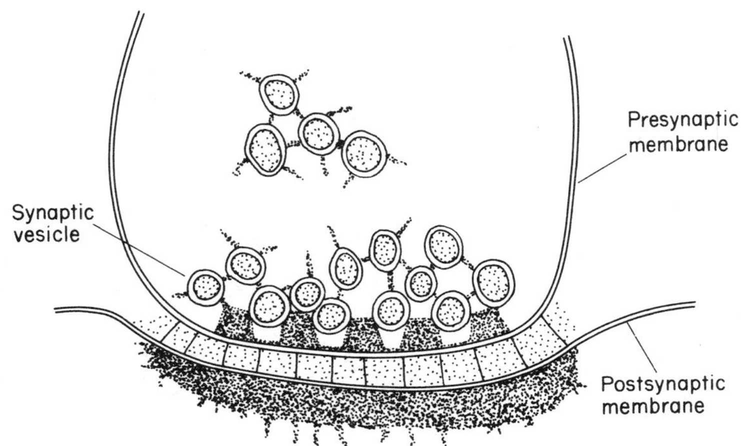


**Fig. 1.18** Diagram to show the structural features of a generalized vertebrate excitatory synapse from the central nervous system. The electron-dense presynaptic structures form a grid over the presynaptic membrane. (After Osborne, M. P. (1975). In *Insect Muscle* (Usherwood, P. N. R., ed.). Academic Press, London.)

At most vertebrate and arthropod synapses the vesicles contain material which is electron-translucent (light-cored vesicles), but at synapses where noradrenaline (norepinephrine) is the neurotransmitter (p. 63), the vesicles have an electron-dense core. Similar dense-cored vesicles are also present at many annelid neuromuscular synapses.

Some of the light-cored vesicles are spherical, others are flattened, and there is evidence from both invertebrates and vertebrates that these are characteristic of excitatory and inhibitory synapses respectively. Larger diameter (80–200 nm), granular vesicles occur at synapses on vertebrate smooth muscle, where ATP has been suggested as the neurotransmitter.

The synaptic vesicles tend to be aggregated rather than distributed homogeneously and, while some do lie against the presynaptic membrane, at many synapses the majority are generally associated with an electron-dense structure or structures of about 50–60 nm diameter, which are juxtaposed to the presynaptic membrane and physically separate the vesicles from the latter (Fig. 1.18). When more than one electron-dense body occurs they tend to be interconnected, and in vertebrate interneurons the electron-dense bodies are arranged in a triagonal array over the presynaptic membrane, with a spacing of about 80 nm. The vesicles appear to be connected to the electron-dense material and, in insects at least, to each other. In dipteran insects the electron-dense structure(s) is joined to an electron-dense plaque, with which the synaptic vesicles are associated. At the synapses between the receptor cells and the sensory axons in the vertebrate eye and ear there is a large electron-dense structure connected to the electron-dense bodies. In vertebrates there is evidence that the presynaptic dense material is more prominent at excitatory synapses, and that hexagonally arranged pits or protuberances (synaptosomes) occur on the presynaptic membrane.

Other organelles found in the presynaptic terminals include mitochondria, which tend to be fairly numerous, and often endoplasmic reticulum. Recently, using appropriate fixation techniques, microtubules (neurotubules) have been observed associated with the vesicles.

**The postsynaptic cell**

There tends to be little obvious ultrastructural specialization of the postsynaptic region, except that at many synapses there is a layer of electron-dense material on the inner surface of the postsynaptic membrane, and there are indications that this layer is wider at excitatory junctions.

The neurotransmitter released from the presynaptic terminals does not enter the postsynaptic cell. Receptor sites for the neurotransmitter exist on the postsynaptic membrane, although they have not been located ultrastructurally. At the vertebrate motor end-plate these receptors occupy the crests of the junctional folds and also extend part of the way down into them, while the enzyme responsible for the breakdown of the neurotransmitter (see Chapter 5) occurs in the synaptic cleft and on the walls of the junctional folds.

In developing mammalian skeletal muscle, acetylcholine (ACh) (Chapter 5) receptors appear when the myoblasts start to fuse to form multinucleate muscle cells. At this stage the muscle cells have a general sensitivity to ACh and the receptors are evenly distributed over their surface. Subsequently, the receptors become progressively localized into a specific area or areas and hence it would appear that they determine the site of synapse formation (Fig. 1.19). Furthermore, when a denervated muscle is re-innervated by the same nerve fibres, the original pattern of innervation is re-established.

However, it is also apparent that the nerve fibres have a marked trophic (neurotrophic) effect on the postsynaptic cell, as regards controlling the distribution (and possibly the type; see Chapter 5) of the postsynaptic receptors and the physiological characteristics of the cell. In fully developed mammalian skeletal muscle, most of the

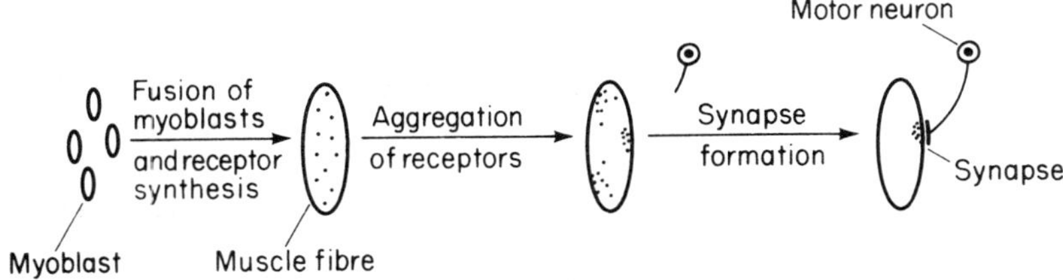


**Fig. 1.19** Diagram showing the development of a vertebrate muscle fibre and its innervation. (After Sytkowski, A. J., Vogel, Z. and Nirenberg, M. W. (1973). *Proceedings of the National Academy of Science*, **70,** 270–74.)

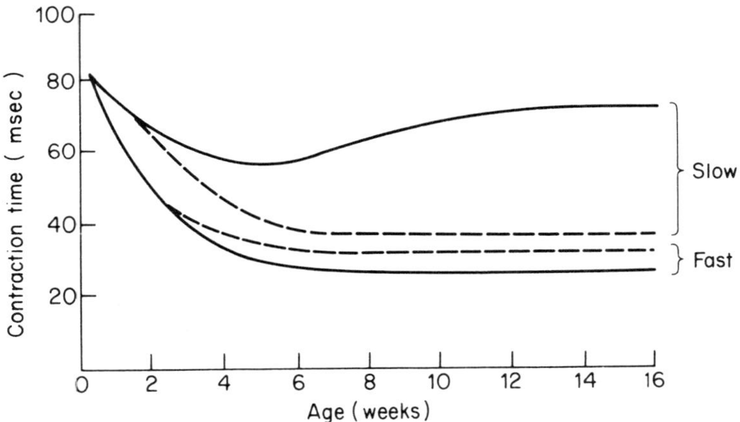


**Fig. 1.20** The development of contraction time with age for slow and fast vertebrate skeletal muscles (continuous lines), and the postulated curves for these muscles when denervated (dashed lines). (After Buller, A. J., Eccles, J. C. and Eccles, R. M. (1960). *Journal of Physiology*, **150,** 399–416.)

receptors are located at the synaptic junction (i.e. they are junctional receptors). However, if the muscle is subsequently denervated, there is a marked increase in the number of extra-junctional receptors, which is *not* caused by a simple redistribution of the junctional receptors, and there is a concomitant overall increase in the sensitivity of the muscle cells to ACh (i.e. there is a situation which resembles the pre-innervated state). Other changes include an increase in protein synthesis.

In the early developmental stages of mammalian skeletal muscles, all the muscles have basically the characteristics of the fast twitch type and early denervation prevents their complete differentiation into slow and fast twitch muscles (p. 106). This is particularly apparent for the slow twitch muscles (Fig. 1.20). If fully developed fast and slow twitch muscles are denervated and the nerves are allowed to innervate muscles of the opposite physiological type (cross-innervation), the fast twitch muscles are converted into slow twitch muscles and vice versa.

Neurons can also affect the pattern of synapse formation since, once a synapse has been established, it seems that the surrounding area of postsynaptic membrane cannot support a synapse. This helps to fix the spacing between synapses.

## SIZE SPECTRA OF AXONS

The motor axons of vertebrates are divisible into two main groups on the basis of their diameter (Fig. 1.21) and conduction velocity.

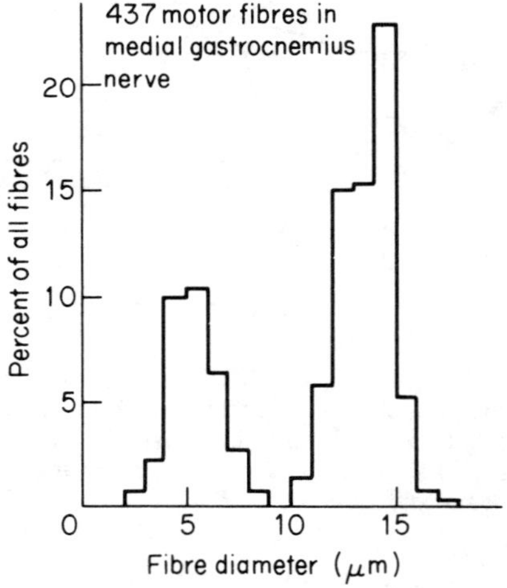


**Fig. 1.21** The distribution of the diameters of the motor fibres innervating the medial head of cat gastrocnemius muscle. The diameter includes the myelin sheath. (From Matthews, P. B. C. (1972). *Mammalian Muscle Receptors and their Central Actions.* Edward Arnold, London; after Eccles, J. C. and Sherrington, C. S. (1930). *Proceedings of the Royal Society of London, B,* **106,** 326–57.)

The larger, more rapidly conducting axons are termed $\alpha$ fibres, and the smaller, more slowly conducting axons are called $\gamma$ fibres. In mammals the $\alpha$ fibres are 8–20 $\mu$m in diameter with conduction velocities of 50–150 $\text{ms}^{-1}$ (Table 1.1) and primarily innervate the ordinary (extrafusal muscle fibres. Some also innervate the muscle fibres of the muscle spindles (p. 135), when they are referred

**Table 1.1** The classification of mammalian* peripheral nerve fibres.

| | Motor (Efferent) | | Sensory (Afferent) | | | |
|---|---|---|---|---|---|---|
| | $\alpha$ | $\gamma$ | I | II | III | IV |
| Diameter ($\mu$m) | 8–20 | 2–8 | 12–20 | 4–12 | 1–4 | $<1$ |
| Conduction velocity ($ms^{-1}$) | 50–120 | 10–50 | 72–120 | 24–72 | 6–24 | $<2$ |
| Innervation | Extrafusal muscle fibres (some ($\beta$) fibres also innervate muscle spindles) | Muscle spindles | Ia Muscle spindle—primary endings; Ib Golgi tendon organs | Muscle spindle—secondary endings; free nerve endings; some Golgi endings; Ruffini endings | Free nerve endings | Free nerve endings |

* Based on the main nerve trunks in the hind limb of the cat. There is some overlap between the size categories. Furthermore the diameters and conduction velocities become less towards the periphery. For details of the sense organs see Chapter 8. (Partly after Mattthews, P. B. C. (1972) *Mammalian Muscle Receptors and their Central Actions*. Edward Arnold, London.)

to as $\beta$ fibres! The $\gamma$ fibres have a diameter of 2–8 $\mu$m and conduction velocities of 10–50 $ms^{-1}$ in mammals (Table 1.1), and exclusively innervate the muscle spindles. This functional distinction between the $\alpha$ and $\gamma$ fibres does not exist in frogs.

The classification of sensory fibres in vertebrates is more complex than that of motor fibres. Nevertheless, they can be divided into four groups I–IV, on the basis of their diameter, conduction velocity and function. Group I contains the largest diameter, and hence most rapidly conducting, fibres and, in the cat, has been subdivided into group Ia which contains the fibres providing the primary innervation

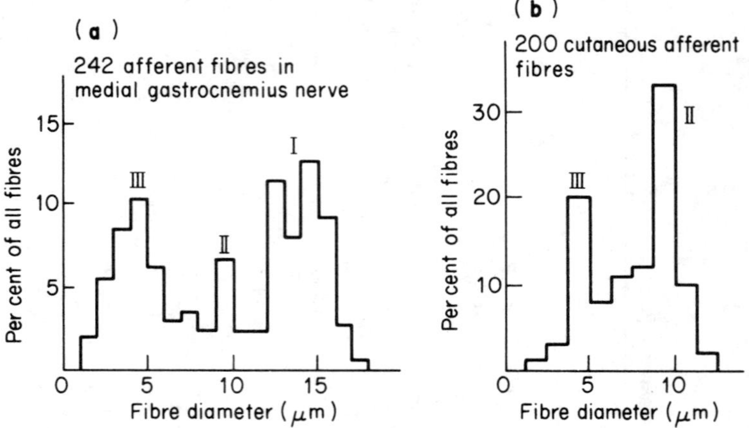


**Fig. 1.22** The distribution of the diameters of (**a**) the medullated sensory fibres from the cat gastrocnemius muscle and (**b**) the sensory fibres from a largely cutaneous nerve in the cat hindlimb. (From Matthews, P. B. C. (1972). *Mammalian Muscle Receptors and their Central Actions*. Edward Arnold, London; after Eccles, J. C. and Sherrington, C. S. (1930). *Proceedings of the Royal Society of London, B*, **106**, 326–57.)

of the muscle spindles (p. 135) and group Ib which contains those innervating the Golgi tendon organs (p. 145). The fibres in groups I–III are all medullated, while group IV contains small non-medullated fibres. Table 1.1 shows the correlation between diameter, conduction velocity and function for these groups in the hind limb of the cat. Different sensory nerves contain different proportions of the four groups, depending on which sense organs they innervate. Thus the sensory component of the nerve innervating the gastrocnemius muscle (which contains various sense organs, see Chapter 8) contains mainly group I and group III fibres, with just a few group II fibres (Fig. 1.22a); whereas the size spectrum of the cutaneous (skin) nerve illustrated in Fig. 1.22b indicates almost exclusively group II and group III fibres.

It can be seen that, in mammals at least, the sensory and motor axons cover a similar size range. This does not appear to be the case in invertebrates, nor do the axons of invertebrates separate out into

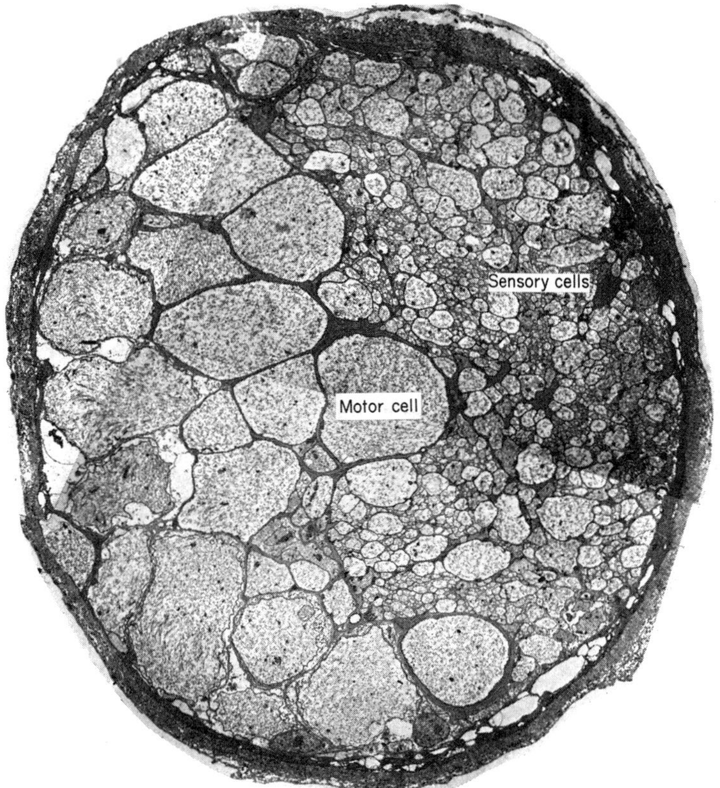


**Fig. 1.23** An electron micrograph of a transverse section through a segmental nerve of a dragonfly larva. (Photograph by C. A. Whittles, Department of Pure and Applied Zoology, University of Leeds.)

obvious size classes. The range varies from diameters of less than 1.0 $\mu$m to the giant axons of the squid which are several hundred $\mu$m in diameter. In arthropods the majority of the larger axons are motor, although a few are sensory, such as those innervating the stretch receptors (Chapter 8). However, the smaller axons are exclusively sensory. A mixed nerve root is shown in Fig. 1.23. The majority of axons are less than 1 $\mu$m in diameter.

# 2

# *The Resting Cell*

All nerve and muscle cells have in common the capability of maintaining a potential difference of, normally, between 30 mV and 90 mV across their surface membrane, so that the inside of the resting cell is negative compared to the outside (Fig. 2.1). Furthermore, they

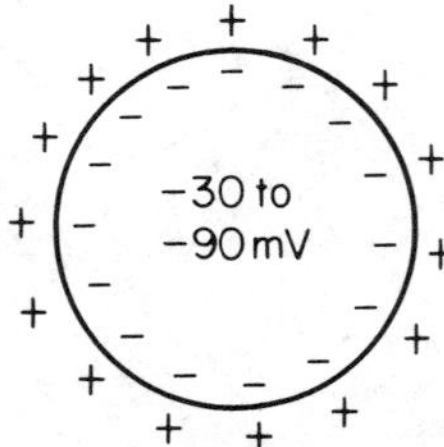


**Fig. 2.1** Diagram illustrating the potential difference across the surface membrane of a nerve or muscle cell.

are capable of restoring this ***resting potential*** when, as we shall see later, this potential is altered in some way.

Typically, excitable cells contain less sodium and chloride ions than the surrounding medium, but an excess of potassium ions and large amino acids such as glutamate and isethionate (Fig. 2.2). These latter, negatively charged, anions are incapable of passing across the surface membrane and provide a basis for the internal negativity of the cell. However, it is the distribution of the other ions and the permeability of the cell membrane to them which are the primary factors responsible for establishing the existence and magnitude of the potential difference and which provide the basis for the restorative mechanism discussed below. Some typical values of the relative concentrations of these ions are given in Table 2.1.

**Table 2.1** The concentrations of various ions for squid giant axons (interneurons) and frog muscle fibres.

| Ion | Concentration (mM) | | | |
|---|---|---|---|---|
| | Squid axon | | Frog muscle | |
| | Inside | Outside | Inside | Outside |
| K | 400 | 20 | 124 | 2.25 |
| Na | 50 | 440 | 10.4 | 109 |
| Cl | 40–150 | 560 | 1.5 | 77.5 |
| Ca | 0.4 | 10 | 4.9 | 2.1 |
| Mg | 10 | 54 | 14.0 | 1.25 |
| $HCO_3$ | ? | ? | 12.4 | 26.6 |
| Organic anions | Isethionate 250<br>Other *c.* 110 | —<br>— | *c.*74 | *c.*13 |

(From Aidley, D. J. (1971). *The Physiology of Excitable Cells.* Cambridge University Press, Cambridge. Squid axon values after Hodgkin, A. L. (1958). *Proceedings of the Royal Society B,* **148,** 1–37. Frog muscle values after Conway, E. J. (1957). *Physiological Reviews,* **37,** 84–132.)

Ions can move across a semi-permeable membrane either passively by diffusion or actively by being pumped across. The net passive movement depends on several factors: the mobility of the ions, the permeability of the membrane to them, the difference in their concentration on the two sides of the membrane (net ion movement

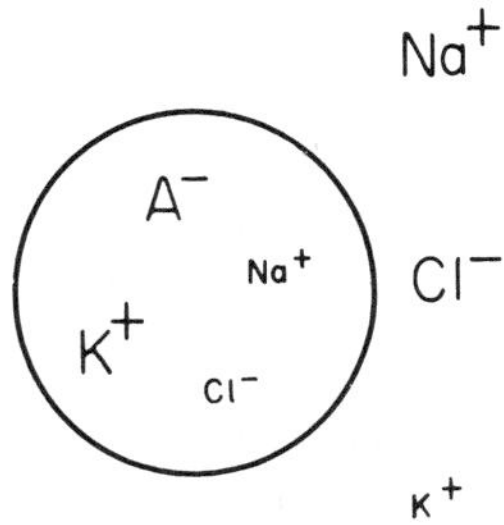


**Fig. 2.2** Diagram illustrating the distribution across the surface membrane of nerve and muscle cells of those ions which are important in determining the membrane potential. The size of the symbols represents the difference in concentrations on opposite sides of the membrane.

is from high to low concentration) and the electrical charge which exists between the two sides of the membrane (net movement is towards a region of opposite charge) (Fig. 2.3). The ionic movements

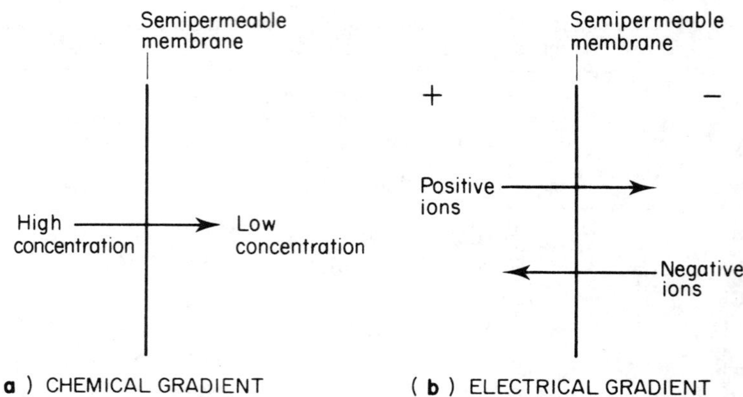


**Fig. 2.3** Diagrams to illustrate (**a**) the chemical gradient and (**b**) the electrical gradient which can exist across a semipermeable membrane. The combination of the two is the electrochemical gradient.

produced by the differences in concentration and electrical charge may be in the same or opposite directions. The resultant of these two factors is called the ***electrochemical gradient*** and the net movement of ions is down their electrochemical gradients. The relationship between the net passive distribution of an ion species on either side of a semipermeable membrane and the potential difference across the membrane is given by an equation of the form:

$$E = k \log_{10} \text{concentration ratio} \qquad \text{at } T^{\circ}$$

where E is the potential difference and k (a constant at any given temperature) increases with temperature. It follows that, for passive diffusion, E is the potential difference that exists across a membrane for an observed difference in concentration for a particular ion species, and hence it is termed the ***equilibrium potential*** for that ion species. Therefore, the distribution of any ion species can be explained in terms of simple diffusion, if it has an equilibrium potential for the observed difference in concentration across the surface membrane which is equal to the resting potential of the cell.

The sign of E can be determined by inspection. Thus, if the ratio inside:outside is used for negative ions and the ratio outside:inside is used for positive ions, the sign of the answer will indicate the equilibrium potential difference of the inside of the cell with respect to the outside. If we take, as an example, the chloride distribution about the membrane of the mammalian motor neuron (Table 2.2) then, at 38°C

$$\begin{aligned} E_{Cl} &= 61.5 \log_{10} \frac{Cl_i}{Cl_o} \\ &= 61.5 \log_{10} \frac{9}{125} \\ &= 61.5 \times -1.1427 \\ &= -70.3 \text{ mV} \end{aligned}$$

(i.e. the inside is negative with respect to the outside). Reference to Table 2.2 shows that the equilibrium potential for the observed

**Table 2.2** The concentrations of sodium, potassium and chloride ions, and their equilibrium potentials (inside with respect to outside) for cat motor neurons. The resting membrane potential is −70mV.

| Ion | Concentration (mM) | | Equilibrium potential (mv) |
|---|---|---|---|
| | Inside | Outside | |
| Na | *c.*15 | 150 | *c.*+60 |
| K | 150 | 5.5 | −90 |
| Cl | 9 | 125 | −70 |

(From Eccles, J. C. (1957). *The Physiology of Nerve Cells.* The Johns Hopkins Press, Baltimore.)

concentration difference is indeed the same as the resting potential of the cell; the distribution of the chloride ions can therefore be explained in terms of simple diffusion. Thus a Donnan equilibrium exists in which the inflow of chloride ions down their concentration gradient is exactly balanced by their repulsion due to the large internal negativity of the cell.

However, if the same treatment is applied to the potassium and sodium ions, equilibrium potentials of 90 mV (inside *negative*) and 60 mV (inside *positive*) respectively are obtained for the observed differences in concentrations. In other words, the inside of the cell is 20 mV too positive for the observed distribution of potassium ions and 130 mV too negative for the observed distribution of sodium ions to be achieved by simple diffusion. Hence these two ion species must be actively pumped against their electrochemical gradients (Fig. 2.4). At equilibrium potentials identical with the resting potential, the

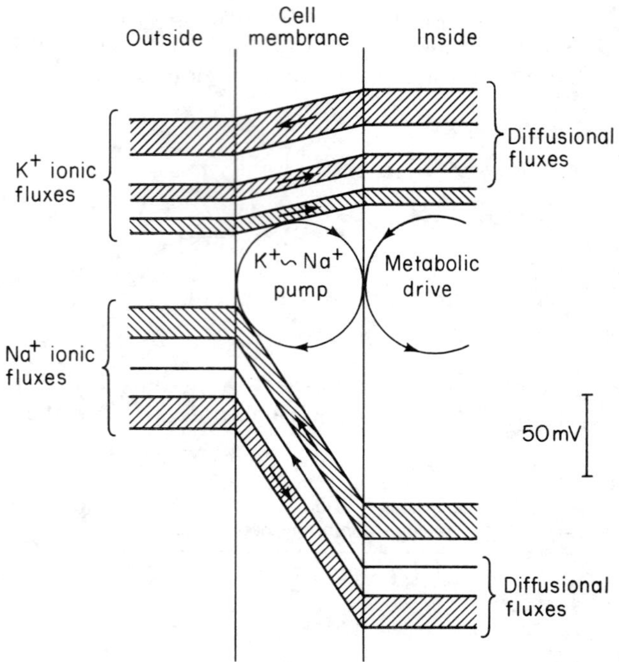


**Fig. 2.4** Diagram illustrating the potassium and sodium fluxes across the surface membrane of a mammalian motor neuron in the resting state. The direction and magnitude of the slopes in the flux channels across the membrane represent the electrochemical gradients. At a resting membrane potential of −70 mV these correspond to potassium and sodium equilibrium potentials which are 20 mV more negative and 130 mV more positive, respectively, than the resting potential. The magnitudes of the fluxes are indicated by the widths of the channels. (After Eccles, J. C. (1957). *The Physiology of Nerve Cells*. The Johns Hopkins Press, Baltimore.)

concentration ratio for potassium ions would be halved and the distribution of sodium ions would be almost exactly reversed. Thus, under the conditions pertaining in the resting cell, the outward diffusional flux of potassium ions will be about twice the inward diffusional flux, and hence the pump must double the inward flux. In the case of sodium ions the outward diffusional flux is negligible compared to the inward diffusional flux, and hence the pump must remove sodium ions from the cell as fast as they diffuse in. There is evidence that the potassium and sodium pumps are coupled, so producing an electrically neutral system with, probably, one potassium ion being pumped into the cell for every sodium ion removed. Although it may seem that sodium has to be pumped at a greater rate than potassium, this is not necessarily the case since the resting cell membrane is considerably less permeable to sodium ions. In the mammalian motor neuron, typical resting values for the specific membrane conductances for sodium and potassium are, respectively, 0.01 mmhos.cm$^{-2}$ and 0.5 mmhos.cm$^{-2}$ (mho—ohm written backwards—is the unit of conductance). Thus, although the electrochemical gradient for sodium ions is steeper than that for potassium ions, the *net* rate of diffusion of the two ions is probably similar. Energy, derived from metabolic activity in the cell, is of course required to drive the ionic pumping mechanism.

Since the potassium ions can move much more freely across the membrane than can the sodium ions, the magnitude of the resting potential is determined largely by the potassium concentration gradient. It has been shown experimentally that, except at very low potassium concentrations, the level of the resting potential is directly dependent on the external potassium concentration (Fig. 2.5). Hence

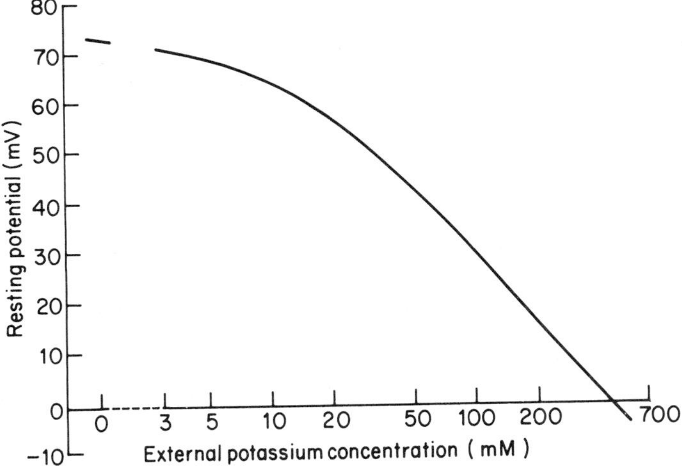


**Fig. 2.5** The relationship between the resting potential of a nerve cell and the external potassium concentration. (After Hodgkin, A. L. and Keynes, R. D. (1955). *Journal of Physiology*, **128,** 61–88.)

the resting potential is close to the potassium equilibrium potential.

The situation in frog skeletal muscle is very similar to that in the mammalian motor neuron, but in the squid giant axon the ratio of the concentration of chloride ions inside and outside the cell is low, giving an equilibrium potential for the chloride ions of only about 39 mV (inside negative) compared with a resting potential of about

60 mV (inside negative). In this case chloride ions must be actively pumped into the cell.

The surface membrane of an excitable cell can be described in electrical terms (Fig. 2.6). It has a variable resistance for each ion species, each of which has an electromotive force. Also, since a

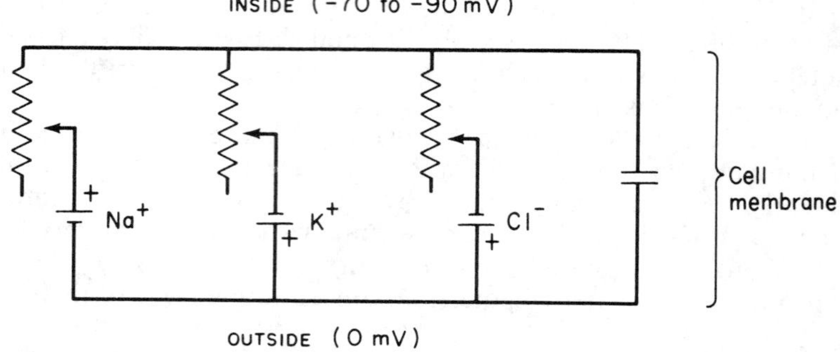


**Fig. 2.6** An electrical representation of the surface membrane of a nerve or muscle cell. $R_{Na^+}$, $R_{K^+}$ and $R_{Cl^-}$ are variable while the capacitance is constant. Note that in the mammalian motor neuron $R_{Cl^-}$ is constant. (After Hodgkin, A. L., and Huxley, A. F. (1952). *Journal of Physiology*, **117**, 500–44.)

potential difference is established across the membrane, it has capacitance. Average values for the specific membrane resistance and capacitance of a mammalian motor neuron are, respectively, 400 ohms $cm^2$ and $6\mu F\ cm^{-2}$. If a current pulse is applied across such a membrane, a new potential difference will be established gradually, as it would be across any circuit which contains resistive and capacitive elements in parallel. The electrical time constant of such a circuit, defined as the time taken to reach within 1/e ($\simeq 0.63$) of the final value, is dependent solely on the resistance and capacitance, and indeed is their product. The average time constant for a mammalian motor neuron is 2.4 msec (i.e. $400 \times 6 \times 10^{-6}$ sec).

# 3

# *The Active Cell: Introduction*

## GRADED AND ACTION POTENTIALS

In all excitable cells the resting potential is capable of being altered transiently and it is this property which enables information to be transduced and transmitted in coded form. Basically there are two types of potential change—the decremental, non-propagated ***graded potential*** and the all-or-none, propagated ***action potential*** (Fig. 3.1).

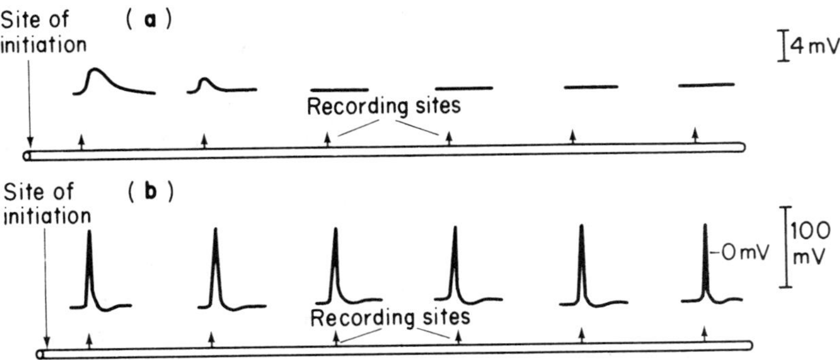


**Fig. 3.1** Diagrams illustrating the difference between (**a**) a graded potential and (**b**) an action potential.

Since graded potentials are not actively propagated, they can only have an effect over short distances, this effect diminishing with increase in distance from the source of the potential (Fig. 3.1a). Once initiated, however, they do not require any transfer of energy. Their effect, therefore, is virtually instantaneous. Graded potentials rarely exceed a change in membrane potential of more than a few millivolts, but this change may make the inside of the cell less negative or more negative. Changes which make the inside of the cell less negative are called depolarizing; those which make it more negative, hyperpolarizing (Fig. 3.2, see also Chapter 4).

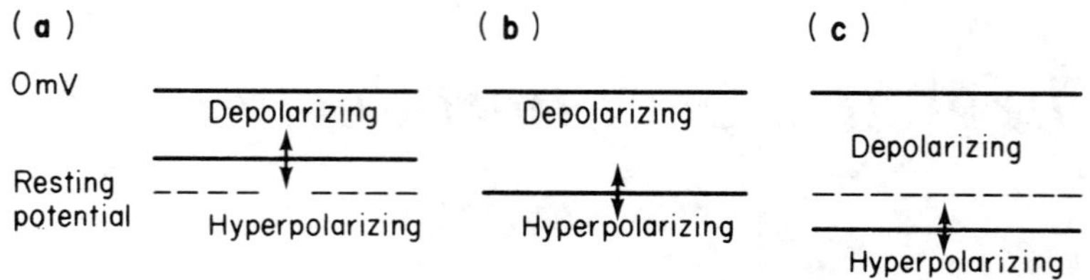


**Fig. 3.2** Diagrams illustrating the use of the terms 'depolarizing' and 'hyperpolarizing'. Note that these terms imply directionality and are not used solely with reference to the resting level of a cell (**b**). Thus a neuron may already have a membrane potential which has been depolarized by a previous event (**a**), such as stretch applied to a tonic stretch receptor (see p. 132), or one which has been hyperpolarized (**c**).

Action potentials, often referred to simply as 'spikes', are the means by which information is transmitted over greater distances (Fig. 3.1b). They are always depolarizing and involve an active *reversal* of the membrane potential; hence they may have amplitudes in the order of 100 mV. This reversal of the membrane potential means, of course, that the outside of the membrane becomes momentarily negative with respect to the inside; an action potential passing along, say, an axon, may therefore be envisaged as a travelling wave of external negativity (Fig. 3.3). *Action potentials are initiated by depolarizing graded potentials*. Since they are transmitted by a regenerative process requiring energy (see Chapter 6), they travel comparatively slowly, although their local electrotonic effect is instantaneous.

In some excitable cells no part of the membrane is capable of supporting an action potential and information transmission in these cells is solely by means of graded potentials. This is the case in the primary sensory cells in sense organs such as the eye, and in a few arthropod sensory neurons which have short axons, notably the thoracic-coxal receptors of decapod crustaceans (p. 133). It also applies to many multiterminally innervated muscle cells and probably to many (if not most) of the amacrine cells. In each of these examples transmission of information is over a short distance only.

In other cells a considerable proportion of the cell membrane is capable of supporting an action potential (Fig. 3.4). This applies to

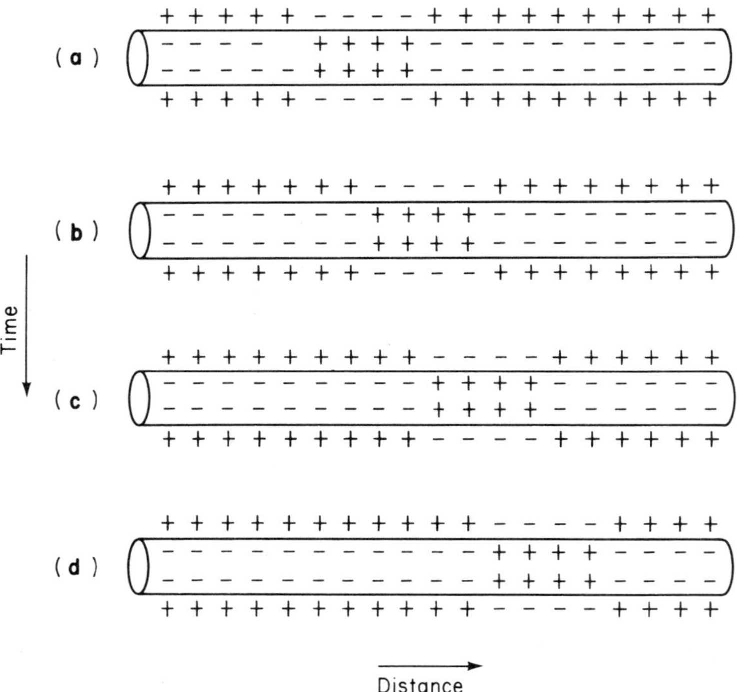


**Fig. 3.3** Diagrams illustrating the passaage of an action potential along an axon as a wave of external negativity. (**a**)–(**d**) represent successive time intervals.

neurons with long axons, such as most sensory neurons and motor neurons; also to vertebrate fast muscle cells, where there is only a single synaptic region on each muscle cell and where the information has therefore to be transmitted a considerable distance if the whole cell is to be involved in contraction.

Graded potentials occur in the dendrites of sensory neurons and in the postsynaptic regions of motor neurons and muscle cells. In all these cells there is a specific region of the cell membrane where action potentials are normally initiated, called the ***spike-initiating zone***. If a depolarizing graded potential reaches a sufficient magnitude in this region, then an action potential will be induced. The level of depolarization at which an action potential is initiated is known as the ***threshold level***. The areas of these cells which support graded potentials either have a spike threshold which is considerably higher than at the spike-initiating zone, or do not support action potentials at all. In the former case an action potential, once initiated, will invade this region; in the latter an action potential will just have an electronic effect on it.

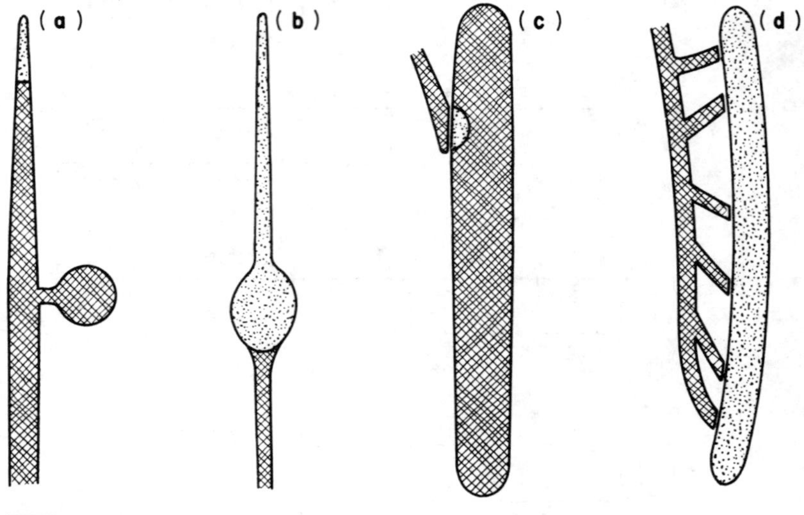


**Fig. 3.4** The distribution of graded and all-or-none conducting membrane in a selection of cells. (**a**) Invertebrate unipolar neuron with active soma; (**b**) lobster cardiac ganglion cell; (**c**) vertebrate fast muscle and its innervation; (**d**) arthropod slow muscle and its innervation. (After Bishop, G. H. (1958). *Electroencephalography and Clinical Neurophysiology, Supplement* **10,** 12–21; and Bullock, T. H. and Horridge, G. A. (1965). *Structure and Function in the Nervous System of Invertebrates.* W. H. Freeman, San Francisco.)

## RECORDING TECHNIQUES

It is not the intention of this book to serve as a laboratory guide to neurophysiology, but it will be helpful at this point to consider briefly how records of the potential differences and potential changes which occur in excitable cells are obtained.

By far the most convenient parameter to measure is potential difference and there are two types of technique which are utilized to achieve this—intracellular recording and extracellular recording.

With the intracellular method of recording, the actual difference in potential across the membrane is measured by placing one electrode (a microelectrode) inside the cell, and the other, the reference (or indifferent) electrode, on the outside, either on the surface of the cell or some distance away. This method has the advantage that the full potential difference of a resting cell can be observed (Fig. 3.5) as well as details of the shape and time course of even small potential changes, and is the method which must be used to gain accurate

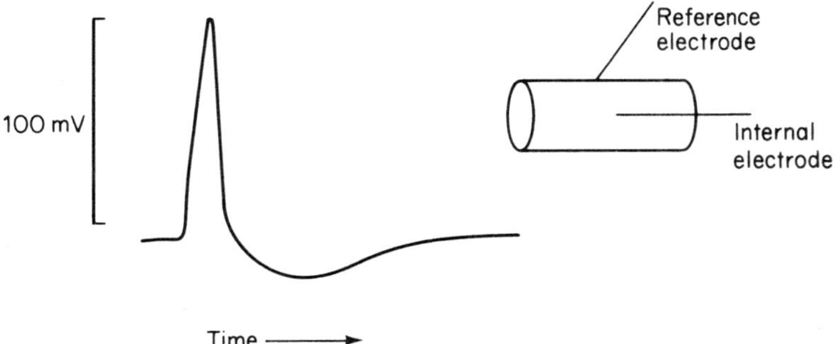


**Fig. 3.5** Diagram of a 'typical' action potential as recorded using an internal microelectrode.

measurements of these parameters. However, the intracellular method is restricted in use to those cells, or parts of cells, which are sufficiently large to allow penetration by a microelectrode without undue damage being caused to the cell.

Extracellular recording, on the other hand, involves comparing the potential difference between two electrodes, both of which are external to the cell under investigation. This can be achieved in two ways. One electrode can be placed on the surface of the cell in the region from which it is desired to record (usually the axon in the case

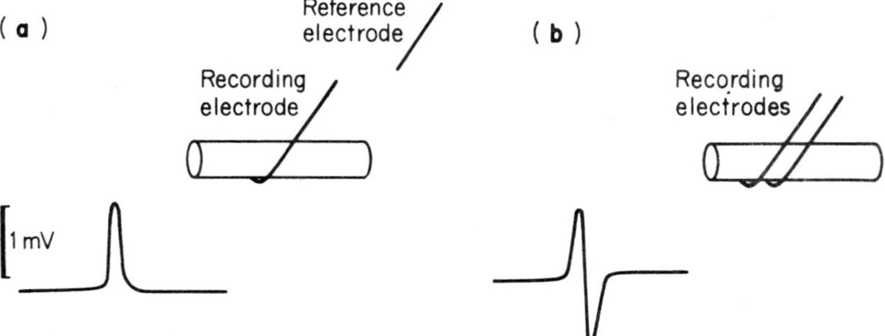


**Fig. 3.6** (**a**) Monophasic and (**b**) biphasic methods of extracellular recording, showing the theoretical shapes of an action potential recorded by the two methods.

of neurons), with the other electrode at some distance from it to provide a zero reference point. Alternatively, both electrodes can be placed slightly apart on the surface of the cell, so that events in one region can be compared with an adjacent, inactive region. If an action potential is recorded from an axon with only a single electrode placed on it, a negative monophasic spike will be recorded as the wave of negativity passes under the electrode (Fig. 3.6a). If both electrodes are on the axon a biphasic spike will be seen as the wave of negativity passes first under one electrode and then under the other. Because of the design of the amplifying system, the negative wave recorded at one electrode will be amplified with opposite sign to that recorded at the other (Fig. 3.6b). Changes in potential are severely attenuated by the extracellular method of recording and an action potential of 100 mV may be represented by a recorded spike of only a few hundred microvolts. Hence it is impossible to record graded potentials in this manner, unless they are of reasonably large magnitude. The main advantage of extracellular techniques is that they do allow recordings to be obtained from a considerably greater number of cells and parts of cells than would otherwise be possible using intracellular methods. Unfortunately, the attenuation of the extracellularly recorded potentials increases with decrease in axon diameter and there are still no techniques available for measuring activity in the smallest neurons. However, this size effect does have one advantage since it helps to differentiate between the responses in different axons.

With both methods, intracellular and extracellular, it is essential to use electrodes which interfere as little as possible with the cells from which recordings are being made and to use conductors which do not become polarized. Intracellular and extracellular electrodes are also both used to stimulate excitable cells to produce action potentials.

With both types of recording technique the potential differences are amplified and displayed, usually on an oscilloscope, when they can be photographed to make permanent records. If the potential differences are reasonably large and of sufficient duration, an ultraviolet or pen recorder may be used instead of an oscilloscope and camera. However, this inevitably involves some attenuation of the recorded signals. Often it is convenient to store the information on magnetic tape: for intracellular work an FM tape recorder is essential.

The above account is only a simple outline of the main types of technique utilized and there are, of course, numerous variations and many sophisticated adaptations of these.

# 4

# *Graded Potentials*

Graded potentials can be classified into a variety of types, depending on how they are produced, where they occur, and what their functions are.

## RECEPTOR AND GENERATOR POTENTIALS

Sense organs are concerned with transducing into electrical energy the information which they receive; this, after transduction, is in the form of graded, depolarizing potentials. In a sense organ such as the vertebrate eye, where the primary receptor cells have a non-nervous origin, the graded potential which occurs in them is called the ***receptor potential***. This elicits another graded potential, the ***generator potential***, in the dendritic terminations of the sensory neuron (Fig. 4.1a). The generator potential is thus a postsynaptic potential. If it is sufficiently large, an action potential, or a series of action potentials, will be produced at the spike-initiating zone of the sensory neuron. In mechanoreceptors, the sensory neuron is itself the receptor cell and, although the graded potential produced in its dendritic terminations is generally referred to as a receptor potential, it is functionally synonymous with both the receptor and the generator potentials as described above (Fig. 4.1b).

The site of the spike-initiating zone has been investigated in several sense organs. In the sensory neuron of the lobster abdominal muscle receptor organ (see Chapter 8) it is located some 500$\mu$m along the axon from the cell body. When the threshold in this region is reached, the action potential(s) so produced is transmitted both along the axon

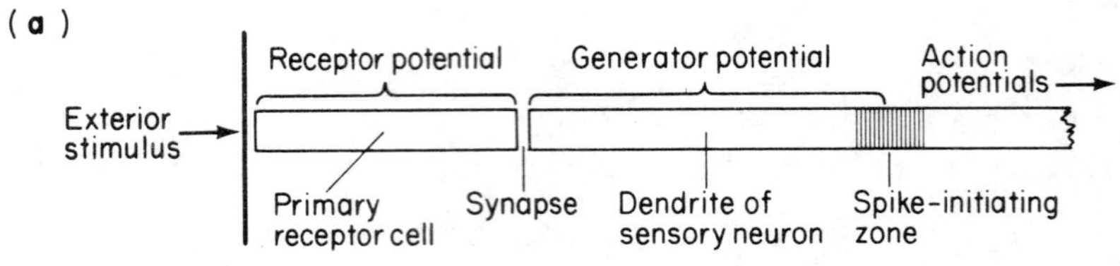


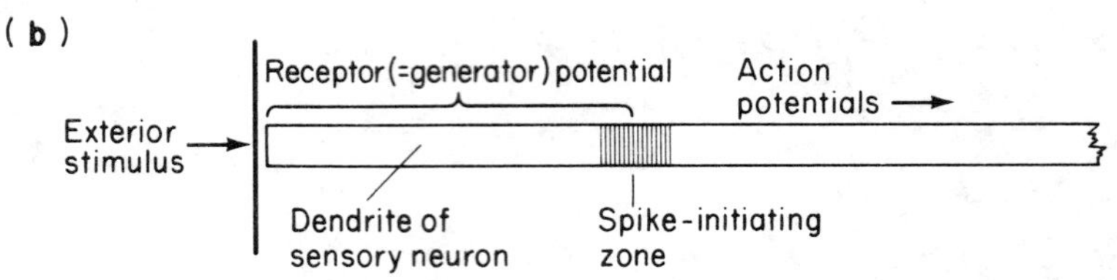


**Fig. 4.1** Diagrams of (**a**) a receptor with a primary receptor cell and (**b**) a receptor comprising a modified dendrite, to illustrate the terminology used.

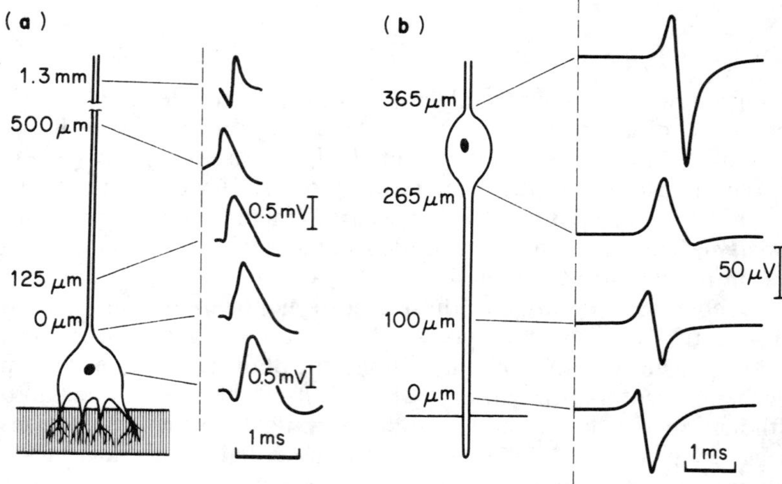


**Fig. 4.2** Tracings of an impulse set up by stretch in (**a**) a lobster abdominal muscle receptor organ and (**b**) a crab joint chordotonal organ, recorded with external electrodes at the various indicated points along the neuron. Negative is upwards in (**a**) and downwards in (**b**). In (**a**) the upper four records were recorded at the same amplification. ((**a**) After Edwards, C. and Ottoson, D. (1958). *Journal of Physiology*, **143,** 138–48; (**b**) after Hartman, H. B. and Boettiger, E. G. (1967). *Comparative Biochemistry and Physiology*, **22,** 651–63.)

towards the central nervous system, and backwards (i.e. distally) to invade the membrane of the cell body which, although it has a very high threshold, is capable of supporting an action potential (Fig. 4.2a). The action potential possibly also invades the bases of the dendrites, but probably not their distal regions where the receptor potential is produced, although there will presumably be a transient electrotonic depolarization here.

In contrast, the spike-initiating zone in the sensory cells of the joint chordotonal organs of the crustacean limb (see Chapter 8) is in the

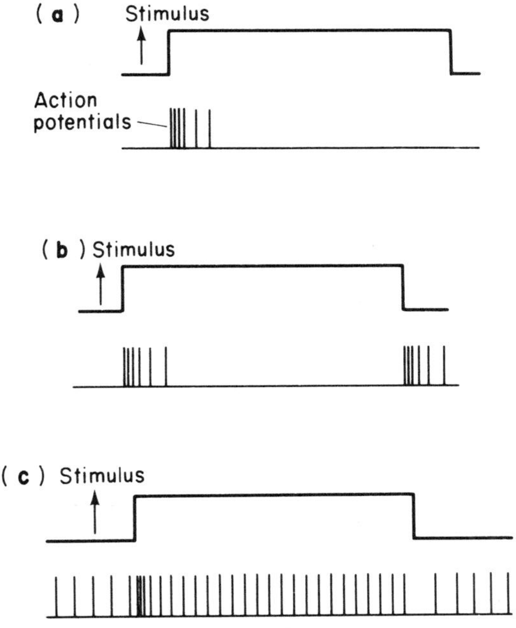


**Fig. 4.3** The relationship between a 'step' stimulus maintained for some time and the production of action potentials in (**a**) an 'on' type phasic neuron, (**b**) an 'on-off' type phasic neuron and (**c**) a tonic neuron.

dendrite instead of in the axon. It is located in the region of the scolopale (p. 143) and the action potentials pass centripetally to the cell body and thence to the axon (Fig. 4.2b). Again there will be a resultant transient depolarization of the dendritic terminal.

In the vast majority of cases the axons of sensory neurons transmit information to the central nervous system in the form of action potentials, and receptors can be divided into two categories—those which produce a brief and rapidly adapting burst of action potentials in response to an applied stimulus (***phasic receptors***) (Fig. 4.3a), and those in which adaptation is relatively slight and in which action potentials continue to be produced at a frequency related to the magnitude of the stimulus, however long the stimulus is maintained (***tonic receptors***) (Fig. 4.3c). In the latter the initial burst—the dynamic (phasic) component—varies in magnitude in different receptors. On

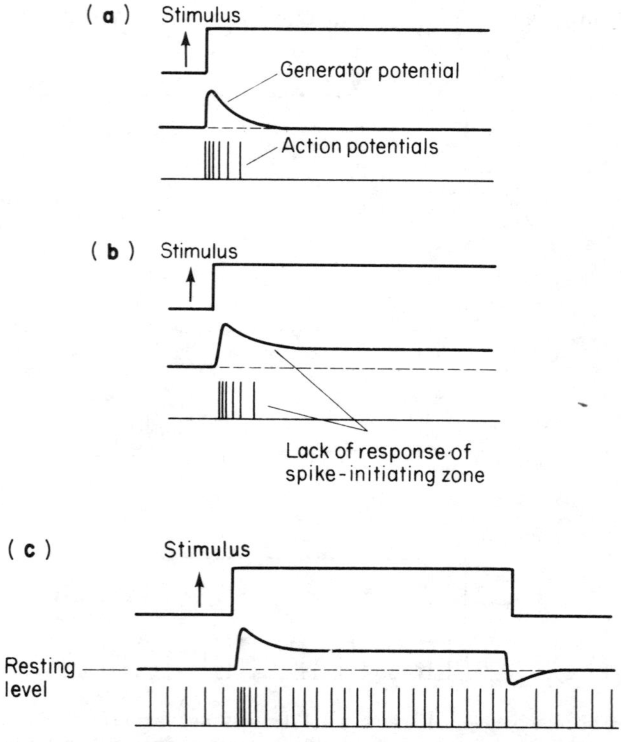


**Fig. 4.4** The relationship between the stimulus and the production of a generator potential and action potentials in (**a**) a phasic receptor with a phasic generator potential, (**b**) a phasic receptor with a tonic receptor potential and (**c**) a tonic receptor.

removal of the stimulus many phasic receptors remain quiescent ('on' receptors Fig. 4.3a), others respond with another brief burst of action potentials ('on-off' receptors, Fig. 4.3b); yet others only fire on removal of the stimulus ('off' receptors). Removal of the stimulus from a tonic receptor produces a reduction in the firing frequency, followed by recovery to the original (pre-stimulus) level. A number of receptors are intermediate between phasic and tonic in their response characteristics, and are referred to as phaso-tonic receptors.

In some phasic receptors the receptor potential is itself phasic, rapidly falling below the threshold for action potential production (Fig. 4.4a); for example the Pacinian corpuscle of the cat (a touch or pressure receptor; see Chapter 8). In this receptor the very rapid adaptation of the receptor potential is primarily a mechanical property of the capsule ensheathing the dendritic termination. If the sheath is removed, the receptor potential adapts less rapidly. However, in the muscle receptor organs of the crayfish abdomen, the receptor potential of the phasic receptor is similar to that of the tonic receptor, and in both the receptor potential shows a brief initial adaptation (dynamic component) after which it remains at a constant level (static component) throughout the period during which the stimulus is maintained. Hence, in these receptors, the pattern of firing is solely a function of the spike-initiating zone (Fig. 4.4b). It may be that the threshold of the spike-initiating zone in the phasic receptor is considerably higher than that in the tonic receptor and that the former is only exceeded during the initial dynamic phase. Alternatively, the spike-initiating zone in the phasic receptor may 'fatigue' and only be re-activated when there is another sudden depolarization. Whichever is the case, in the phasic receptor the spike-initiating zone is incapable of producing a long-lasting train of action potentials, whereas it can produce such a train in the tonic receptor (Fig. 4.4c). In phaso-tonic receptors there is usually a steady decline in the receptor potential to a maintained stimulus and a consequent gradual decrease in the frequency of action potentials.

The size of the receptor potential is generally some function of the amplitude of the stimulus, with increase in stimulus intensity producing an increase in the size of the receptor potential and hence, where relevant, in the size of the generator potential. Once the threshold of the spike-initiating zone is reached an action potential will be produced. As will be seen in Chapter 6, the recovery phase of the action potential has a hyperpolarizing effect on the cell membrane. In a receptor such as the tonic stretch receptor of the crayfish abdomen, where the receptor potential is maintained at a steady level for a maintained stretch of the receptor, the depolarizing effect of the receptor potential and the hyperpolarizing effect of the action potential recovery phase are mutually antagonistic, and it is the interaction between the two at the spike-initiating zone which determines the firing rate. Thus, if the amount of stretch, and hence the receptor potential, is small, the recovery phase will be completed before the depolarization effect of the receptor potential can drive the spike-initiating zone up to its threshold level again (Fig. 4.5a). However, with increase in the magnitude of the stimulus, the larger and more dominant the receptor potential becomes; less hyperpolarization therefore occurs and there is a shorter period before the threshold is reached and the next action potential is produced (Fig.

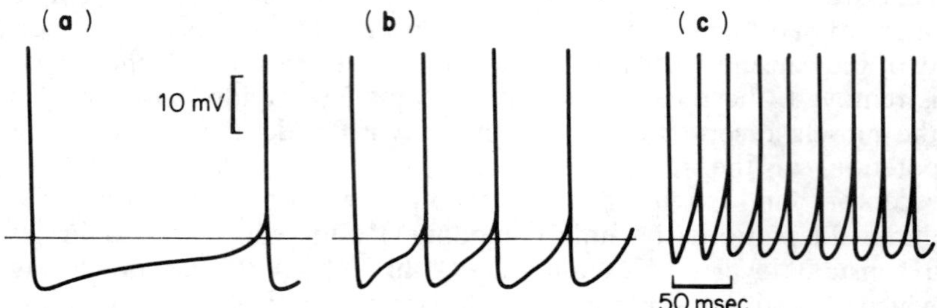


**Fig. 4.5** Intracellular recordings from the neuron innervating the tonic crustacean abdominal muscle receptor organ at different levels of stretch. (**a**) The effect of a near threshold stretch; (**b**), (**c**) two greater degrees of stretch. Note the increase in firing frequency, the increase in rate of rise of the pre-potential, the raising of the threshold level (the inflection between the pre-potential and the spike) and the reduction of the repolarization phase to increased amounts of maintained stretch. (From Eyzaguirre, C. and Kufflere, S. W. (1955). *Journal of General Physiology*, **39,** 87–119.)

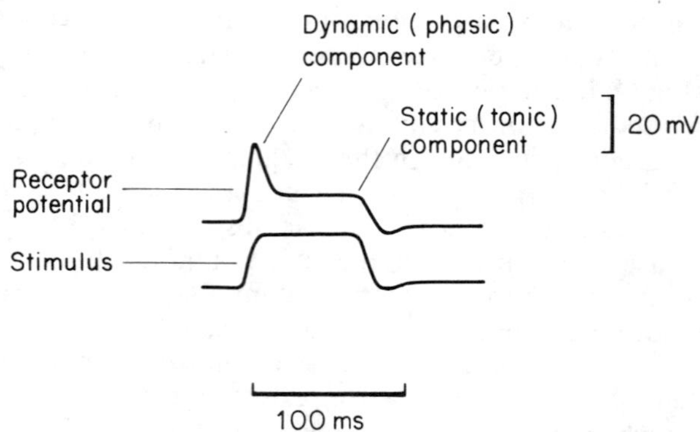


**Fig. 4.6** Intracellular recording from the T-fibre of a crustacean thoracic-coxal receptor showing the dynamic and static components of the receptor potential in response to a brief maintained stretch. (After Bush, B. M. H. and Roberts, A. (1971). *Journal of Experimental Biology*, **55,** 813–32.)

4.5b, c). Hence increase in the size of the receptor potential leads to an increase in the firing rate of the sensory cell. The rapid depolarization immediately preceding spike-initiation is called the pre-potential.

There are a few sensory cells in which information is transmitted to the central nervous system by means of graded potentials rather than action potentials, and indeed their membranes are incapable of supporting action potentials. In each case the axon is comparatively short and the sensory cell body is located within the central nervous system. The best known examples are the thoracic-coxal receptors of decapod crustaceans. These comprise a muscle receptor organ and two elastic receptors at the base of each leg (see Chapter 8). The receptor potential elicited by stimulation of such a receptor has a dynamic and a static component (Fig. 4.6), both of which are proportional to the rate and amplitude of the applied stimulus.

### Transduction

The ***transduction*** process, whereby the information content of a stimulus is changed into electrical potentials, varies according to the stimulus modality to which the receptor is sensitive, although there are probably some common underlying ionic changes. Visual receptors respond to changes in light intensity, chemoreceptors to variations in the chemical environment, electroreceptors to changes in the electric field surrounding an animal, mechanoreceptors to some form of physical deformation, and so on. In mechanoreceptors, the optimal stimulus appears in some cases to be elongation, in others compression, of some part of the dendritic membrane of the receptor cell, but there are different ways of achieving these deformations.

Some understanding has been reached of the relationship in mechanoreceptors between length and tension changes, the amplitude of the receptor potential and the frequency of action potential production. In the tonic abdominal muscle receptor organ of the crayfish and lobster a linear relationship has been proposed, both between firing frequency and receptor muscle tension, and between firing frequency and receptor muscle length; all researchers agreeing that length and tension are not linearly related. A linear relationship between receptor muscle length and firing frequency seems the more likely since the experimental work on which this proposal is based involved applying stretches to the receptor from the same initial length, thereby avoiding 'overstretch' and the cumulative effects of adaptation (Fig. 4.7).

## POSTSYNAPTIC POTENTIALS

Postsynaptic potentials occur in the postsynaptic membranes of nerve and muscle cells in response to activity in a presynaptic neuron. Two types can be differentiated—those which are electrically trans-

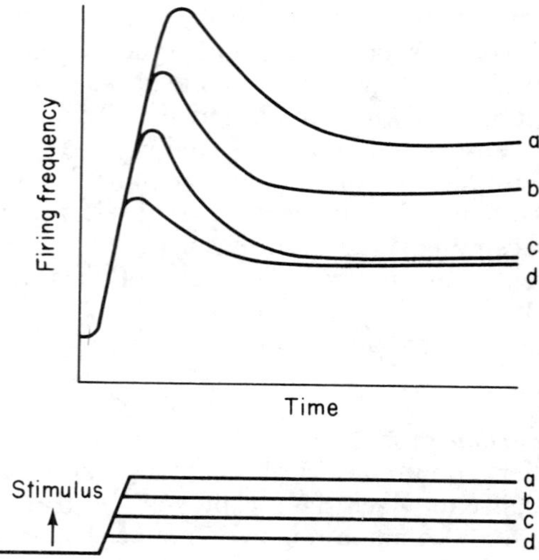


**Fig. 4.7** The relationship between firing frequency and time for four different levels of stretch (**a–d**) applied to the tonic abdominal muscle receptor organ of the crayfish. (From Brown, M. C. and Stein, R. B. (1966). *Kybernetik*, **3**, 175–85.)

mitted across the synapse and those which require the release of an intermediary chemical neurotransmitter.

**Electrical synapses**

The best known electrical synapses are those which occur between various large ('giant') interneurons in the central nervous system of many invertebrates and between these and 'giant' motor neurons. In the earthworm, *Lumbricus*, there is a single median and two lateral giant interneurons. Each consists of segmental units separated by septa which act as electrical synapses. Action potentials are conducted equally well in either direction across these junctions (***non-rectifying synapses***) without any loss in amplitude. The two lateral giant interneurons are also connected to each other via electrical synapses. Like the synapses between segmental units, these conduct in both directions (i.e. are non-rectifying) but the signal is attenuated across the synapse by about a third. The function of the synapses between the lateral giants is thought to be to ensure that they fire synchronously, and the attenuated depolarization is normally quite sufficient to ensure this.

At other electrical synapses, such as those between the lateral giant interneurons and the giant motor neurons of the crayfish, transmission is in one direction only. These are called ***rectifying synapses*** (Fig. 4.8). Electrical synapses also occur between the fibres of smooth muscles.

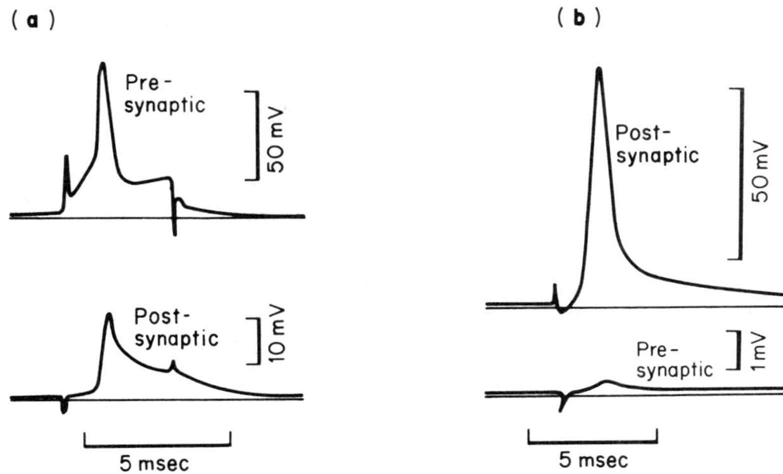


**Fig. 4.8** The effects of (**a**) orthodromic (the direction under natural conditions) and (**b**) antidromic (the reverse direction) stimulation at the rectifying electrical synapse between the lateral and motor giant fibres of the crayfish. Stimulation of the lateral giant (presynaptic) (**a**) produced a large postsynaptic potential in the motor giant; stimulation of the motor giant (postsynaptic) (**b**) elicited only a very small presynaptic potential in the lateral giant. (From Furshpan, E. J. and Potter, D. D. (1959), *Journal of Physiology*, **145,** 289–325.)

**Chemical synapses**

Chemical synapses can be divided into those which are excitatory and those which are inhibitory. However, it is important to note here that the nature of the action potential (see Chapter 6) is *identical in both excitatory and inhibitory neurons* and that it is the nature of the neurotransmitter substance present in the presynaptic axonal terminals and/or the reaction of the postsynaptic membrane to the neurotransmitter which determines the effect on the postsynaptic cell. In both excitatory and inhibitory neurons the action potential in the presynaptic axon invades the axonal terminals, or at least has an electrotonic depolarizing effect on them. This depolarization stimulates release of the neurotransmitter substance from the terminals into the synaptic cleft.

Whilst the majority of neurons are either excitatory or inhibitory in function, there are some, such as the right pedal giant neuron of the snail *Lymnea*, which have both excitatory and inhibitory effects. The available evidence indicates that such ***dual function*** neurons produce only a single neurotransmitter, and hence in these neurons it is presumably the response of the postsynaptic membrane to the neurotransmitter which determines the postsynaptic effect.

It is the chemical nature of synaptic transmission that produces polarization of information flow in the nervous system, with information passing from one 'presynaptic' cell which contains a neurotransmitter to another 'postsynaptic' cell which has receptor sites for this neurotransmitter. Information cannot travel in the reverse direction via a synapse even though parts of a cell (such as the axon) are physically capable of transmitting action potentials in either direction. As mentioned previously (p. 23, Fig. 1.16b), reciprocal synapses can exist between two neurons, but each of these transmit information in one direction only.

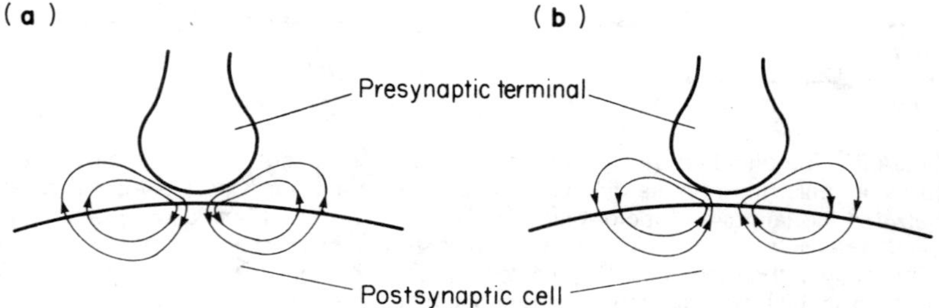


**Fig. 4.9** Diagrams showing the current flow across the postsynaptic membrane at (**a**) an excitatory and (**b**) an inhibitory synapse.

At excitatory synapses, the postsynaptic membrane permeability is altered in such a way that a current flows inwards through the postsynaptic membrane in the region of the synaptic cleft and outwards through the surrounding postsynaptic membrane (Fig. 4.9a). This results in a depolarizing potential in the postsynaptic cell. At inhibitory synapses, however, the postsynaptic potentials may be either hyperpolarizing *or depolarizing*, depending on the relationship between the resting potential of the cell and its inhibitory equilibrium level. In cells in which the inhibitory equilibrium level is more negative than the resting potential, such as the mammalian motor neuron, the inhibitory potential is hyperpolarizing. This is achieved by a current flow across the postsynaptic membrane in the reverse direction to that producing a depolarizing postsynaptic potential (Fig. 4.9b). In contrast, other cells, such as the crayfish muscle receptor organ (which receives both motor excitation and inhibition; p. 132), can have an inhibitory equilibrium level which is less negative than the resting potential. Under these circumstances the inhibitory potential is depolarizing. In the muscle receptor organ this occurs when the receptor is relaxed. However, as the receptor is stretched, the membrane potential becomes less negative (i.e. the cell becomes depolarized) until it passes the inhibitory equilibrium level; whereupon the inhibitory potential becomes hyperpolarizing (Fig. 4.10).

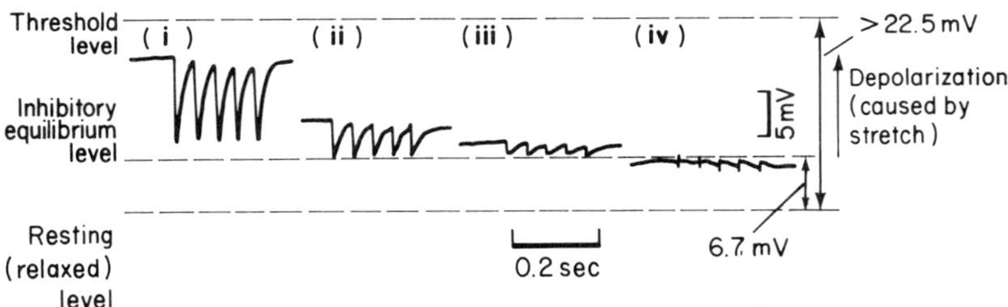


**Fig. 4.10** Intracellular recording from the sensory cell of the phasic abdominal muscle receptor organ of the crayfish to show the effect of the membrane potential on the inhibitory potentials elicited by stimulation of the inhibitory motor neuron at 20 $sec^{-1}$. Initially the cell was depolarized to near the threshold level (**i**) by applying a maintained stretch to the receptor. Progressive reduction of the stretch (**ii–iv**) caused corresponding increased levels of hyperpolarization and smaller inhibitory potentials, until at (**iv**) the inhibitory potentials became depolarizing. At the resting level of the completely relaxed cell the depolarizing inhibitory potentials had an amplitude of about 7 mV (not shown). The level of reversal from hyperpolarizing to depolarizing inhibitory potentials is the inhibitory equilibrium level. (After Kuffler, S. W. and Eyzaguirre, C. (1955). *Journal of General Physiology*, **391**, 155–83.)

Thus the difference between excitatory and inhibitory synapses is that, at the former, the postsynaptic potentials are always driving the cell towards its threshold level for action potential initiation and must therefore always be depolarizing; whereas, at inhibitory synapses, the postsynaptic potentials are always driving the cell towards its inhibitory equilibrium level. This may be either less or more negative than the resting potential, with consequent depolarizing and hyperpolarizing postsynaptic potentials respectively in the resting cell, but must always be more negative than the threshold level.

Before discussing the chemical nature of transmission (Chapter 5), examples of neuro-neuronal and neuromuscular synapses will be described.

## NEURO-NEURONAL SYNAPSES

The mammalian motor neuron has received considerable attention in work on the properties of neuro-neuronal synapses. It is a particularly suitable preparation in view of its large size (which enables penetration of the cell body with microelectrodes) and the number of neurons, both excitatory and inhibitory, which synapse on it. The postsynaptic potentials elicited in the motor neuron by

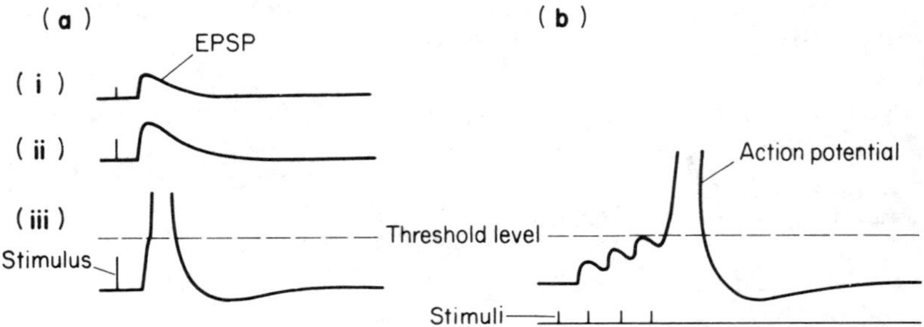


**Fig. 4.11** Diagrams to illustrate (**a**) spatial and (**b**) temporal summation of excitatory postsynaptic potentials (EPSPs) in a mammalian motor neuron. In (**a**) increased strength of stimulation causes the excitation of more presynaptic neurons and hence a larger EPSP which, if large enough to reach the threshold level, elicits a spike (**iii**). In (**b**) sequential stimulation of the same presynaptic neurons produces summation to the threshold level and hence the production of a spike, provided the frequency of stimulation is sufficiently high for each stimulus after the first to elicit an EPSP before that elicited by the previous stimulus has decayed completely away.

stimulation of excitatory and inhibitory presynaptic neurons are referred to respectively as ***excitatory postsynaptic potentials (EPSPs)*** and ***inhibitory postsynaptic potentials (IPSPs)***.

Stimulation of a single excitatory presynaptic neuron produces a small EPSP in the soma-dendritic region of the motor neuron. This depolarization is the sum of the very small individual EPSPs which occur at each of the synapses which the presynaptic axon makes with the motor neuron. Increase in the number of excitatory presynaptic nerves stimulated results in more synaptic regions contributing to the EPSP, and hence causes a larger EPSP (Fig. 4.11a). Since this represents a summation of events occurring at the same time at different sites it is known as ***spatial summation***. The same relationship exists between the inhibitory presynaptic neurons and the IPSP.

If a sufficiently large EPSP occurs, i.e. one which reaches the threshold level, it will initiate an action potential at the spike-initiating zone. In the mammalian motor neuron this is located in the initial segment region at the base of the axon, a region devoid of any synaptic contacts. The action potential is propagated along the axon to the periphery and also backwards (antidromically) into the soma-dendritic region.

An action potential may also be produced in the motor neuron by repetitive stimulation of a single excitatory neuron. This will produce a train of action potentials in the presynaptic neuron, each of which will elicit an EPSP in the motor neuron. If the action potentials in the train are sufficiently close together (i.e. the stimulation rate is reasonably high) so that the EPSP produced as a result of one action potential arriving at the synaptic region has not decayed completely away before the EPSP produced by the next action potential is elicited, then the second EPSP will sum with the remainder of the first and so on until the threshold level is reached (Fig. 4.11b). This summation of events occurring at the same place(s), but successively in time, is called ***temporal summation***.

Under normal circumstances in these cells, IPSPs are always hyperpolarizing potentials since, as mentioned above (p. 54), the inhibitory equilibrium level is below the resting level. However, if the membrane is artificially hyperpolarized (by passing current through an intracellular electrode) by several millivolts so that it is below the inhibitory equilibrium level, the IPSPs become depolarizing since they always try to drive the membrane towards this level.

At first sight one might expect the IPSP to be the exact reverse of the EPSP, but this is not the case. The EPSP decays with a rather longer time constant (over 4 msec) than that of the resting membrane (2.5 msec); whereas the IPSP has a similar time constant of decay to that of the resting membrane. This is a reflection of a difference between the time courses of the generator currents which flow across the postsynaptic membrane. In both cases the generator current achieves maximum intensity in 0.5 msec and then decreases rapidly. Indeed, at inhibitory synapses there is virtually no current flow after about 2 msec have elapsed. However, at excitatory synapses it decreases to about 10% of its maximum after 2 msec and there is then a residual flow of current which declines more slowly for several milliseconds (Fig. 4.12), and it is this which accounts for the longer time constant of decay of the EPSP.

Approximately simultaneous stimulation of excitatory and inhibitory presynaptic neurons produces an interaction between the EPSP and the IPSP. This interaction is dependent on their relative timing. Thus, if an EPSP is elicited when the IPSP is in its late stages there is simple summation (or rather subtraction since the IPSP is a hyperpolarizing potential) of the two potentials where they overlap

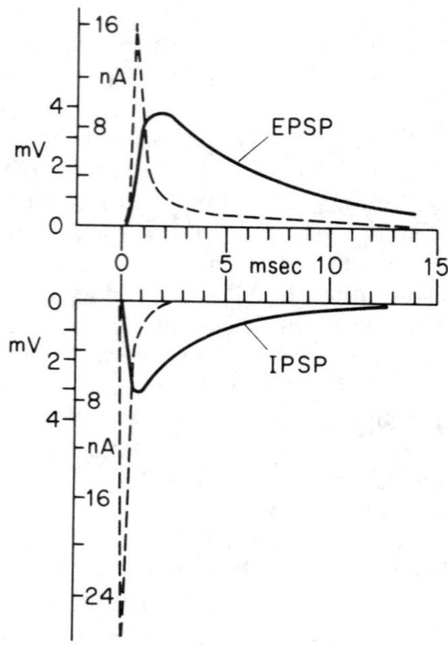


**Fig. 4.12** The mean values of intracellular recordings of EPSPs and IPSPs in a mammalian motor neuron (continuous lines). The dashed lines indicate the time courses of the subsynaptic currents required to generate these potential changes. mV, millivolts; nA, nanoamps. (After Coombs, J. S., Curtis, D. R. and Eccles, J. C. (1956). *Nature, London*, **178,** 1049–50.)

(Fig. 4.13c). However, if the order is reversed so that the EPSP is elicited first and the IPSP elicited in the late stages of the EPSP, then the effect of the IPSP is increased (potentiated) (Fig. 4.13d). This occurs because the effect of the EPSP is to significantly increase the distance of the membrane potential from the inhibitory equilibrium level, and under such conditions the voltage which drives the IPSP generator current is greatly increased. However, whatever the relative timing, the interaction occurs in the postsynaptic cell and the inhibition is hence referred to as postsynaptic inhibition.

Suppression of EPSPs has also been observed when stimulation of a presynaptic inhibitory neuron considerably precedes (by tens of milliseconds) stimulation of a presynaptic excitatory neuron, and indeed may occur in the absence of any detectable IPSPs. The maximum effect occurs with an interval of 15–20 msec, and it has been suggested that it is produced by the inhibitory axons making synaptic contact with the excitatory ones close to the axonal terminals

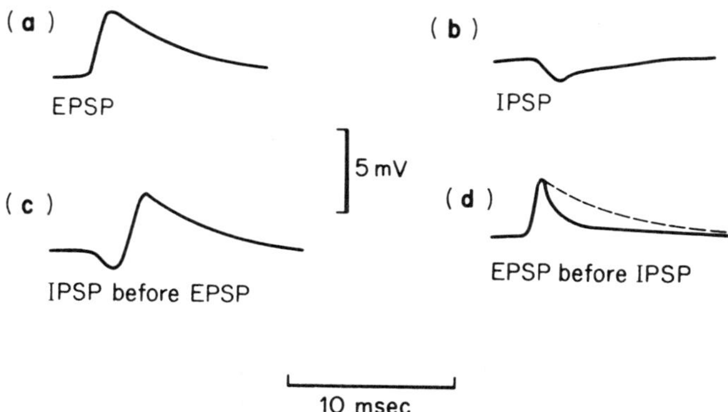


**Fig. 4.13** Tracings of intracellular recordings of EPSPs and IPSPs in a mammalian motor neuron evoked by stimulation of presynaptic neurons. (**a**) EPSP; (**b**) IPSP; (**c**) both, with the EPSP starting at about the time the IPSP has started to decline; (**d**) both, with the IPSP starting at about the time the EPSP has started to decline. In (**c**) there is a simple summation (subtraction) of the two repsonses. In (**d**) there is potentiation (enhancement) of the inhibition, the dotted line indicating the time course if simple summation had occurred. (After Coombs, J. S., Curtis, D. R. and Eccles, J. C. (1955). *Journal of Physiology*, **130,** 396–413.)

of the latter (i.e. a serial synapse arrangement as described in Chapter 1; Fig. 1.16a). Inhibition of the excitatory axon is thus occurring before it makes synaptic contact with the motor neuron, and hence is called presynaptic inhibition.

## NEUROMUSCULAR SYNAPSES

In vertebrates the motor axons are always excitatory and thus any inhibition of muscle activity occurs as a result of inhibition of the motor neurons within the central nervous system, i.e. ***central inhibition***. Hence the postsynaptic muscle potentials are always depolarizing. Since the synaptic region is called a motor end-plate, the postsynaptic potentials are referred to as ***end-plate potentials (EPPs)***. Although central inhibition is also found in arthropods, both excitatory and inhibitory motor axons occur in this group of animals (see Chapter 1) and hence there is ***peripheral inhibition*** in addition. The corresponding postsynaptic potentials are called ***excitatory junction potentials (EJPs)*** and ***inhibitory junction potentials (IJPs)***.

In arthropods, temporal summation of both EJPs and IJPs can occur and, in addition, successive presynaptic impulses may produce a larger postsynaptic response than can be attributed to simple summation; a phenomenon known as ***facilitation*** (Fig. 4.14). Furthermore, activity in one excitatory motor axon may augment a contraction produced soon afterwards by stimulation of a second excitatory motor axon. This is called ***heterofacilitation***.

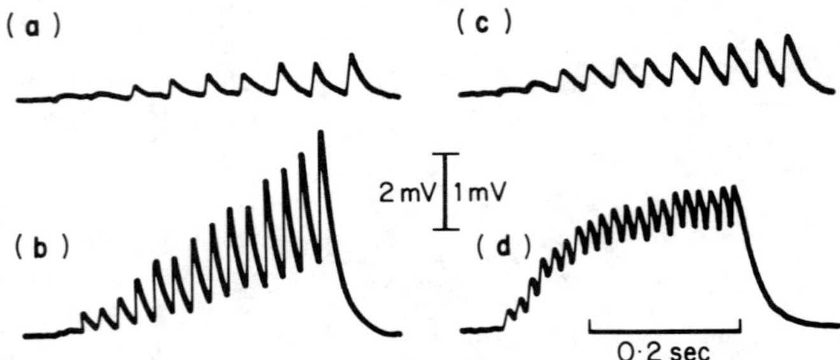


**Fig. 4.14** Tracings of intracellular recordings of excitatory (**a, b**) and inihibitory (**c, d**) junction potentials in the dactylopodite opener muscle in the walking leg of the crayfish *Orconectes virilis* elicited by stimulation of the excitatory and inhibitory motor neurons respectively. Stimulation rates were (**a**) 20 $sec^{-1}$, (**b**) 40 $sec^{-1}$, (**c**) 23 $sec^{-1}$, (**d**) 58 $sec^{-1}$. Note that both the EJPs and the IJPs show facilitation at the higher stimulation rates used. The inhibitory potentials are recorded at a higher amplitude than the excitatory potentials. (From Dudel, J. and Kuffler, S. W. (1961). *Journal of Physiology*, **155,** 531–42.)

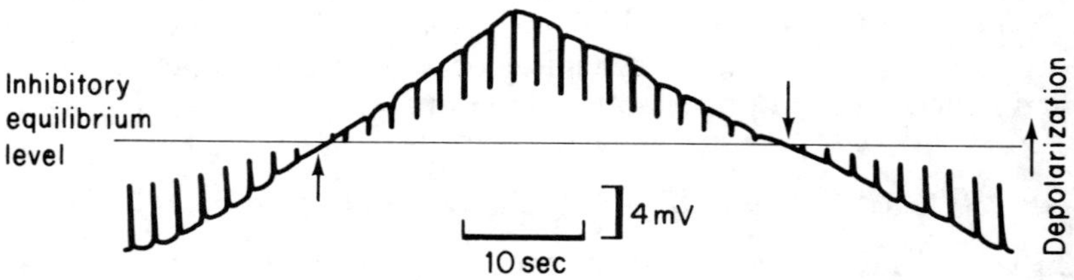


**Fig. 4.15** Tracing of intracellular recording of IJPs in the dactylopodite opener muscle in the walking leg of the crayfish *Orconectes virilis* elicited by stimulation of the inhibitory motor neuron, while the membrane potential was depolarized from −80 mV to −61 mV and back again by passing current through a second intracellular microelectrode. The IJPs were evoked by 0.2 second trains of inhibitory stimuli at 150 $sec^{-1}$, repeated every 2 seconds. The reversal potential (−72 mV) is the inhibitory equilibrium level. (From Dudel, J. and Kuffler, S. W. (1961). *Journal of Physiology*, **155,** 540–42.)

As was noted in discussing the effects of inhibitory stimuli on the membrane potential of the crustacean muscle receptor organ (p. 55), the IJPs always drive the membrane potential towards the inhibitory equilibrium level; in crayfish limb muscles the potential lies, as in the receptors, between the resting and threshold levels (Fig. 4.15).

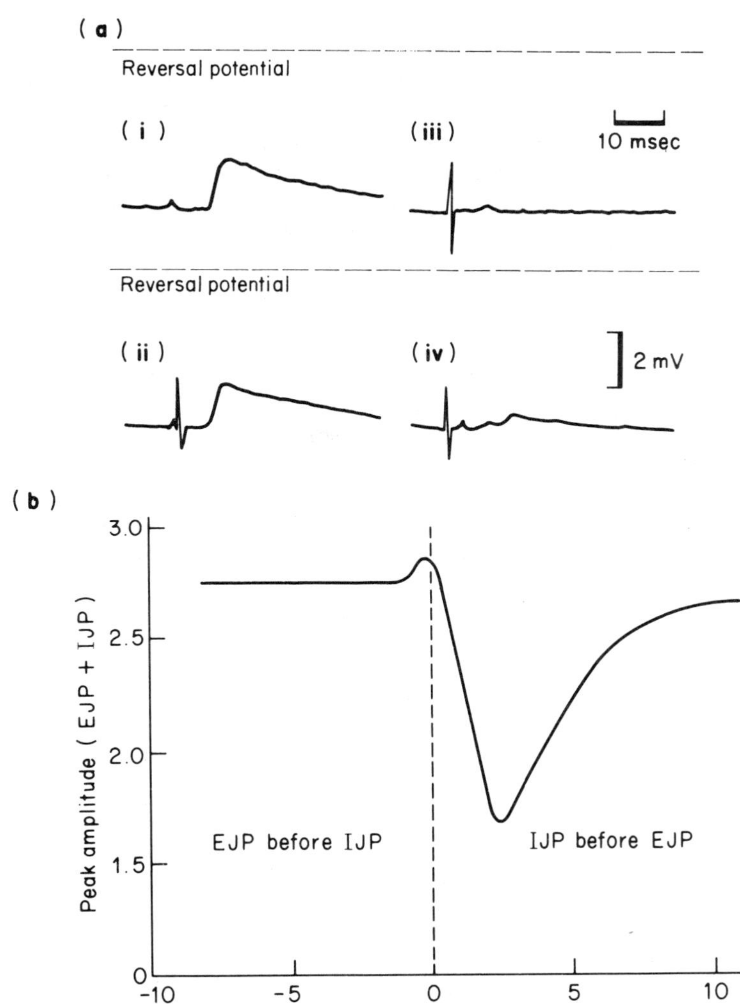


**Fig. 4.16** (**a**) Tracings of intracellular recordings of EJPs and IJPs in the dactylopodite opener muscle in the walking leg of the crayfish *Orconectes virilis* evoked by stimulation of the excitatory and inhibitory motor neurons respectively. (**i**) EJP; (**ii**) IJP occurring when the EJP has reached its peak (the excitatory axon was stimulated 1.5 msec before the inhibitory axon); (**iii**) IJP; (**iv**) IJP immediately preceding the EJP (the inhibitory axon was stimulated 3.0 msec before the excitatory axon). Note the extreme attenuation of the EJP. (**b**) The relationship between the peak amplitude of the EJP plus the IJP and the relative timing of the two potentials, based on an experiment as illustrated in (**a**). Note that in both (**a**) and (**b**) the inhibitory equilibrium level is 6 mV less negative than the resting potential and hence the IJPs are depolarizing. (After Dudel, J. and Kuffler, S. W. (1961). *Journal of Physiology*, **155,** 543–62.)

As at neuro-neuronal synapses, two types of inhibition have been noted at the crayfish neuromuscular junction. If an EJP and an IJP are elicited by presynaptic stimulation so that their peaks coincide, there is simple summation or subtraction, depending on the level of the membrane potential with respect to the inhibitory equilibrium level. This interaction of events in the postsynaptic membrane is postsynaptic inhibition (Fig. 4.16aii, b). However, if the IJP occurs a few milli-seconds before the EJP there is far greater suppression of the latter than can be accounted for by the above mechanism, and indeed optimum inhibition occurs when the IJP precedes the EJP by about 3 msec (Fig. 4.16aiv, b). This can best be explained if the inhibitory axon synapses directly with the excitatory axon close to the neuromuscular synapses of the latter (i.e. a serial synapse arrangement), so suppressing its effect. This is, therefore, presynaptic inhibition. The existence of both types of inhibition means that variations in the pattern of motor output can have a very precise effect on the control of muscular activity, which is presumably a necessity when so few motor axons innervate a muscle.

# 5

# The Pharmacology of Synaptic Transmission

In Chapter 4 it was noted that the transfer of information across the synaptic cleft is elicited by a chemical neurotransmitter substance which is synthesized and stored in the presynaptic cell. A wide variety of chemicals have been identified as neurotransmitters, or as potential (putative) neurotransmitters. Acetylcholine (ACh) is the best known and the most widely documented neurotransmitter. It occurs, for example, at vertebrate and some invertebrate (e.g. annelid) neuromuscular synapses and in the vertebrate parasympathetic system, and is widespread throughout much of the vertebrate central nervous system.

Many neurotransmitters are amines. Thus noradrenaline (norepinephrine) and adrenaline (epinephrine) are the neurotransmitters of the vertebrate sympathetic system. Noradrenaline is found in elasmobranchs, reptiles, birds and mammals; adrenaline occurs in teleosts and amphibians. Noradrenaline, at least, also occurs in brain stem cells which send branches to the cerebellar cortex (see Chapter 10). There is good evidence that dopamine, histamine and octopamine are all neurotransmitters in the vertebrate central nervous system, while 5-hydroxytryptamine (5-HT) (serotonin) is found in the insect central nervous system.

In insect and crustacean neuromuscular synapses there is a strong probability that the excitatory neurotransmitter is L-glutamate, while the inhibitory neurotransmitter at the neuromuscular synapses of insects, crustaceans and annelids is almost certainly $\gamma$-aminobutyric acid (GABA).

Other substances which have a putative neurotransmitter role include adenosine triphosphate (ATP) at vertebrate neuro-(smooth) muscular synapses, aspartate and various small, single chain peptides, including substance P which is widespread in the vertebrate nervous system.

Many of the above neurotransmitters are also found in other regions of the nervous system, with varying degrees of certainty as to their role, and many occur in both invertebrates and vertebrates. While most neurons undoubtedly possess only a single neurotransmitter, there is evidence that some do contain more than one. Furthermore, there are instances, notably in invertebrates, where a single neurotransmitter released from different synaptic endings of a single neuron can elicit different (sometimes opposite) postsynaptic effects. Thus, although in the above account neurotransmitters have been ascribed excitatory or inhibitory functions in relation to specific parts of the nervous system, it is extremely important to realize that the excitatory/inhibitory nature of a synapse may also depend on the type of receptors on the postsynaptic membrane and their response to the neurotransmitter.

## NEUROTRANSMITTER SYNTHESIS AND STORAGE

It is generally accepted that ACh is manufactured in the presynaptic terminals by a process involving the interaction of acetyl-coenzyme A and choline in the presence of the enzyme choline acetyltransferase (Fig. 5.1). Similarly, noradrenaline, adrenaline and GABA are probably produced in the nerve terminals. Adrenaline is derived from tyrosine via dopamine and noradrenaline. The precursor of the inhibitory neurotransmitter GABA is the excitatory neurotransmitter L-glutamate, derived from glucose via the tricarboxylic acid cycle. Hence in arthropods the presence or absence of the enzyme glutamate decarboxylase, which converts L-glutamate to GABA, determines whether the nerve terminals are inhibitory or excitatory respectively. The biosynthetic pathways of a number of neurotransmitters are given in Fig. 5.1.

There is good evidence that ACh, adrenaline, noradrenaline, dopamine, 5-HT and ATP are stored in synaptic vesicles, but probably only some GABA and glycine is stored in this way, the rest being free in the nerve terminal. Some of the amino acid derived neurotransmitters, such as L-glutamate and aspartate, may not be generally associated with vesicles.

There is controversy over the site of production of the synaptic vesicles. The dense-cored noradrenergic vesicles are of two types; the larger ones are thought to be formed by the Golgi apparatus in the

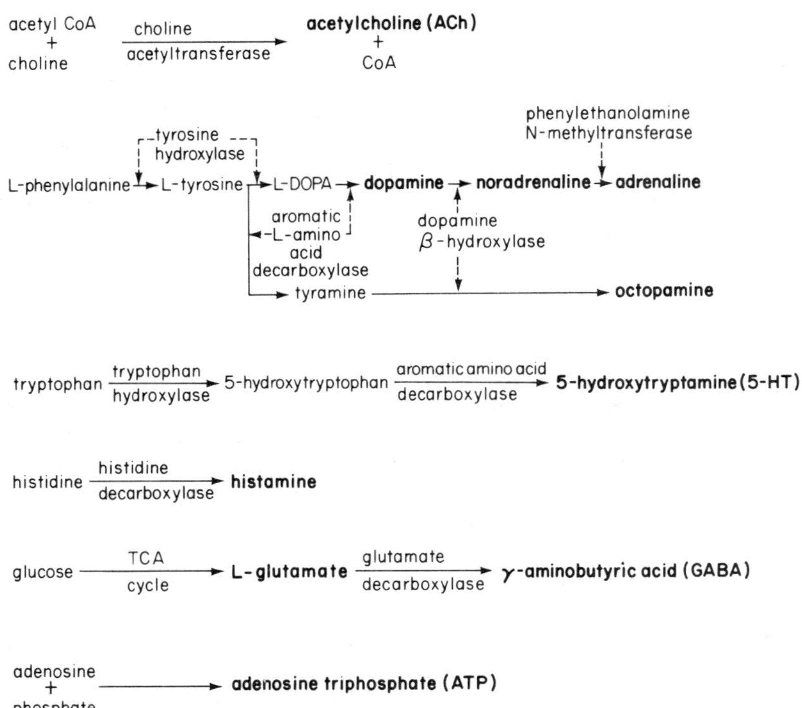


**Fig. 5.1** The biosynthetic pathways of some putative neurotransmitters (bold type).

cell body and transported to the presynaptic terminals, but the site of production of the smaller ones (which are thought to be the main site of noradrenaline storage in the presynaptic terminals) is less certain. There is, however, evidence that they too are produced in the cell body, or possibly formed from the larger ones. As for the vesicles of other neurotransmitter systems, current evidence points towards formation in or near the presynaptic terminals, although an origin in the Golgi apparatus of the cell body has not been ruled out entirely. Various suggestions have been put forward: that they are formed from smooth endoplasmic reticulum, from mitochondria, from the surface membrane by a process of endocytosis, and even from neurotubules. However, it seems that, if neurotubules do play a role, it is more likely to be in the transport of the vesicles to the vicinity of the presynaptic membrane. ACh is probably manufactured in the cytoplasm of the terminals and then taken up into the vesicles. However, dopamine-$\beta$-hydroxylase is present in adrenergic vesicles, suggesting that the final stage in the synthesis of noradrenaline occurs within the vesicles.

In many synapses the vesicles are separated from the presynaptic membrane by electron-dense bodies (see Fig. 1.15) and an alternative theory, arising from this, is that the vesicles convey the neurotransmitter to a store in the region of the presynaptic membrane, the electron-dense bodies adjacent to this membrane perhaps being associated with such a storage function. It is, of course, possible that both types of storage (vesicular and extra-vesicular) occur.

## NEUROTRANSMITTER RELEASE

The most widely adopted hypothesis regarding transmitter release into the synaptic cleft is that the wall of the vesicle fuses with that of the presynaptic surface membrane with subsequent release of the vesicle contents into the synaptic cleft (i.e. a process of exocytosis) and, at the vertebrate motor end-plate, there is evidence that the vesicles fuse with the membrane along a special active zone. If exocytosis does occur, presumably the surface area of the axonal terminal is increased, and it has been suggested that these additional areas of surface membrane move away from the site of transmitter release and are then pinched off internally for re-use as synaptic vesicles. Cyclic nucleotides may play a role in the release of neurotransmitters. The release of ACh, noradrenaline, GABA and L-glutamate is dependent on extracellular calcium, which is taken up into the nerve terminals when they are depolarized. The release of ACh, noradrenaline and dopamine is further controlled by a negative feedback mechanism involving receptors on the presynaptic membrane. Moreover, it seems probable that ACh is involved in the control of noradrenaline release from parasympathetic nerves.

Both the 'exocytosis of vesicles' and the 'extra-vesicular store' theories are compatible with the idea of the quantal release of neurotransmitter which is discussed below. In the case of the exocytosis theory, each vesicle is held to contain a single quantum of neurotransmitter. Alternatively, if there is a presynaptic, extra-vesicular store of neurotransmitter, quantal release could be explained by the presence of a gating mechanism in the presynaptic membrane which allows specific amounts (quanta) of neurotransmitter to pass through.

### Quantal nature of synaptic transmission

The quantal nature of synaptic transmission has been investigated thoroughly in two neuromuscular preparations—frog fast skeletal muscle and the dactylopodite extensor (leg) muscle of the crayfish. In both cases the results obtained support the quantal hypothesis, although variations in detail occur between the two preparations consequent upon their different motor innervation patterns. Frog fast skeletal muscle receives a number of excitatory motor axons but there is only one synaptic region, the motor end-plate, on each muscle fibre. In contrast, the crayfish dactylopodite extensor muscle is innervated by a single excitatory motor axon together with a single inhibitory motor axon and there are numerous synapses on each muscle fibre (see Chapter 1).

In both preparations, spontaneous depolarizing potentials, which are not associated with any motor neuron activity, occur sporadically. These potentials are small and are always of similar amplitude. Their average size is about 500 $\mu$V in the frog muscle and about 70 $\mu$V in the crayfish muscle. They are referred to as ***spontaneous miniature potentials (SMPs)*** (Fig. 5.2) or sometimes as ***miniature end-plate potentials (MEPPs)*** in the frog. They are evidently produced at synapses, since they can only be recorded extracellularly when the recording electrode is at or close to a synapse. They are always recorded by an intracellular electrode. However, in the multiterminally innervated crayfish muscle there are many synapses at which an SMP can arise and the ratio between SMPs recorded intracellularly and those recorded with an extracellular electrode at a single synapse (60:1) is thought to give some indication of the number of excitatory synapses on a single muscle fibre (i.e. about 60), assuming that the SMPs are occurring randomly.

The potentials elicited by stimulation of the excitatory motor axon(s) are called end-plate potentials (EPPs) in the frog and excitatory junction potentials (EJPs) in the crayfish (see Chapter 4); they are considerably larger than the spontaneous potentials (Fig. 5.2).

The idea behind the quantal theory is that the spontaneous potentials are the result of individual packets or quanta of transmitter being released randomly from the presynaptic nerve endings, while the elicited EPPs and EJPs are produced by the release of large numbers of quanta of transmitter at the synapses as a result of their excitation. If this is the case, then the amplitudes of the EPPs and EJPs should be multiples of the amplitudes of the SMPs and this has been shown to be so in both preparations. Some of the evidence is considered below.

In the frog muscle the EPPs are normally all about the same size. However, progressive reduction of calcium in the external bathing medium results in a reduction in the amplitude of the EPPs and, at low external calcium concentrations, the amplitude reductions obviously proceed step-wise, with the smallest EPPs being of similar magnitude to the SMPs. A similar effect can be achieved by increasing the external magnesium concentration (Fig. 5.3).

In the crayfish muscle, the intracellularly recorded EJPs, like the frog EPPs, are all of similar amplitude. However, EJPs recorded extracellularly from a single synaptic zone vary in amplitude and, indeed, may not occur after every stimulus (Figs 5.2b, 5.4). Furthermore, the smallest recorded extracellular EJPs are of a similar

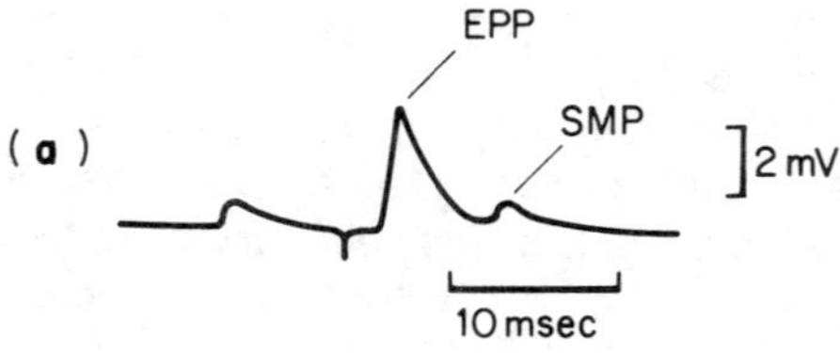


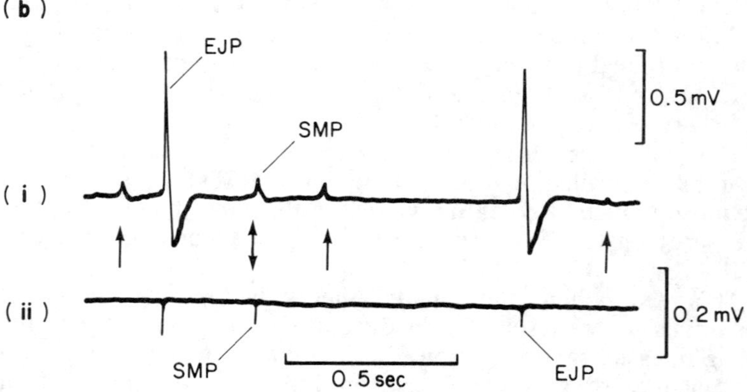


**Fig. 5.2** (**a**) Intracellular recording of two spontaneous miniature potentials (SMPs) and an end-plate potential (EPP) in a mammalian skeletal muscle fibre. (**b**) Recordings from a muscle fibre of a crayfish limb muscle during stimulation of the excitatory motor neuron at a frequency of 1 $sec^{-1}$. Upper trace (**i**) shows an intracellular recording of four SMPs (arrows) and two EJPs. Lower trace (**ii**) shows a simultaneous extracellular recording from a single synaptic region. Note that there is only a single SMP (arrow) and that it is the same amplitude as the second elicited EJP. ((**a**) From Liley, A. W. (1956). *Journal of Physiology*, **133,** 571–87; (**b**) from Dudel, J. and Kuffler, S. W. (1961). *Journal of Physiology*, **155,** 514–29.)

magnitude to the SMPs, while the larger ones tend to be direct multiples of this minimum size.

In both preparations the size distribution of the excited potentials (EPPs and EJPs) has been analysed (Fig. 5.5). The Poisson distribution expresses the probability of an unlikely event occurring. This should apply if there are a large number of quanta available for release from the presynaptic terminals but only comparatively few are released following a single stimulus, i.e. the probability of any one being released is an unlikely event. The Poisson distribution is given by

$$\frac{n_x}{N} = \frac{m^x}{x!} e^{-m}$$

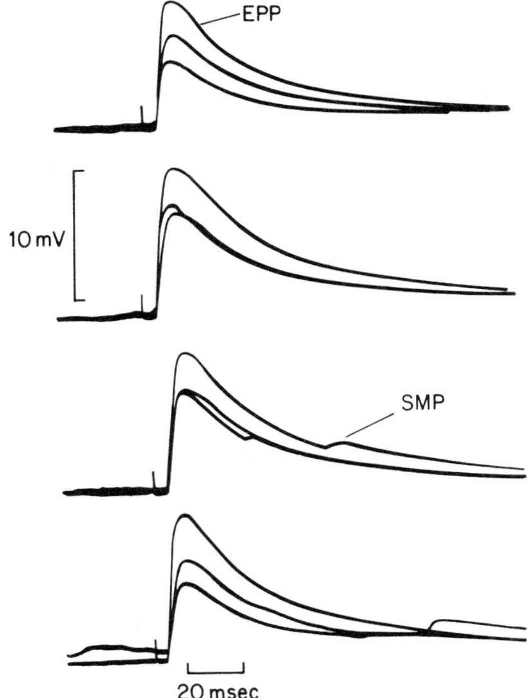


**Fig. 5.3** The effect on EPPs of increasing the concentration of the external magnesium ions. This reduces the amount of acetylcholine released by each action potential. Thus the EPPs are smaller and fluctuate in a step-wise manner. Each recording comprises three superimposed sweeps. Note the occassional spontaneous minature potentials. (From Del Castillo, J. and Katz, B. (1954). *Journal of Physiology*, **124**, 560–73.)

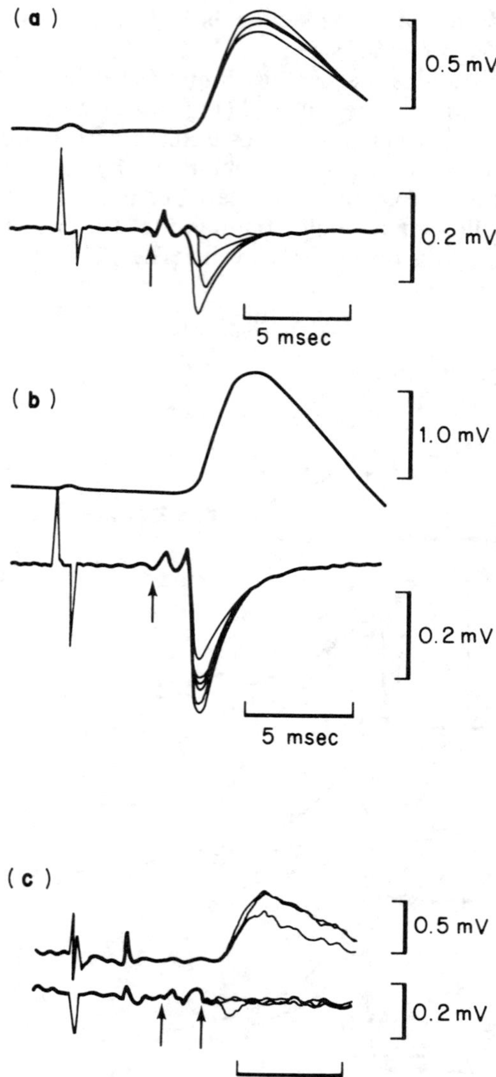


**Fig. 5.4** Simultaneous intracellular (upper traces) and extracellular (lower traces) recordings of evoked EJPs from a muscle fibre of a crayfish limb muscle. (**a**) Stimulation of the excitatory motor neuron at 1 $sec^{-1}$: four superimposed sweeps. (**b**) Stimulation of the excitatory motor axon at 5 $sec^{-1}$, at which frequency facilitation occurs: seven superimposed sweeps. (**c**) Stimulation of both the excitatory and the inhibitor motor axons at 1 $sec^{-1}$, the inhibitory stimulus preceding the excitatory one

where x is the number of quanta in a single response, m is the mean number of quanta in a response (derived from all values of x), N is the total number of responses and $n_x$ is the number of occasions on which x quanta are released by a nerve stimulus. When $x = 0$ we obtain

$$n_0 = Ne^{-m}$$

The number of times when a stimulus does not elicit synaptic transmission ($n_0$) can be counted; also the value of N is known. Hence m can be calculated ($m = \log_e(N/n_0)$). Succeeding terms of the Poisson distribution can then be calculated. Thus

$$n_1 = mn_0$$
$$n_2 = (\tfrac{1}{2}m)n_1$$
$$n_3 = (\tfrac{1}{3}m)n_2$$

and from these a Poisson distribution can be drawn. In both preparations the experimental results showed a good fit with this calculated Poisson distribution derived from the experimental values of $n_0/N$.

The size of the average *unit* potential ($E_1$) can be obtained by dividing the mean amplitude of the elicited potentials ($\bar{E}$) by m, i.e.

$$E_1 = \frac{\bar{E}}{m}$$

If the spontaneous potentials are each caused by the release of a single quantum of neurotransmitter, their mean amplitude ($\bar{M}$) should be the same as that of the average unit potential. The value of m calculated by dividing the mean amplitude of the elicited potentials by the mean amplitude of the spontaneous potentials, i.e.

$$m = \frac{\bar{E}}{\bar{M}}$$

should be the same as that calculated from $m = \log_e(N/n_0)$. The above have been shown to be the case in both preparations.

In summary, the evidence shows that, following motor nerve stimulation, the current flow across the postsynaptic membrane is

---

by 2 msec: three superimposed sweeps. The extracellular recordings are from a single synaptic region and the arrows indicate the action potentials in the motor axons. In comparison with (**a**) the number of failures of transmission is less in (**b**) and more in (**c**); similarly the EJPs tend to be larger in (**b**) and smaller in (**c**). Arrows indicate nerve potentials. ((**a**), (**b**) After Dudel, J. and Kuffler, S. W. (1961). *Journal of Physiology*, **155,** 530–42; (**c**) after Dudel, J. and Kuffler, S. W. (1961). *Journal of Physiology*, **155,** 543–62.)

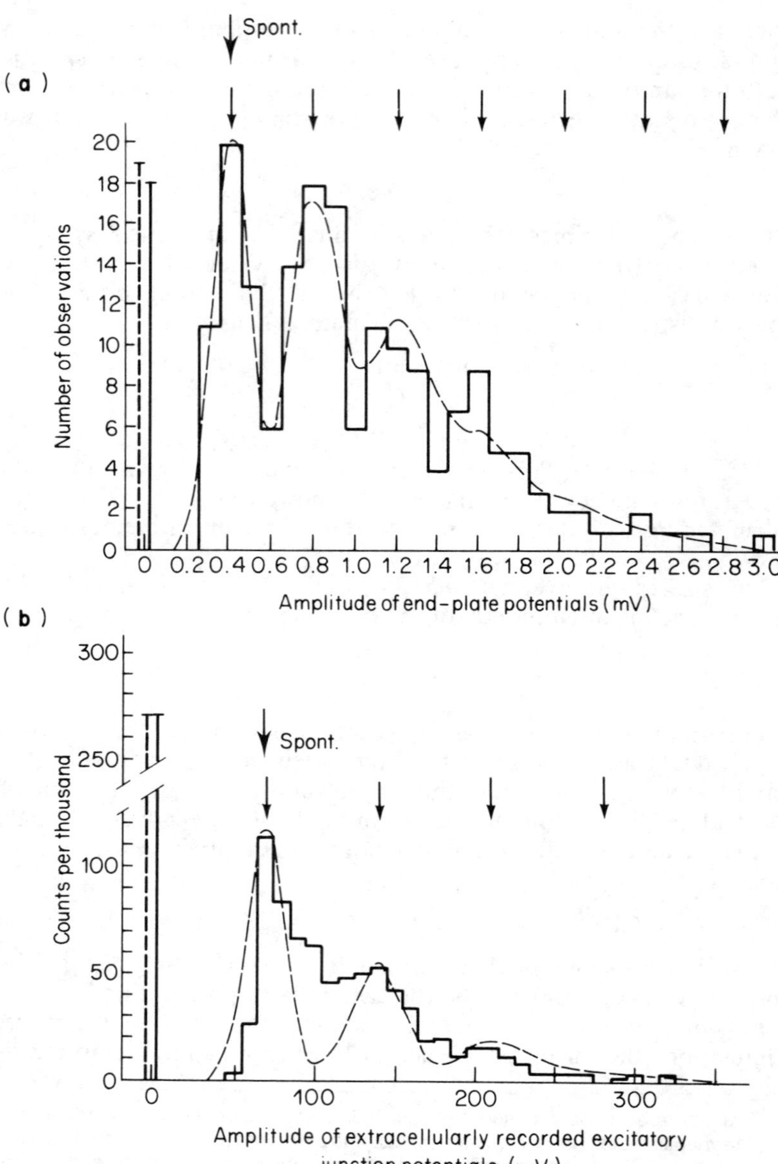


**Fig. 5.5** Histograms of the size distribution of (**a**) intracellularly recorded EPPs from a frog skeletal muscle fibre in which neuronmuscular transmission was blocked by an increased external magnesium concentration, and (**b**) extracellularly recorded EJPs

quantal in nature and that this is probably a result of the neurotransmitter being released from the nerve terminals in discrete packets or quanta. In the frog muscle there is normally a large number of packets (probably about 250) liberated at the end-plate as a result of a single presynaptic impulse. In the crayfish muscle the number liberated at any given synapse is low (1 or 2); although the total number liberated at all of the synapses on any one fibre is quite high.

*Facilitaton and inhibition*

In the crayfish, if the frequency of excitatory motor neuron stimulation is sufficiently high, facilitation of the EJPs occurs at each synapse. This is seen, recorded extracellularly at a single synapse, as an increase in the number of larger potentials and a reduction in the number of occasions when synaptic transmission does not occur (Fig. 5.4b). Thus the average size of the potentials is increased and hence m is increased.

Stimulation of the inhibitory motor axon elicits inhibitory junction potentials (IJPs) (Chapter 4) and these can also be facilitated by increasing the stimulation frequency (see Fig. 4.14). However, if both the excitatory and the inhibitory axons are stimulated repetitively at a frequency below that which causes facilitation and so that each EJP is immediately preceded by an IJP to obtain an effective level of presynaptic inhibition (Chapter 4), there is a reduction in the average amplitude of the extracellularly recorded EJPs and an increase in the number of occasions when synaptic transmission does not occur (Fig. 5.4c), and hence m is decreased.

Analysis of facilitation and inhibition, using the techniques described above, shows that they can be explained in terms of an increase and a decrease respectively in the probability of transmitter being released at any given synapse. Thus the effect is presynaptic. There is no indication of any change either in the quantum size or in the sensitivity of the postsynaptic membrane.

This is further confirmed by the effect on the SMPs, the frequency of which increases during facilitation and decreases during optimal presynaptic inhibition, while maintaining a similar average amplitude.

---

from a single synaptic area on a crustacean limb muscle fibre. The dashed lines are theoretical curves derived from Gaussian curves fitted to a distribution calculated using the Poisson equation. Large arrows indicate the average size of the SMPs; small arrows indicate multiples of the unit size. ((**a**) After Boyd, I. A. and Martin, A. R. (1956). *Journal of Physiology*, **132,** 74–91; (**b**) from Dudel, J. and Kuffler, S. W. (1961). *Journal of Physiology*, **155,** 514–29.)

Facilitation also occurs in vertebrate muscle and has been demonstrated in, for example, rat diaphragm muscle when decrease in the external calcium ion concentration is followed by repetitive stimulation.

## ACTIVATION OF THE POSTSYNAPTIC MEMBRANE

The time taken for the neurotransmitter to be released and to diffuse to the postsynaptic membrane determines the synaptic delay time. Once the neurotransmitter reaches the postsynaptic membrane it combines with receptor sites on it. Not only does each neurotransmitter interact with a specific receptor, but some at least interact with two or more different types of receptor and thereby produce different postsynaptic effects. Thus, in vertebrates, there are two types of ACh receptor—nicotinic and muscarinic—which are characterized by their responses to nicotine and the alkaloid muscarine respectively. Nicotinic receptors occur at synapses between pre- and postganglionic fibres in the autonomic nervous system, at neuro(skeletal)muscular synapses, and in the mammalian motor neuron—Renshaw cell system; muscarinic receptors occur at most other cholinergic synapses, such as those formed by the postganglionic fibres of the parasympathetic system. In some cases both types of receptor occur on a single cell and, in mammalian ganglion cells for instance, the fast and slow components of the response can be ascribed to the separate receptors.

Similarly, there are two main receptor types for noradrenaline (the $\alpha$- and $\beta$-receptors), two for glutamate (the D- and H-receptors) and at least two for 5-HT (the D- and M(morphine)-receptors). There are indications that in ganglion cells in the molluscs *Helix* and *Aplysia* there may be as many as six 5-HT receptor types.

Receptors are classified in terms of the chemical specificity of the ligand recognition process, rather than by their physiological postsynaptic effects. Hence, in visceral ganglion cells of *Aplysia* three ACh receptors can occur on a single cell, two of which are nicotinic, one mediating a fast depolarization, the other a fast hyperpolarization. The third receptor type, which mediates a slow hyperpolarization, is neither nicotinic nor muscarinic. Different ACh receptors may affect conductance changes of $Na^+$, $K^+$ or $Cl^-$ ions individually or in various combinations. This indicates that the receptors are composed of a neurotransmitter recognition component and a catalytic component to mediate the physiological function.

The effect of ACh on vertebrate skeletal muscle will be described to illustrate one of the conductance-change mechanisms by which depolarization of the postsynaptic cell may be brought about. In this case the effect is to markedly increase the permeability of the postsynaptic membrane to both sodium and potassium ions, the former moving into the cell, the latter outwards. Hence the membrane potential of this region tends towards a value in between the equilibrium potentials of these two ions (p. 34). Thus there is a depolarization in the order of tens of millivolts. Although the immediate postsynaptic membrane cannot support an action potential, current flows inwards across this region and outwards through the surrounding postsynaptic membrane, so that the latter is depolarized. In frog fast skeletal muscle fibres, where there is only a single synapse per fibre, this depolarization of the surrounding membrane is usually sufficient to elicit an action potential in the muscle fibre. Other ways in which depolarization can be achieved are by increasing the membrane permeability to sodium ions alone, or by decreasing the membrane permeability to potassium ions.

At inhibitory synapses the permeability of the postsynaptic membrane is increased to potassium and/or chloride ions, both of which have equilibrium levels close to the resting potential of the cell. Depending on the membrane potential of the cell, on the equilibrium potentials of these two ions, and on the changes in membrane permeability to them, the membrane of the postsynaptic cell is *either hyperpolarized or depolarized* towards its inhibitory equilibrium level (see Chapter 4).

Membrane permeability could presumably be increased, either by altering the configuration of certain membrane proteins so that ion channels are opened, or by directly affecting the enzyme-controlled ionic pump mechanism; or perhaps by a combination of both.

Neurotransmitters are unable to penetrate the membrane of the postsynaptic cell and hence must produce their effect on the permeability of the postsynaptic membrane by binding to and activating the receptors on this membrane. These receptors are large protein molecules and are specific for individual neurotransmitters. Considerable insight has been gained into the mechanism of receptor activation by using various substances which act like the neurotransmitter and activate the receptors (agonists), and other substances which also bind with the receptors but block their activity (antagonists).

At least two suggestions have been put forward as to how the interaction of the neurotransmitter with the receptor operates. It is possible that the receptor is directly activated by the neurotransmitter (or an agonist) binding to it, and that antagonists also bind to the receptor but in such a way that activation does not occur (Fig. 5.6).

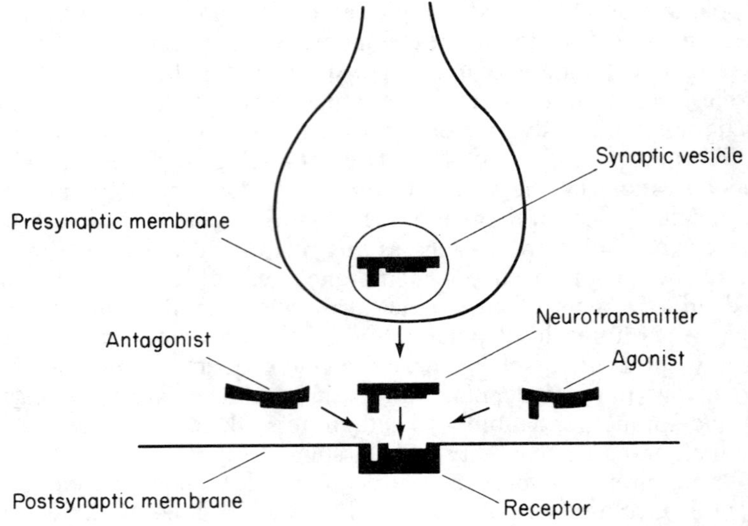


**Fig. 5.6** Theoretical model of the binding of the neurotransmitter and its agonists and antagonists to the postsynaptic receptor. (After Nathanson, J. A. and Greengard, P. (1977). *Scientific American*, **237** (Aug.), 108–19.)

An alternative possibility is that the receptor protein can exist in either of two conformations, resting and active, and that most receptors are in the resting state in the absence of neurotransmitter. The neurotransmitter (or an agonist) binds preferentially to the active conformation. In order to restore the equilibrium between unbound active and resting receptors there is a shift from resting to active states, and this continues while there is sufficient neurotransmitter present to bind with the active receptors. Antagonists, on the other hand, bind preferentially to the resting conformation and hence result in a shift towards the resting state (Fig. 5.7). There is evidence that long exposure to the neurotransmitter results in desensitization. This condition could be brought about by the neurotransmitter becoming more lightly bound to the receptor and producing a third 'desensitized' conformation of the receptor protein.

There appear to be at least two types of synaptic mechanism, related to different speeds and durations of activity. Voluntary (skeletal) muscle needs to be able to react rapidly to information arriving at the neuromuscular synapses and so the effect of the neurotransmitter released from the axonal terminals on the permeability of the postsynaptic membrane must be very rapid. In

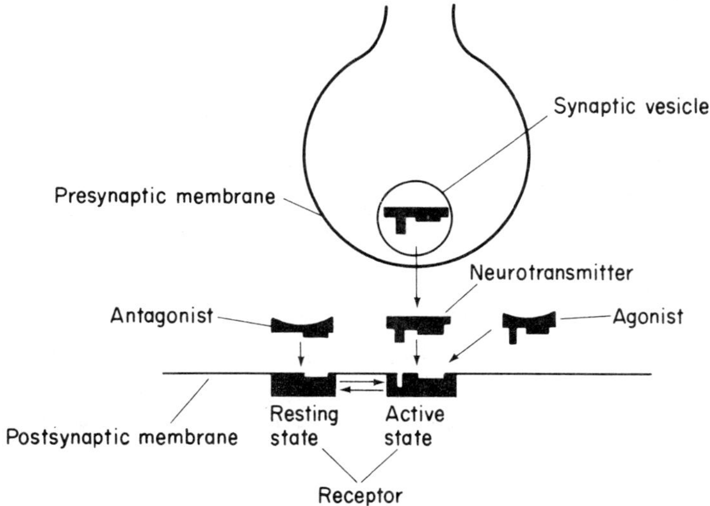


**Fig. 5.7** Rather more elaborate theoretical model than that shown in Fig. 5.6, in which the postsynaptic receptor protein exists in different conformational states. (After Lester, H. A. (1977). *Scientific American*, **236** (Feb.), 106–18 and Nathanson, J. A. and Greengard, P. (1977). *Scientific American*, **237** (Aug.), 108–19 (based partly on a theoretical model proposed by J.-P. Changeux).)

contrast, there is evidence of a much slower mechanism, with a longer lasting effect, at many synapses within the mammalian central nervous system; notably at some of those which are concerned with a modulatory role. These two systems are discussed below.

**Fast transmission system**

Much of the information on this system has been obtained from the electric organs of certain teleost fishes. These consist of modified muscle cells (electroplaques) and are particularly well-endowed with postsynaptic receptors. As mentioned in Chapter 1, the receptors at the end-plate of vertebrate voluntary muscle are located on the crests of the junctional folds and also extend part of the way down into them. The neurotransmitter at these synapses is acetylcholine and it has been calculated that one presynaptic nerve impulse releases the contents of about 100 synaptic vesicles at the end-plate and that the neurotransmitter contained in one vesicle can open some 2000 ion channels in the postsynaptic membrane in about 0.3 msec—a very rapid process. Each open channel is associated with an approximately square pulse of current which lasts for a few milliseconds. The acetylcholine is rapidly broken down into choline and acetate by acetylcholinesterase, which occurs in the synaptic cleft and lines the junctional folds.

It has been suggested that each receptor opens a channel directly when it has been activated, and that it has functionally distinct parts

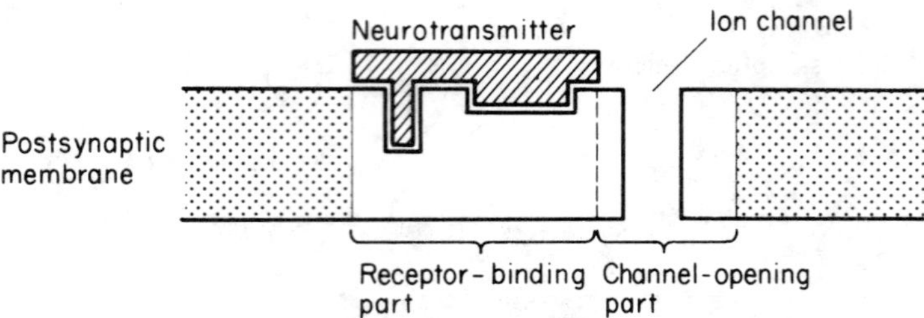


**Fig. 5.8** Simple theoretical model for the fast-acting postsynaptic receptor system, with the ion channel comprising part of the receptor.

for binding the neurotransmitter and for opening the channel (Fig. 5.8).

**Slow transmission system**

This type of system involves the use of cyclases and cyclic nucleotides to transfer information from the activated receptors to the permeability controlling mechanism of the cell. The best documented examples are those which involve adenylate cyclase and cyclic adenosine monophosphate (cyclic AMP). Thus, when the neurotransmitter becomes bound to a receptor, adenylate cyclase is activated to convert adenosine triphosphate (ATP) into cyclic AMP. Those hormones which cannot penetrate cell membranes use the same mechanism to transfer information to the internal biochemical machinery of the target cells.

In the postsynaptic cell the cyclic AMP binds with the inhibitory subunit of protein kinase, thus freeing the catalytic subunit of this enzyme to transfer a phosphate group from ATP to a membrane protein. The latter is thereby altered so as to increase the membrane permeability, either by opening up an ion channel or by affecting the ionic pump mechanism (see Chapter 2). The cyclic AMP is inactivated by phosphodiesterase, while phosphoprotein phosphatase removes the phosphate group from the membrane protein, again reducing membrane permeability (Fig. 5.9).

In support of this interpretation of the mechanism, adenylate cyclase, cyclic-AMP-dependent protein kinase, phosphorylated proteins, phosphodiesterase and phosphoprotein phosphatase have all

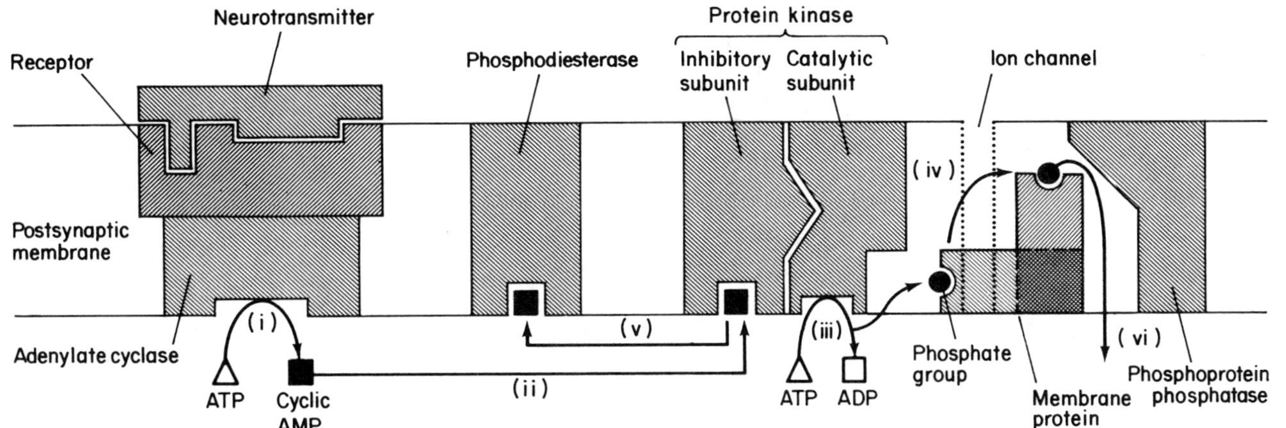


**Fig. 5.9** Theoretical model for the slow-acting postsynaptic receptor system, involving cyclic AMP. Several stages are envisaged in the functioning of this model. Binding of the neurotransmitter to the receptor activates adenylate cyclase to convert ATP to cyclic AMP (**i**); the cyclic AMP binds to the inhibitory subunit of a protein kinase (**ii**), thereby freeing the catalytic subunit to transfer a phosphate molecule from ATP to a membrane protein (**iii**), the molecular configuration of which is thereby altered to open an ion channel (**iv**); the reaction is stopped when the neurotransmitter dissociates from the receptor and any remaining cyclic AMP is deactivated by phosphodiesterase (**v**); the molecular configuration of the membrane protein is restored and the ion channel closed when phosphoprotein phosphatase removes the phosphate molecule from the membrane protein (vi). (After Nathanson, J. A. and Greengard, P. (1977). *Scientific American*, **237** (Aug.), 108–19.)

been found in those fractions of homogenized mammalian brain tissue which contain most of the synaptic membrane fragments, and dopamine-sensitive adenylate cyclase has been located specifically in the caudate nucleus. Furthermore, the concentration of cyclic AMP in brain tissue is sufficient to activate the protein kinase, and stimulation of the appropriate nerves results in an increase in cyclic AMP in the nerve tissue. Also, protein kinase has been found to transfer a phosphate group to certain proteins and those proteins phosphorylated to the greatest extent occur in the synaptic membrane fragments fraction of homogenized brain tissue. Only two or three of the several dozen proteins in this fraction are phosphorylated to any marked degree. Thus the necessary constituents and reactions which would enable this mechanism to operate are present. There is, however, no direct proof that phosphorylation is a definite precursor of membrane permeability changes and it may, itself, be a secondary effect.

The neurotransmitters dopamine, noradrenaline, histamine, octopamine and 5-HT (serotonin) have all been shown to activate specific neurotransmitter-sensitive adenylate cyclases. While there is evidence that acetylcholine, noradrenaline and histamine, at certain synapses (i.e. not the motor nerve–voluntary muscle synapses in the case of acetylcholine, and cyclic AMP synapses in the cases of noradrenaline and histamine), activate a different specific neurotransmitter-sensitive cyclase, guanylate cyclase. This enzyme converts guanosine triphosphate (GTP) into cyclic guanosine monophosphate (cyclic GMP).

## INACTIVATION OF NEUROTRANSMITTERS

Once the neurotransmitter has had its appropriate effect on the postsynaptic membrane it must be inactivated or removed from the cleft; otherwise the postsynaptic membrane would be permanently stimulated.

Many neurotransmitters (e.g. noradrenaline, dopamine, 5-HT, GABA, L-glutamate, aspartate and glycine) are inactivated by being taken back into the nerve terminal through the presynaptic membrane (Fig. 5.10b, c). Others, such as ACh and ATP, are first broken down in the cleft (Fig. 5.10a, d). Thus ACh is acted upon by acetylcholinesterase to produce choline and acetate. The choline is taken into the nerve terminal for resynthesis into ACh while the acetate diffuses out of the cleft and enters the circulatory system (Fig. 5.10a). ATP is broken down by ATPase and the resulting adenosine is taken up into the nerve terminal (Fig. 5.10d). In all cases re-uptake

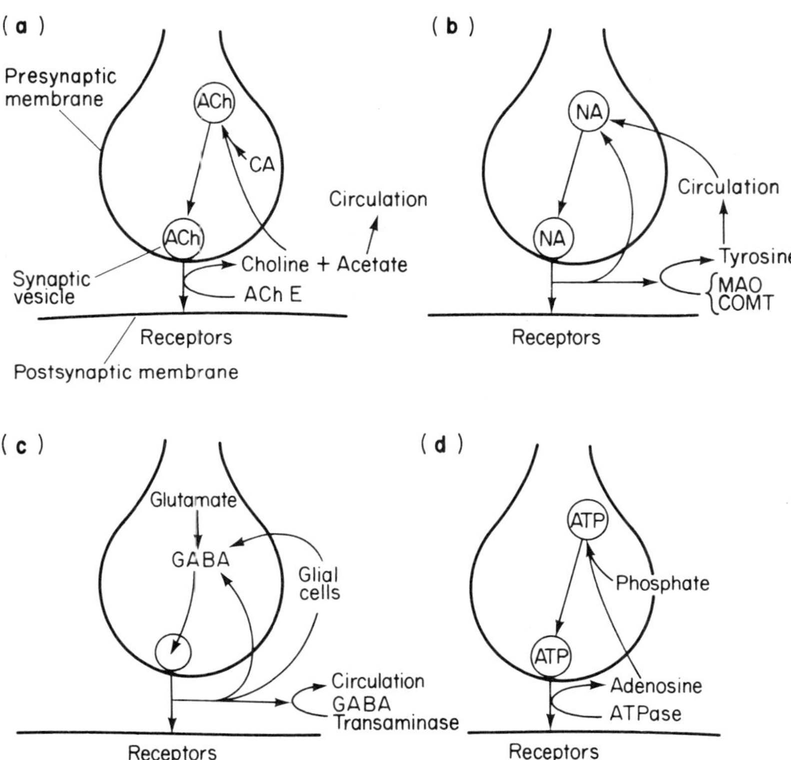


**Fig. 5.10** Diagrams illustrating the method of inactivation in the synaptic cleft of (**a**) acetylcholine; (**b**) noradrenaline; (**c**) $\gamma$-aminobutyric acid (GABA); (**d**) adenosine triphosphate (ATP). (After Triggle, C. R. and Triggle, D. J. (1976). In *Chemical Pharmacology of the Synapse* (Triggle, D. J. and Triggle, C. R., eds), pp. 1–127. Academic Press, London.)

of a neurotransmitter (or one of its metabolic breakdown products) into the nerve terminal is effected by a high-affinity uptake mechanism which is dependent on extracellular sodium.

The above methods of inactivation are the primary ones for those neurotransmitters concerned. However, some have additional inactivation pathways of secondary importance. For example, some noradrenaline and dopamine is broken down by monoamine oxidase (MAO) and catechol-O-methyl transferase (COMT) into tyrosine (Fig. 5.10b). Initially this probably diffuses out of the cleft, but can be utilized ultimately for resynthesis of the neurotransmitters. Also, some GABA and L-glutamate is taken up into the glial cells by a high-affinity uptake system similar to that in the nerve terminals, while some is broken down by GABA (glutamate) transaminase and enters the circulatory system (Fig. 5.10c).

## THE EFFECTS OF DRUGS ON SYNAPTIC TRANSMISSION

Drugs can be divided into various categories, depending on their effect and on which part of the system they operate. They may act

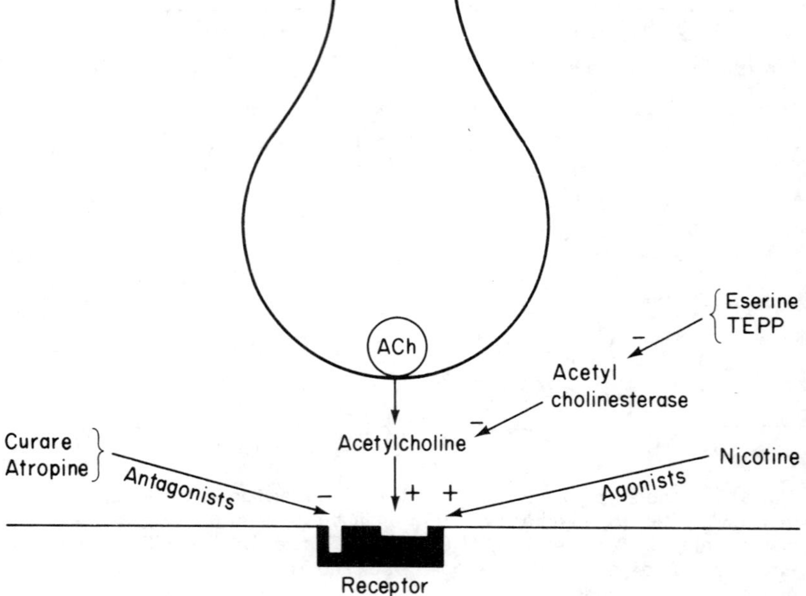


**Fig. 5.11** Diagram illustrating the site of action of various drugs at a cholinergic synapse. +, excitatory effect; −, inhibitory effect.

directly on the postsynaptic receptors. For example, at the acetylcholine-sensitive synapses on vertebrate voluntary muscle nicotine acts as an agonist by activating the receptors, while curare and atropine have the reverse effect (antagonists) by competing with the acetylcholine for the receptors and so blocking the effect of the neurotransmitter (Fig. 5.11). Chlorpromazine acts in a similar antagonistic way to block the effect of dopamine.

Various drugs increase the level of available neurotransmitter. The anticholinesterase group of drugs, which includes eserine and tetraethylpyrophosphate (TEPP), do this at cholinergic synapses by inactivating the acetylcholinesterase. This allows a build up of acetylcholine in the synaptic cleft and, at vertebrate neuromuscular synapses, causes tetanus of the muscle fibres. L-DOPA, which is a precursor of dopamine, directly increases the synthesis of this neurotransmitter but amphetamine, which has a similar effect to L-DOPA at dopamine-sensitive synapses, acts by stimulating the release of neurotransmitter. Other drugs decrease the level of available neurotransmitter.

# 6

# *The Action Potential*

An action potential, or a train of action potentials, will be initiated in those cells capable of supporting an action potential if the depolarizing (or admix of depolarizing and hyperpolarizing) input(s) is sufficient to depolarize the spike-initiating zone to its threshold level (p. 41). The characteristics of the action potential are:

(a) it is self-regenerating and is thus propagated throughout those regions of the cell capable of supporting it;
(b) it has an all-or-nothing nature, in so far as it has a specific magnitude which, although dependent on a variety of factors, is always the same under constant physical conditions for any given region of the cell;
(c) it involves a reversal of the membrane potential, the cell briefly becoming positive inside with respect to the outside.

Figure 6.1 shows an action potential as it passes a point on an axon. The resultant picture is the conventional one, showing the amplitude of the potential change plotted against time. Typically there is an initial depolarization of the cell, involving reversal of the membrane potential, followed by re-polarization of the membrane with an undershoot of the resting level. The total duration of these two phases is usually in the order of 2–4 msec. There is then a slow recovery with the membrane gradually returning to its resting level. Various other small potential changes (after-potentials) occur in some cells during the recovery phase.

To understand the nature of the action potential it is useful to consider the conductance changes of the cell membrane for sodium

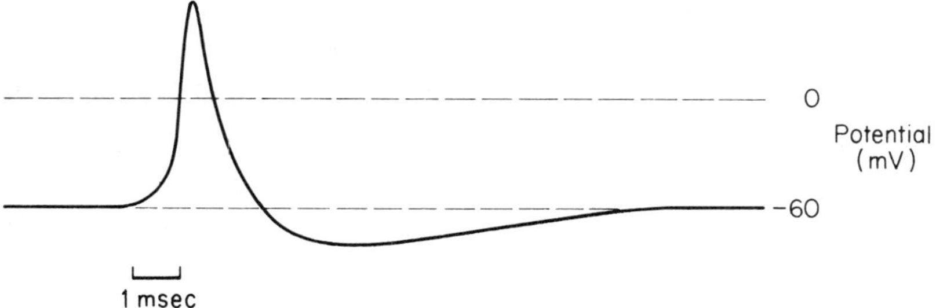


**Fig. 6.1** The time course of a 'typical' action potential, recorded intracellularly.

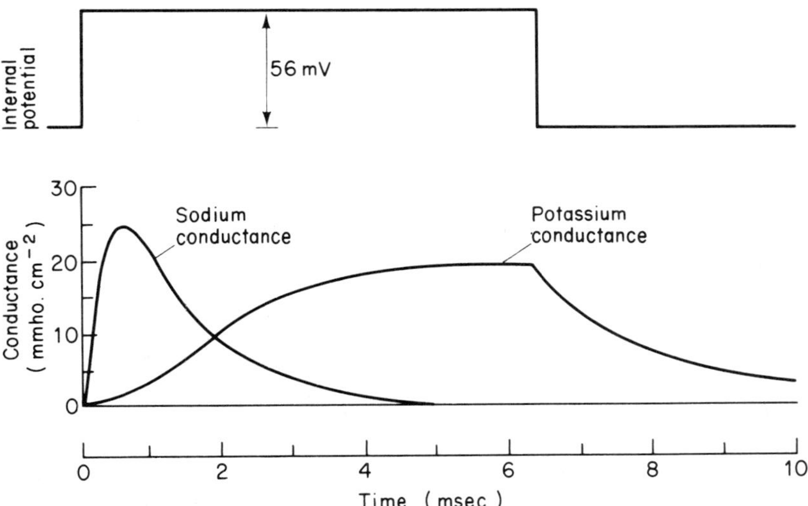


**Fig. 6.2** Changes in sodium and potassium conductance associated with a 6.3 msec duration depolarization (voltage clamp) of the membrane of the squid giant axon by about 60 mV. (From Hodgkin, A. L. (1958). *Proceedings of the Royal Society, B,* **148,** 1–37.)

and potassium ions when the membrane is abruptly depolarized (artificially) to some pre-determined level, held at this level for a short period of time and then returned (again abruptly) to its resting level (Fig. 6.2). This procedure involves the use of the 'voltage-clamp' technique, in which the potential across the membrane is held or 'clamped'. Under these conditions there is an initial, rapid increase in sodium conductance and hence an increase in the diffusion of sodium ions down their electrochemical gradient, i.e. into the cell. However, even with a maintained depolarization, the increase in sodium conductance is not maintained; it soon reaches a maximum value and then declines rapidly. The membrane conductance for potassium ions, on the other hand, increases much more slowly, only reaching a maximum when the sodium conductance has returned almost to its original (resting) level. Furthermore, the maximum potassium conductance level, with its corresponding increase in the

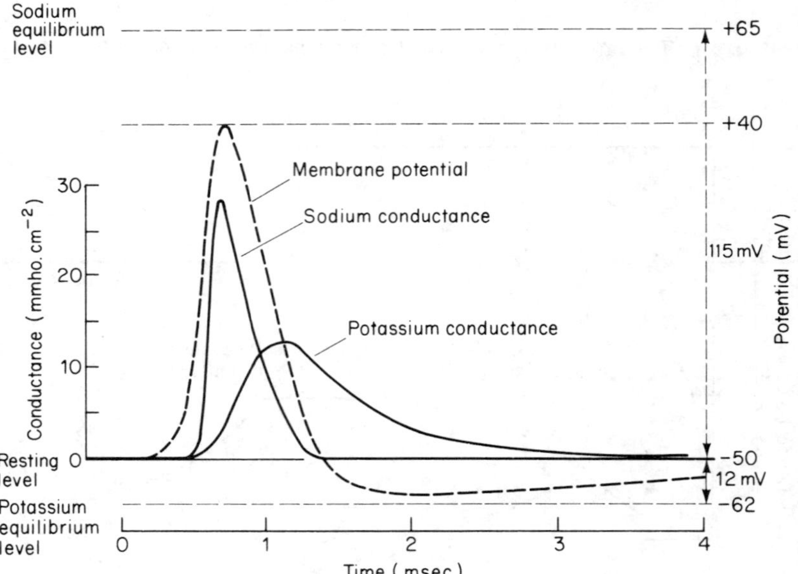


**Fig. 6.3** Theoretical action potential and associated sodium and potassium conductance changes in a squid giant axon. (After Hodgkin, A. L. and Huxley, A. F. (1952). *Journal of Physiology*, **117**, 500–44.)

diffusion of potassium ions out of the cell, is maintained for as long as the potential change is maintained. On restoration of the resting potential, the potassium conductance decreases exponentially to its low resting level.

Perhaps the easiest example to understand is an action potential in a non-medullated axon. Figure 6.3 shows how the conductance changes for sodium and potassium ions affect the shape of the action potential curve. Initially, the cell membrane in the region of the recording electrodes starts to be depolarized by the approaching action potential. This small depolarization elicits an increase in sodium ion conductance and sodium ions start to diffuse in increasing numbers inwards across the cell membrane, carrying positive charge with them. This depolarizes the membrane still further, the sodium conductance increases, more sodium ions move inwards, and so on. If this region of the membrane is capable of supporting an action potential then, if its threshold level is reached, this positive feedback cycle will continue until the membrane attains some maximal level of depolarization. If the sodium ions were the only ones involved, this maximum would theoretically be at the sodium equilibrium level (see p. 35) which, in the example shown in Fig. 6.3, is at +65 mV. However, as noted in the voltage-clamp experiment described above, the potassium conductance is meantime very slowly but significantly increasing. Hence an increase in the outward flow of potassium ions is beginning, which starts to counteract the effect of the increased inward movement of sodium ions. This slows down the rate of depolarization, which in turn has the effect of curtailing the increase in sodium conductance and this, consequently, starts to fall. However, since there is still an appreciable level of depolarization, the potassium conductance continues to increase. The combined effect of decreasing sodium conductance and increasing potassium conductance is that the membrane potential starts to be pulled back towards its resting level, without it ever reaching the sodium equilibrium level. The repolarization phase is dominated by the outward flow of potassium ions. Ultimately, however, the level of depolarization becomes so low as to cause the potassium conductance to start decreasing. By the time the membrane potential has reached its resting level again, the sodium conductance is back at its very low resting level but there is still an appreciable potassium conductance. If the latter were to be maintained, the increased outward diffusion of potassium ions would eventually hyperpolarize the cell to the potassium equilibrium level (−62 mV in the example shown in Fig. 6.3). However, because the membrane potential is now in the region of its resting level, the potassium conductance continues to decline and reaches its low resting value before this happens. Nevertheless, there is a period of sufficiently high potassium conductance to cause the membrane to undershoot its resting level and approach the potassium equilibrium level.

Whether the sodium–potassium pump is overridden during the preceding sequence of events, or whether it ceases to function, is not known. However, as the potassium conductance approaches its resting level, the pump starts to restore the ionic balance of the cell (p. 35).

It is also possible to look, theoretically at least, at an action potential at a given instant of time along an axon (Fig. 6.4). In this diagram the action potential is travelling along the axon from left to right. There is a region on the extreme right, (i), which has yet to be depolarized. Region (ii) is just being depolarized by the advancing action potential, at (iv) the action potential is maximal and at (vi) it

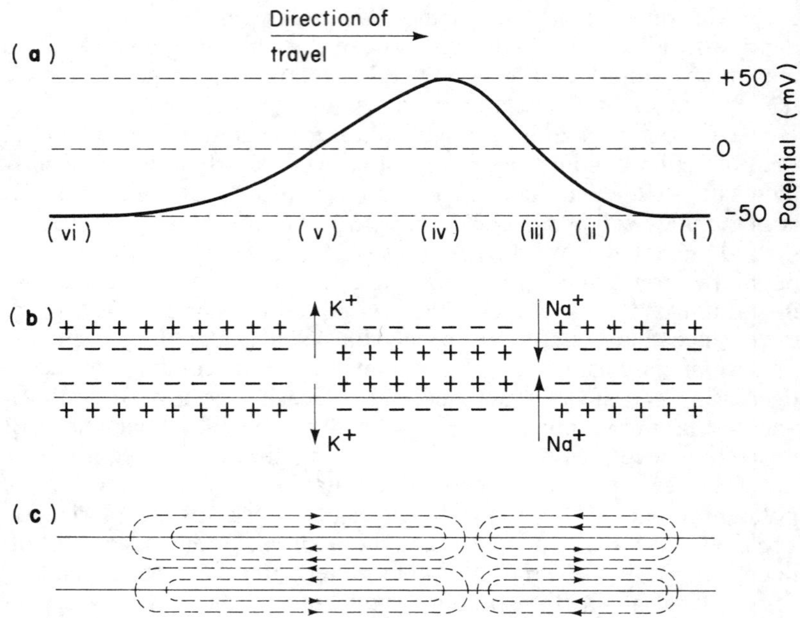


**Fig. 6.4** Diagrams showing various parameters of an action potential in an axon at one instant of time. (**a**) The spatial distribution of the membrane potential; (**b**) the net membrane potential, and the nature and direction of the dominant ion fluxes during the rising (depolarizing) and falling (hyperpolarizing) phases of the action potential; (**c**) the current flow through the axon. The action potential would be moving in the direction of the arrow. See also Fig. 3.3. (After Eccles, J. C. (1959). In *Handbook of Physiology*, Section 1, Vol. 1 (Field, J., Magoun, H. W. and Hall, V. E., eds), pp. 59–74. American Physiological Society.)

has already passed by. Thus the action potential is displayed as amplitude of depolarization against position along the axon (Fig. 6.4a). This looks similar to the more conventional picture shown in Fig. 6.1 and Fig. 6.3. As mentioned in Chapter 3, the action potential can be considered as a wave of negativity passing along the axon; this is demonstrated in Fig. 6.4b, which shows the state of the membrane potential in different regions of the axon. By comparing Fig. 6.4a with Fig. 6.4b it can be seen that the region of the axon between (iii) and (v) has its inside positive with respect to the outside. As the action potential moves from left to right, so also will this negative region (see Fig. 3.3). The ionic movements and the associated potential differences result in current flowing across the membrane, with an outwards direction in front of and behind the region of reversed polarity (and correspondingly inwards in the region where the depolarization is at a peak) (Fig. 6.4c). The outward current flow in front of the advancing action potential is instrumental in depolarizing the next piece of membrane and hence effects the smooth propagation of the potential along the axon. The outward flow behind the action potential does not have this effect as this region of the membrane is still recovering and is thus incapable of supporting an action potential immediately (i.e. it is in its refractory period, see p. 91). Thus conduction is maintained in one direction.

## CONDUCTION VELOCITY

Once initiated, an action potential will travel along an axon with constant velocity, provided that the physical parameters remain constant. Increase in axon diameter, the degree of axon insulation and temperature all produce an increase in conduction velocity (Figs 6.5, 6.6).

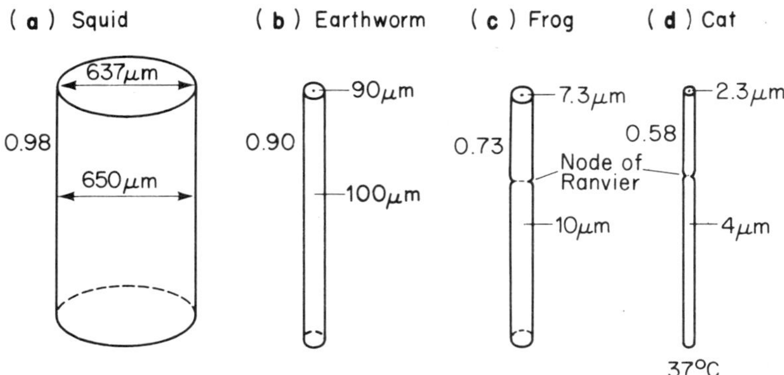


**Fig. 6.5** Four axons with the same velocity of conduction (25 m $sec^{-1}$), showing their different diameters and degrees of sheathing (insulation). (**c**) and (**d**) are drawn on a scale 10× that of (**a**) and (**b**). Two diameters are given for each axon – the upper is the axon diameter, the lower is the overall diameter including the sheath. The figure to the left of each axon is the ratio of these two figures. The recorded velocity refers to 20°C in (**a**), (**b**) and (**c**) but was 37°C in (**d**). (**c**) and (**d**) possess nodes of Ranvier. (From Muralt, A. von. (1958). *Neue Ergebnisse der Nervenphysiologie*. Springer, Berlin.)

Increase in conduction velocity in invertebrates is achieved primarily by increase in the diameter of the nerve axons; the so-called 'giant' axons of squids attain several hundred $\mu$m in diameter (Fig. 6.5a). The ratio of the total width of an axon plus its sheath cell to axon width alone, gives a measure of the amount of insulation afforded by the sheath cells. Reference to Fig. 6.5 illustrates that this mechanism of increasing conduction velocity can be used to a limited extent in invertebrates. Vertebrates, on the other hand, do not have very large diameter axons, but often show a considerable degree of

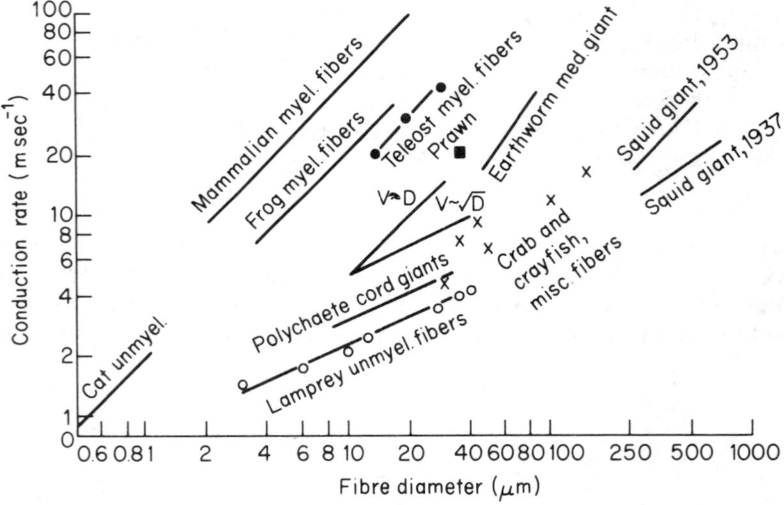


**Fig. 6.6** Velocity of nerve impulse conduction plotted against fibre diameter. The two lines in the centre of the figure indicate the slopes if the velocity is directly proportional to the diameter (V ~ D) or is proportional to the square root of the diameter (V ~ $\sqrt{}$D). (From Bullock, T. H. (1965). In *Structure and Function in the Nervous Systems of Invertebrates*, Vol. 1. (Bullock, T. H. and Horridge, G. S., eds.) Freeman, San Francisco and London, Copyright © 1965.)

sheath cell insulation. As a result of this increase in insulation a non-myelinated vertebrate axon can conduct as rapidly as an invertebrate axon several times its diameter (Fig. 6.5). However, the fastest conducting vertebrate axons are those which have a myelin sheath (myelinated fibres) interrupted by nodes of Ranvier (see Chapter 1). In these axons the insulation afforded by the myelin sheath is such that the axon is only depolarized at the nodes. This results in the action potential 'jumping' along the axon from node to node, rather than running smoothly along it as described above. This is known as

***saltatory conduction***. It is a very effective means of increasing the conduction velocity for a given axon diameter, since most of the conduction time is accounted for by the time taken to depolarize the nodes to their threshold level. For example, in a 10$\mu$m diameter frog axon with nodes 1.6 mm apart, a conduction velocity of 20 m sec$^{-1}$ (1.6 mm per 0.08 msec) has been recorded. The delay at each node in such an axon is 0.06 msec, i.e. 75% of the conduction time.

The effect of temperature becomes noticeable when comparing conduction velocities in axons of homeothermic and poikilothermic vertebrates. For axons of the same diameter the conduction velocity is two or three times greater in the former, presumably reflecting their higher internal temperature (Fig. 6.6).

## THE REFRACTORY PERIOD

Following the depolarization caused by an action potential, there is a short period of time when the cell membrane is incapable of supporting a second action potential. This is the ***absolute refractory***

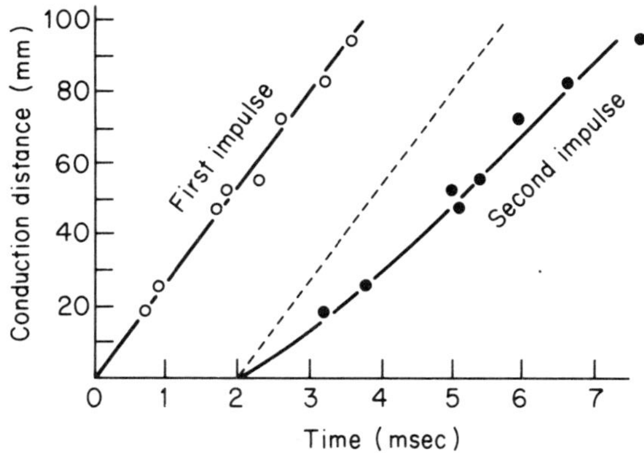


**Fig. 6.7** Relationship between the conduction distance and the stimulus response interval for two action potentials elicited at an interval of 2 msec in a toad motor axon of 11 $\mu$m diameter. The total refractory period is a 4 msec. (From Tasaki, I. (1959). In *Handbook of Physiology*, Section 1, Vol. 1. (Field, J., Magoun, H. W. and Hall, V. E., eds.) American Physiological Society, Washington, D.C.)

***period***. In some mammalian axons ($\alpha$ fibres) it may be as brief as 0.4 msec, in squid giant axons it is about 3.0 msec, and in some cell bodies in the ganglia of the mollusc *Aplysia* it is as long as 10 msec. This is followed by a period, the ***relative refractory period***, during which a second action potential is not normally carried, but may be elicited by electrical stimulation. However, the threshold is higher than normal. Thus, if an action potential is elicted in an axon with a stimulus which is just sufficient to raise the membrane to its threshold level (p. 41), a second stimulus delivered during the relative refractory period will have to be slightly larger if it also is to produce an action potential.

If an action potential is produced during the relative refractory period, it is propagated more slowly than the first action potential and only reaches the normal propagation velocity for the axon when it has been slowed down sufficiently to be just outside this period (Fig. 6.7). The duration of the relative refractory period is usually longer than that of the absolute refractory period; approximately 3.0 msec in mammalian $\alpha$ fibres, and as long as 12 msec in the large diameter axons of the frog sciatic nerve. The total refractory period imposes a limit to the frequency at which axons can propagate action potentials.

Immediately following the refractory period there is often a period of increased excitability, i.e. lowered threshold. This is called the ***supernormal period*** and this, in turn, may be followed by a lengthy period of decreased excitability, the ***subnormal period***.

## EXTRACELLULAR RECORDINGS

With extracellular recording techniques the recorded action potential is very much attenuated. It rarely exceeds a few millivolts and is often of the order of tens or hundreds of microvolts. This is due to the low resistance between the two electrodes, resulting in a certain amount of short-circuiting of the signal. The larger the axon diameter, the greater the contact with the electrodes and thus the less short-circuiting and the greater the proportion of the potential change recorded. This is why larger diameter axons appear to have larger action potentials when extracellular recording is employed. However, it is not quite as simple as this, since the depth of the axon within the nerve (i.e. its distance from the recording electrodes) probably also reduces the size of the recorded signal. Furthermore, there are real differences between axons in the amplitudes of action potentials.

## ACTION POTENTIALS IN CELL BODIES

In many insect motor neurons the cell body is not invaded by action potentials, but nevertheless an all-or-nothing potential is often recorded from them. However, this potential is of comparatively small size and does not involve a reversal of the membrane potential. It represents the electrotonic spread of the action potential from an adjacent region of the cell (the axon) which is conducting it (Fig. 6.8a). On the other hand, the cell body membrane of probably all

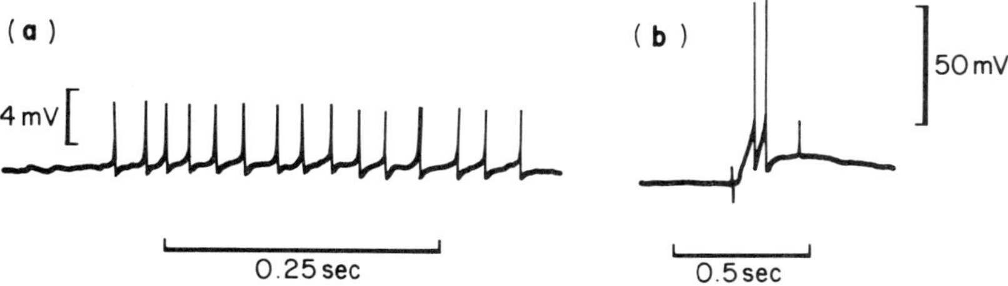


**Fig. 6.8** Intracellular recordings of action potentials from (**a**) the cell body of a locust ventilatory motor neuron and (**b**) a cell body in the central nervous system of the mollusc *Aplysia*. ((**a**) From Miller, P. L. and Mills, P. S. (1976). In *Perspectives in Experimental Biology*, Vol. 1. (Spencer-Davies, P., ed.) Pergamon, Oxford; (**b**) from Kandel, E. R. and Tauc, L. (1965). *Journal of Physiology*, **181**, 1–27.)

vertebrate motor neurons, and at least the larger molluscan motor neurons and some insect motor neurons, for example, does support action potentials (Fig. 6.8b).

Recordings from the cell bodies of mammalian motor neurons show an inflection on the rising phase (Fig. 6.9a). This is a result of the spike-initiating zone being in the initial segment region (the non-myelinated base of the axon and the immediately adjacent region of the cell body membrane which is devoid of synaptic contents). Thus the EPSP(s) produced by presynaptic activity elicits an action potential by depolarizing the initial segment region to its threshold level. Since the cell body (soma-dendritic region) is nearer to the presynaptic activity, it is depolarized to an even greater extent than the initial segment. However, since its threshold level is so much higher than that of the latter region, this level is not reached before an action potential is produced in the initial segment. The action potential, once initiated, is propagated along the axon, but also further depolarizes the cell body, bringing it to its threshold level. This takes time because of the increase in surface area which the cell body presents to the invading action potential. Hence, a recording from the cell body reveals an EPSP giving rise to an action potential in the initial segment (the IS spike). This is recorded immediately it is produced due to electronic spread to the recording site in the cell body. As mentioned above, it appears smaller than a full action potential because it is recorded at a distance from its site of production. The IS spike is normally capped a fraction of a millisecond later by the full action potential as it invades the cell body (soma-dendritic) membrane. This SD spike is recorded full size because it is produced in the same region as the recording electrode is situated. The junction between the IS and SD spikes is shown by the inflection on the rising phase of the intracellularly recorded action potential (Fig. 6.9a).

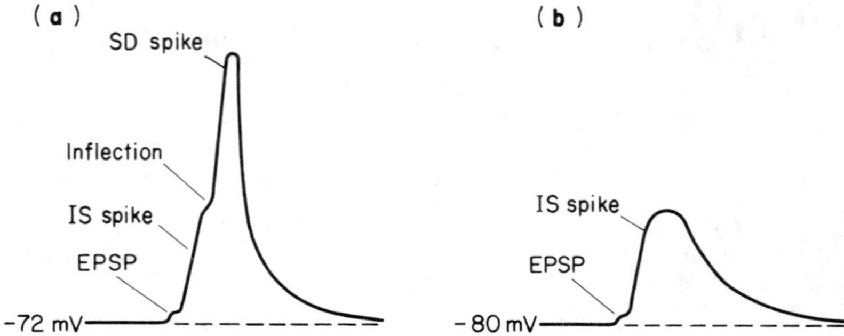


**Fig. 6.9** (**a**) Intracellular recording of an action potential from the soma of a mammalian motor neuron. The small EPSP gives rise to a spike with an inflection on its rising phase. This inflection occurs because the spike is initiated in the initial segment region at the base of the axon and takes a short time to invade the soma. Thus the initial segment (IS) spike can be distinguished from the soma-dendritic (SD) spike. (**b**) Hyperpolarization of the soma prevents the spike from invading it and hence only the IS spike is seen. It appears smaller than the SD spike because it occurs in a region distant to the recording electrode in the soma. The values on the base-lines are the membrane potentials. (After Coombs, J. S., Eccles, J. C. and Fatt, P. (1955). *Journal of Physiology*, **130,** 291–325.)

If the cell body is hyperpolarized artificially by passing a current through an intracellular microelectrode, the soma-dendritic invasion can be suppressed, and then only the distant IS spike is recorded (Fig. 6.9b), much as is the normal situation in many insect motor neuron cell bodies (Fig. 6.8a).

## ELECTRICAL STIMULATION

Having considered the nature of the action potential it is opportune to digress and discuss the means by which the membrane potential can be artificially altered and action potentials elicited by electrical stimulation, a technique which has many implications. As with recording techniques (p. 42), electrical stimulation can be effected

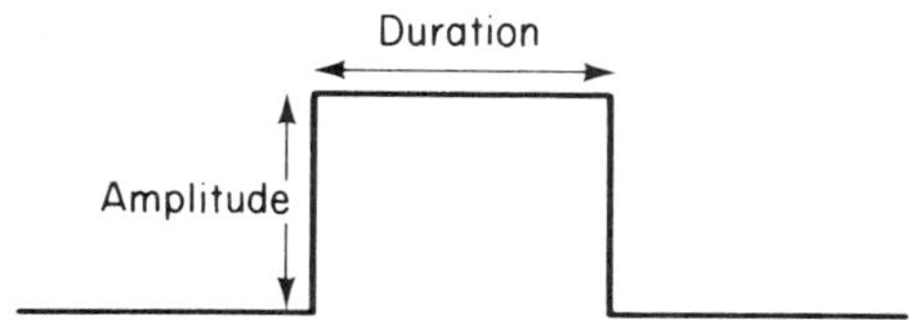


**Fig. 6.10** The parameters of a square wave stimulus.

with either extracellular or intracellular electrodes. The most widely used stimulus is the square-wave voltage (or current) pulse (Fig. 6.10), but ramp stimuli and long term DC level changes are also often used.

Extracellular electrodes are used when the cell, or region of a cell, is too small to be penetrated with a microelectrode. A pair of electrodes is placed against the nerve and the square-wave stimulating pulse causes one electrode to become transiently negative with respect to the other. This causes current to flow through the cell membrane so that the region immediately adjacent to the negative electrode is depolarized (because the outside is made more negative). If its threshold is reached, the resultant action potential is propagated away from the negative electrode. It may not be able to pass the region of hyperpolarization produced at the positive electrode, and hence may travel in one direction only. Often, however, the action potential does 'jump over' the hyperpolarized region and then proceeds in both directions (Fig. 6.11).

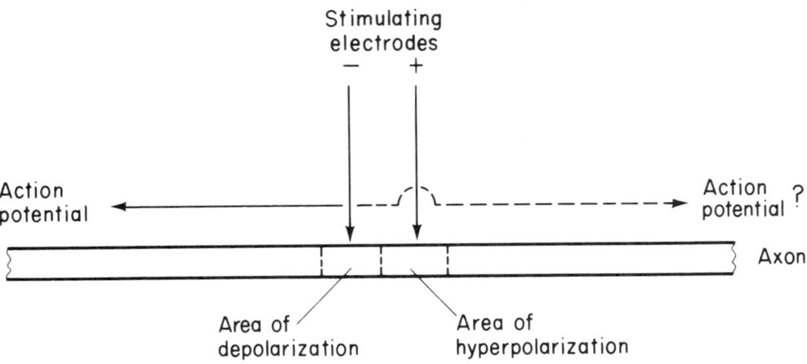


**Fig. 6.11** A method for initiating an action potential in an axon. Although there is a clear threshold for producing an action potential on the side of the negative stimulating electrode, the production of an action potential on the other (positive) side is a more variable event because of the region of hyperpolarization around the positive stimulating electrode.

If the cell is large enough to be penetrated with a microelectrode, a current can be passed through the electrode to either depolarize or hyperpolarize the cell. In the former case an action potential is produced when the threshold is reached.

When using electrical stimuli it is important to ensure that both the amplitude and the duration of the stimulating pulse are of the correct order of magnitude. Neither a very short, high voltage pulse nor a

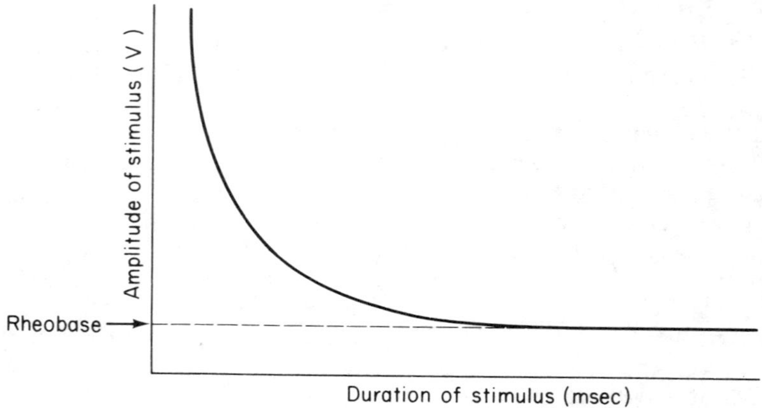


**Fig. 6.12** Strength-duration curve showing the relationship between the amplitude and duration of a just-threshold square wave stimulus. Note that any effective stimulus must possess sufficient amplitude (strength) and duration to fall on, or to the right of, the curve. The threshold amplitude of an infintely long (20–30 msec in practice) square wave stimulus pulse is called the rheobase.

very long, low voltage pulse will be effective. Figure 6.12 illustrates the relationship between these two stimulus parameters for a square-wave stimulating pulse. The amplitude of an infinitely long pulse (30–40 msec in practice) which just elicits an action potential is referred to as the ***rheobase***.

# 7

# *Muscle Physiology*

## THE SLIDING FILAMENT MECHANISM OF SHORTENING

The organization of cross-striated muscle has been described in Chapter 1. When a muscle shortens the myosin and actin filaments slide over one another as depicted in Fig. 7.1 and Fig. 7.2, with a resultant change in their degree of overlap and hence in the relative lengths of the A- and I-bands. Thus, when a muscle fibre is fully extended there is little or no overlap between the myosin and actin filaments (Fig. 7.1a). As contraction proceeds the overlap steadily increases (Fig. 7.1b–d). This sliding mechanism is thought to be brought about by a sequential making-and-breaking of cross-bridges between the myosin and actin filaments, initiated by activation of the muscle.

A simple model to show how this mechanism could operate is shown in Fig. 7.3. The myosin has active sites (M), probably on the heavy meromyosin, each of which oscilates backwards and forwards with respect to its equilibrium position (O). The reactive sites can combine temporarily with projections (A) from the backbone of the thin filaments with a rate constant f:

$$A + M \xrightarrow{\quad f \quad} AM \tag{1}$$

The resultant connection is called a cross-bridge and is broken by reaction with a high-energy phosphate compound with a rate constant g:

$$AM + XP \xrightarrow{\quad g \quad} AXP + M \tag{2}$$

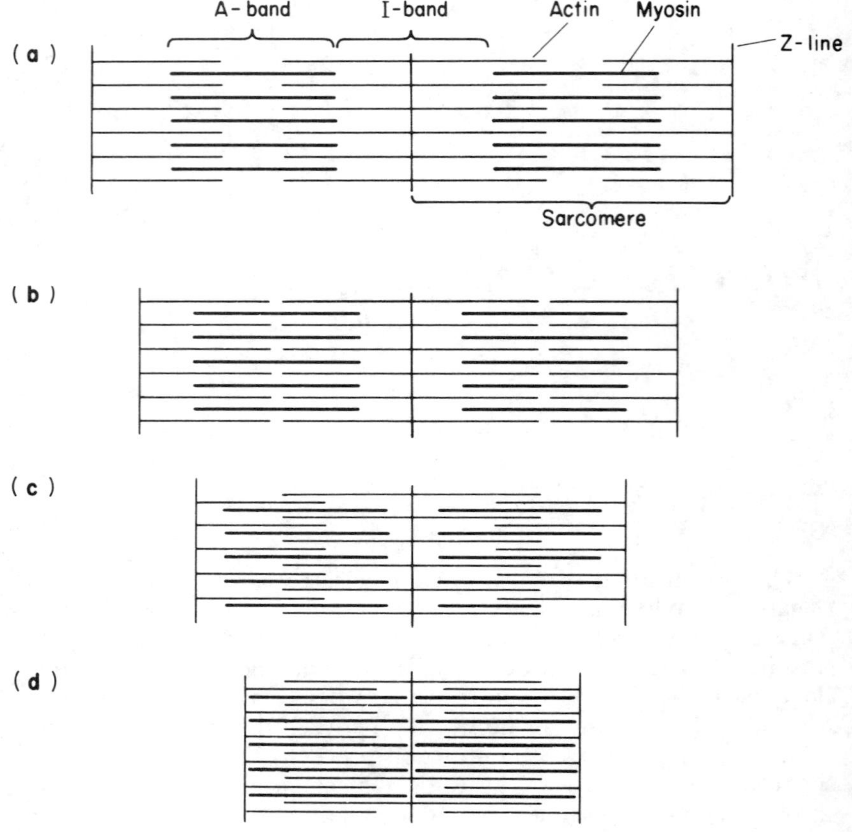


**Fig. 7.1** Diagram illustrating the sliding filament theory of contraction of cross-striated muscle. The longitudinal sliding of the actin and myosin filaments with respect to each other results in a reduction in the length of the I-bands (**a, b, c**) until they finally disappear (**d**).

The initial conditions are restored by splitting the high-energy phosphate bond:

$$\text{AXP} \longrightarrow \text{A} + \text{X} + \text{phosphate} \qquad (3)$$

The rates at which (1) and (2) occur are assumed to depend on the relative position of M with respect to its equilibrium position.

When shortening is initiated the actin filament depicted in Fig. 7.3b will slide to the left with respect to the myosin filament. Only when A is to the right of O can it combine with M. If we consider reaction (1) at

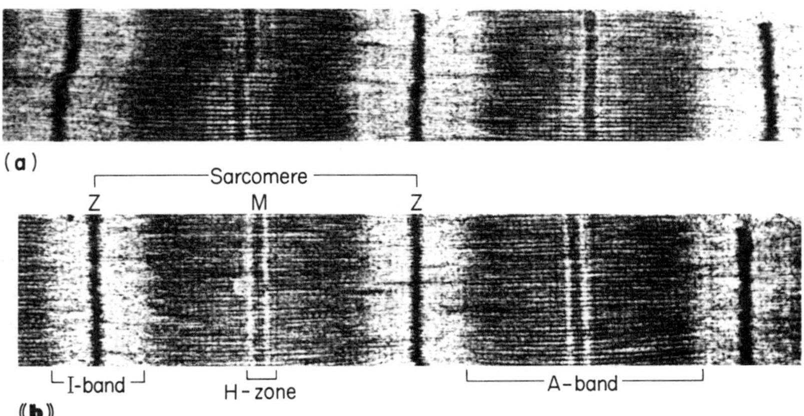


**Fig. 7.2** Cross-striated muscle. Electron micrographs of longitudinal sections of (**a**) relaxed muscle and (**b**) contracted muscle to show the changes in band pattern depicted in Fig. 7.1a, b. Note the narrower H-band in (**b**). (From Huxley, H. E. (1972). In *The Structure and Function of Muscle*, Vol. 1, (Bourne, G. H., ed.) pp. 301–87. Academic Press, London.)

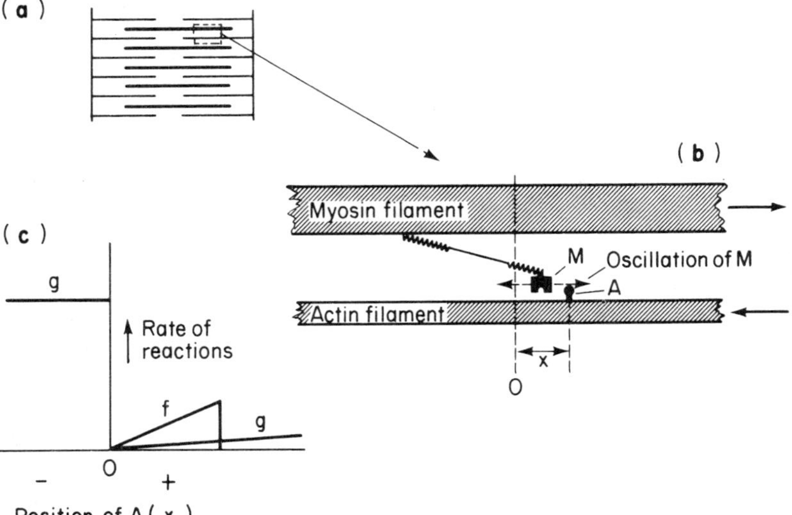


**Fig. 7.3** The tension-generating mechanism in A. F. Huxley's sliding filament model of muscle contraction. (**a**) Indicates the region of the sarcomere from which (**b**) is taken. (**b**) M corresponds to the $S_1$ part of the heavy meromyosin molecule (see Fig. 1.9). A is the cross-bridge attachment site on the actin filament. O is the equilibrium position of M. (**c**) Illustrates the dependence of the rate constants f and g (see text) on x (**b**). (After Huxley, A. F. (1957). *Progress in Biophysics*, **7**, 255–318.)

a large number of sites, the overall rate constant, f, will decrease as A becomes closer to M because increasingly more combinations will have already been made. Once a cross-bridge is established it will move towards O, thereby producing shortening of the muscle. Once it passes to the left of O it must be broken down rapidly to prevent any back-tension from developing, and hence g must be high (Fig. 7.3c). Indeed, at high rates of shortening, the cross-bridges will not be broken down in time to prevent some back-tension from developing, thus providing a limit to the possible rate of shortening. The rate constant g must also have a positive value to the right of O so as to prevent any cross-bridges remaining when activation ceases; otherwise the muscle would stay in a state of partial rigor. The value of g to the right of O must, of course, be less than that of f, so that the probability to the right of O is higher for reaction (1) than for reaction (2) when the muscle is activated.

Once released, A is moved towards the region of another M by the activity of other cross-bridges. For a smooth contraction to occur, this sequence of events must take place asynchronously at a large number of sites. There is evidence that this is achieved by a different spacing of the M sites (42.9 nm) and the A sites (less than the spacing of the M sites).

As shortening continues, the actin filaments from opposite ends of the sarcomere start to overlap in the centre (Fig. 7.1c). Ultimately, the myosin filaments come to abut against the Z-line (Fig. 7.1d). A small amount of shortening is still possible after this stage is reached, whereupon the myosin filaments buckle at their ends, but it reaches a maximum when the ends of the actin filaments reach the opposing Z-lines. In frog skeletal muscle the relaxed sarcomere has a length of approximately 3.5 $\mu$m; the fully contracted sarcomere just over 1.0 $\mu$m. Hence this muscle can contract by, at most, 60–70% of its relaxed length. In a few muscles, such as those of the large barnacle (Crustacea) (which are composed of giant muscle fibres) and the skeletal muscles of blowflies, there are holes in the Z-lines through which the myosin and actin filaments can pass. This allows a greater degree of shortening—approximately 80%; a phenomenon known as 'supercontraction'. In blowfly larvae this is presumably necessary as the method of locomotion of these soft-bodied animals involves considerable length changes.

## THE SHEARING MECHANISM OF SHORTENING

Locomotion in many annelids involves very marked changes in the lengths of individual body segments; more than can be attained by the sliding filament mechanism alone. Hence, while it is almost certain that the obliquely striated body wall muscles of these animals do shorten by means of this mechanism, there is evidence that further shortening is produced by the thick (paramyosin) filaments shearing with respect to one another. The changes in length effected by sliding and shearing are illustrated in Fig. 7.4. Although the sliding filament mechanism does not produce any change in the angle of the striations, shearing causes an increase in their angle with respect to the longitudinal axis of the fibre; this has been observed. As in cross-striated muscle, one effect of shortening is to reduce the extent of the I-bands (Fig. 7.5), presumably due to the sliding filament mechanism.

## ISOTONIC AND ISOMETRIC CONTRACTION

The term 'shortening' has so far been used to denote the sequence of events which occurs in an activated muscle fibre, but under certain circumstances no change in length may occur as a result of activation. In experimental work with muscles, the muscle is often made to shorten (contract) against a constant load and this is known as an ***isotonic* ('same force') *contraction*.** If the load on the muscle is increased, the tension developed by the muscle will increase. If the muscle is not allowed to shorten the contraction is called an ***isometric* ('same length') *contraction*.**

## MUSCLE TENSION

With the sliding filament mechanism, tension is produced by movement of the A projections by the M projections, Hence, under isometric conditions, where the developed tension is not allowed to produce any shortening of the muscle, the amount of tension should be directly proportional to the number of cross-bridges that can be formed and hence to the degree of overlap of the actin and myosin filaments.

Figure 7.6 shows the isometric tension of a frog skeletal muscle at various sarcomere lengths (Fig. 7.6a), the latter being a reflection of the degree of overlap of the filaments (Fig. 7.6b). At a sarcomere length of 3.65 $\mu$m there is no overlap, hence no cross-bridges can be formed, and there should, therefore, be no tension. In fact a very small amount of tension is developed, possibly because of some slight stagger in the alignment of the filaments. Progressive shortening of the sarcomere to 2.20 $\mu$m produces a steady increase, both in the degree of overlap of the filaments and in the tension developed. Between sarcomere lengths of 2.20 and 2.05 $\mu$m there is no increase

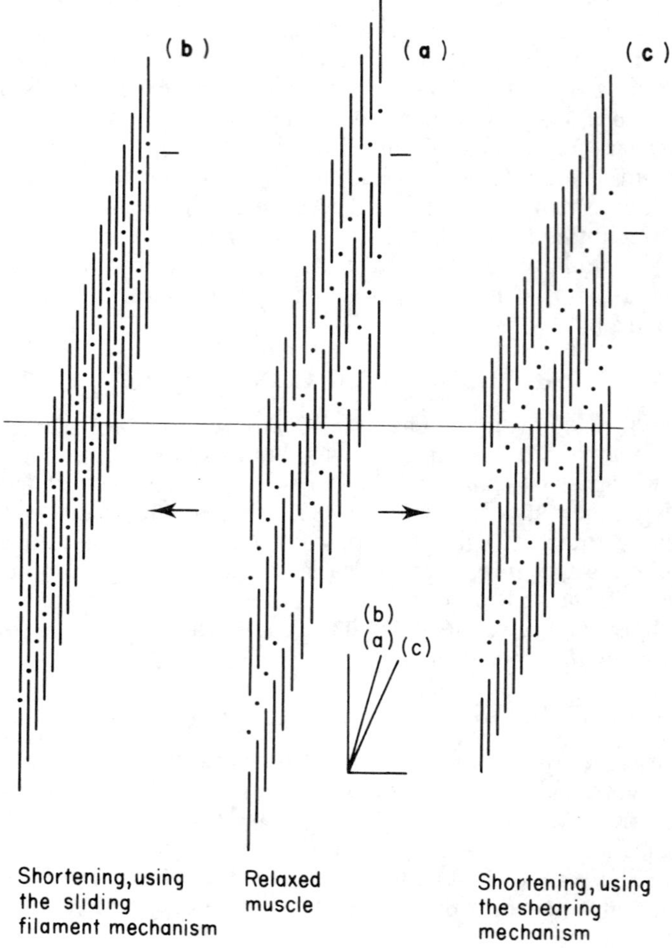


**Fig. 7.4** Diagram illustrating the sliding filament and shearing mechanism of contraction of obliquely striated muscle. The effects of the two mechanisms are shown in the *xz* plane (refer to Fig. 1.13). (**a**) Relaxed fibre; (**b**) fibre contracted by the sliding filament mechanism; (**c**) fibre contracted by the shearing mechanism. The thick vertical lines represent the paramyosin filaments and the dots represent sections through Z-rods. The middle paramyosin filament in the central row is marked by the long horizontal line. The short horizontal lines mark the right hand paramyosin filament of the central row. The angle of the striations is exaggerated for clarity. The inset shows the angle of striation, which is the same in (**a**) and (**b**) but is increased with respect to the longitudinal fibre axis in (**c**). (From Knapp, M. F. and Mill, P. J. (1971). *Journal of Cell Science*, **8,** 413–25.)

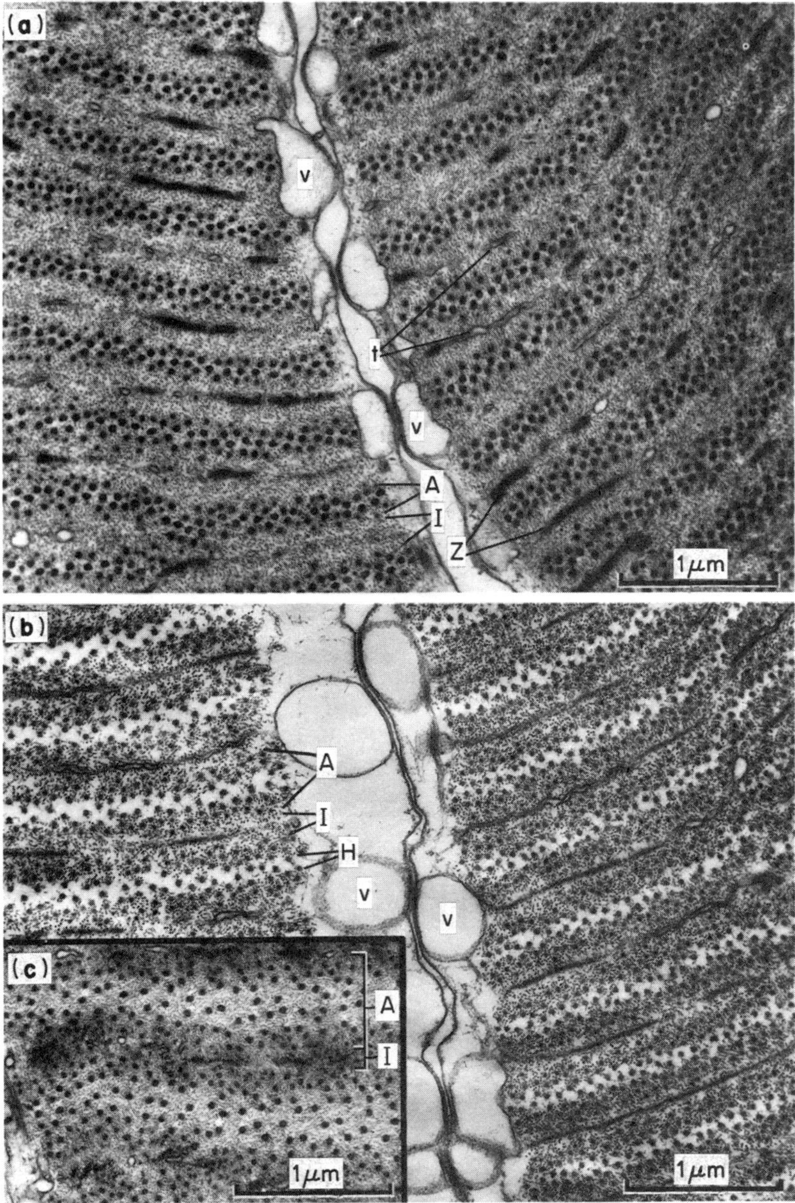


**Fig. 7.5** Obliquely striated muscle. Electron micrographs of transverse sections of earthworm body wall muscle. (**a**) Extended muscle, with the A- and I-bands of approximately equal width. (**b**), (**c**) Contracted muscles, with the I-bands much narrower than the A-bands and with more thick myofilaments in the A-bands than in those of extended muscle. In (**b**) there is an H-zone in the centre of the A-band. A, A-band; H, H-zone; I, I-band; t, tubule of sarcoplasmic reticulum; v, peripheral vesicle of sarcoplasmic reticulum; Z, Z-rod. (From Knapp, M. F. and Mill, P. J. (1971). *Journal of Cell Science*, **8,** 413–25.)

(a)

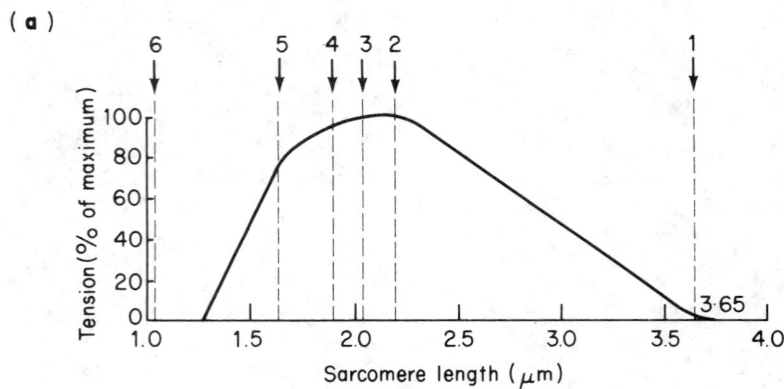


(b)

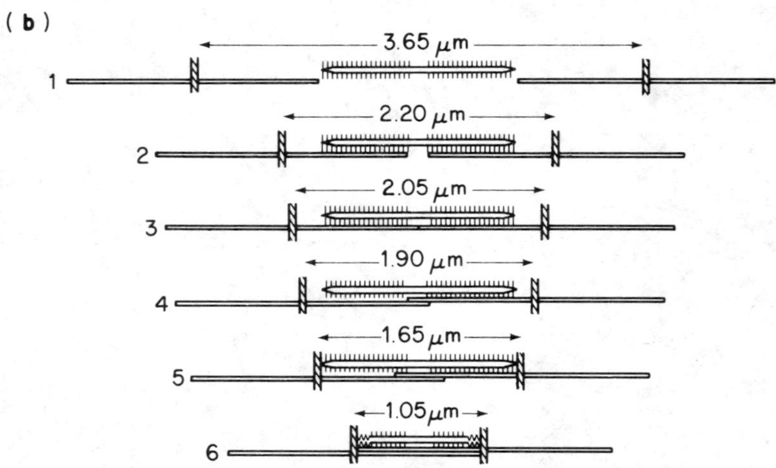


**Fig. 7.6** (**a**) The relationship between tension and sarcomere length in a vertebrate cross-striated muscle fibre. The critical stages of overlap of the filaments are indicated by numbers (1–6). Diagrams of the overlap of actin and myosin filaments are shown in (**b**). (After Gordon, A. M., Huxley, A. F. and Julian, F. J. (1966). *Journal of Physiology*, **184**, 170–92.)

in the number of available cross-bridges as the central zone of the myosin filaments is devoid of M groups. Consequently, the tension remains unchanged over this zone. Below 2.05 $\mu$m there is overlap of opposing actin filaments. Down to 1.90 $\mu$m this has a negligible effect because it is occurring in the central region of the myosin filaments. However, below 1.90 $\mu$m this overlap presumably produces a steady reduction in the number of cross-bridges that can be formed, and this is reflected in a steady fall in tension down to 1.65 $\mu$m. At 1.65 $\mu$m the myosin filaments abut against the Z-lines, and so below this length the internal resistance increases and the number of available cross-bridges is probably reduced still further because of buckling of the ends of the myosin filaments. Hence tension falls sharply, reaching zero at a sarcomere length of about 1.30 $\mu$m, i.e. before the actin filaments reach the Z-lines. These results are very much in accord with the idea that the cross-bridges are instrumental in producing tension.

If a muscle is stimulated to move a load the tension will increase initially as the muscle contracts isometrically. Once the tension is

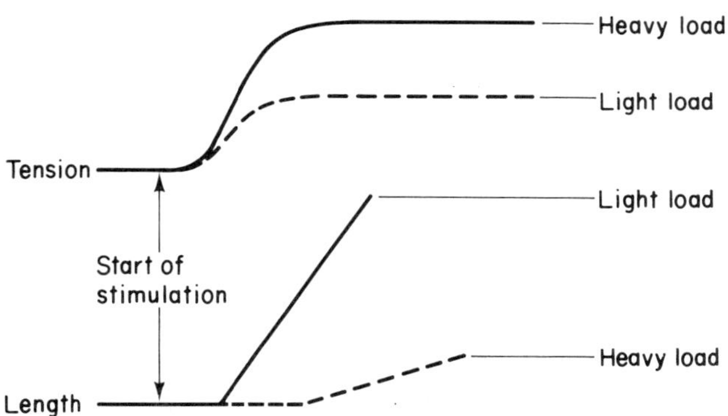


**Fig. 7.7** Tension and length changes in after-loaded isotonic contractions of a vertebrate muscle (i.e. the muscle has to lift a load in order to shorten). The arrow indicates the start of repetitive stimulation. Increase in tension and shortening are shown by upward deflections of the traces. Note the rapid initial increase in tension followed by shortening; also the increase in maximum tension and the increased delay before shortening with a larger load. (After Aidley, D. J. (1978). *The Physiology of Excitable Cells*, second edition. University Press, Cambridge.)

equal to the load it will remain constant and shortening will occur. With increase in load a greater tension has to be developed before shortening can occur. The velocity of contraction is also dependent on the load (force) applied to the muscle, a smaller load allowing a faster contraction (Fig. 7.7).

Muscle contraction is quite complex as the load tends to vary during shortening and there is normally sensory feedback elicited by proprioceptors (see Chapter 8).

## HEAT PRODUCTION BY MUSCLE

There is a basal level of heat production in a resting muscle as a consequence of its metabolic processes. Additional heat is produced during contraction and relaxation (initial heat) and also during the resynthesis of high energy compounds after the muscle has relaxed (recovery heat). Under isometric conditions initial heat can be subdivided into 'activation (maintenance)' heat and 'relaxation' heat. The latter is also appreciable under isotonic conditions if the load is allowed to extend the muscle during relaxation. If the muscle is allowed to shorten, still more heat is produced.

## THE RELATIONSHIP BETWEEN STIMULATION AND CONTRACTION

In all muscles the strength of the contraction is determined, in part, by the frequency of action potentials in the excited motor neurons. In vertebrate muscles the number of axons activated is also important. In arthropods, the latter is considerably less significant since the muscles are innervated by very few axons; rather it is the type of axon innervated which is important (see Chapter 1).

In the fast muscles of vertebrates a single action potential in one of the motor neurons normally elicits a twitch, and repetitive stimulation above a threshold frequency produces summation of successive twitches and hence an increase in the degree of contraction (Fig. 7.8). Contraction increases up to a maximum with further increase in stimulus frequency. The frequency of stimulation at which individual contractions are no longer discernible (i.e. above which there is a smooth contraction or tetanus) is known as the 'fusion frequency' (Fig. 7.8b). In arthropod skeletal muscles the response to stimulation of a fast motor neuron is similar (except that the muscle potentials are non-propagating). In most fast systems there is no facilitation of the postsynaptic potentials (Fig. 7.9), although in some decapod crustacean muscles considerable facilitation does occur.

In mammals the duration of an individual twitch is shorter in the fast twitch muscles than in the slow twitch muscles (Fig. 7.10) and hence mechanical summation starts to occur at a much lower stimulation frequency in the latter. (As mentioned in Chapter 1, the fast twitch and slow twitch muscles of mammals are both fast muscles in the broad sense of the term.)

In slow systems, also, the contractions can summate. Indeed, in arthropods a train of impulses is required to produce even a small contraction and the mechanical response is always a smooth tetanus

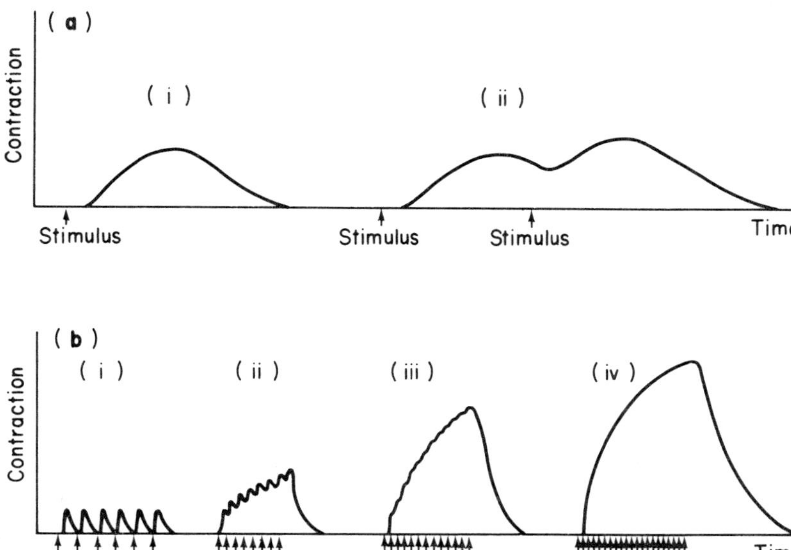


**Fig. 7.8** The contraction of vertebrate fast skeletal muscle. (**a**) A single maximal twitch (**i**) achieved by a stimulus to the motor nerve of sufficient magnitude to elicit action potentials in all of the motor neurons. If the twitch response to a second stimulus starts before the muscle has completely relaxed, summation occurs (**ii**). (**b**) The effect of a train of stimuli to the motor nerve. (**i**) The frequency is too low for summation to occur and so a series of individual twitches occurs. Increasing the frequency of stimuli in the train causes summation (**ii**), (**iii**) and eventually leads to a smooth contraction or tetanus (**iv**) at the fusion frequency.

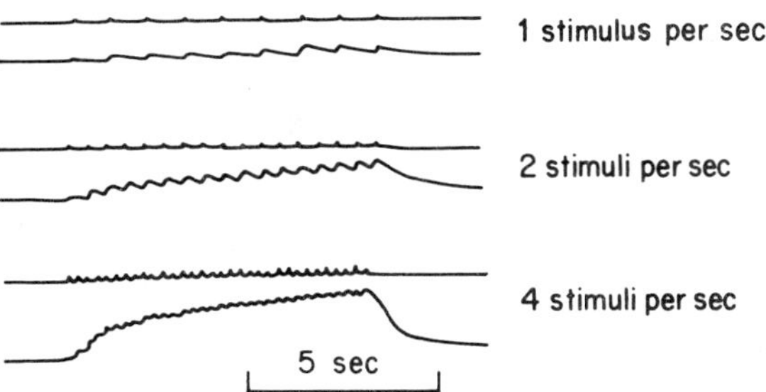


**Fig. 7.9** Recordings from fast muscle fibres of the king crab at three different frequencies of stimulation. Upper traces, electrical recordings; lower traces, mechanical recordings. Note the absence of facilitation; also the individual responses at a stimulation frequency of 4 Hz (cf. Fig. 7.11). (From Lang, F., Sutterlin, A. and Prosser, C. L. (1970). *Comparative Biochemistry and Physiology*, **32,** 615–28.)

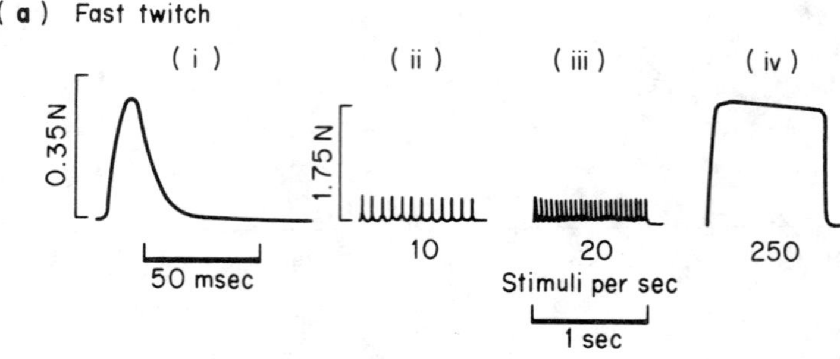


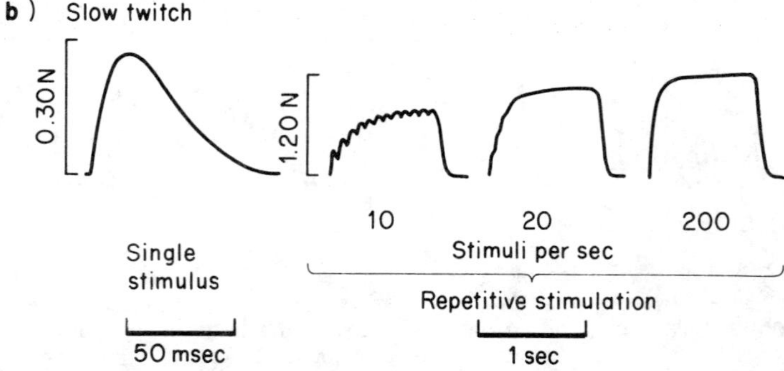


**Fig. 7.10** Isometric recordings from (**a**) fast twitch (extensor digitorum longus) and (**b**) slow twitch (soleus) muscles of the rat. (**i**) The responses to a single stimulus. (**ii**)–(**iv**) The responses to different frequencies of stimulation. (From Close, R. (1967). *Journal of Physiology*, **193**, 45–55.)

(Fig. 7.11). Slow fibres exhibit a lower electrical responsiveness as compared to fast fibres and the postsynaptic potential is always smaller than in fast fibres. Repetitive stimulation of a slow axon in arthropods normally elicits facilitation and, at higher frequencies, summation of the postsynaptic potentials (Fig. 7.11). Similarly, in some slow (multiterminally innervated) vertebrate muscles there is facilitation and summation of the postsynaptic potentials. Tension develops more slowly in slow muscles as compared to fast muscles (Fig. 7.12).

In the inhibitory systems of arthropods, facilitation and summation of the inhibitory postsynaptic potentials can occur (see Fig. 4.14), and this peripheral inhibition has a greater effect on the slow excitatory system than on the fast excitatory system (Fig. 7.13). In many cases the ratio of inhibitory to excitatory stimulation frequency at which

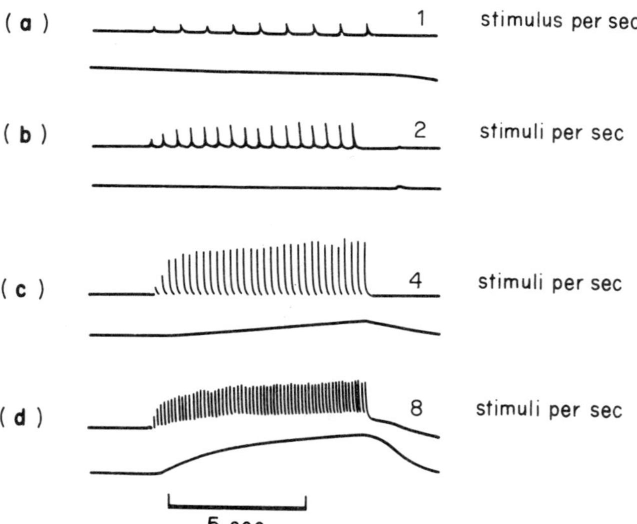


**Fig. 7.11** Recordings from slow muscle fibres of the king crab at different frequencies of stimulation (**a–d**). Upper traces, electrical recordings; lower traces, mechanical recordings. Note the facilitation; also that the mechanical response is always a smooth tetanus (cf. Fig. 7.9). (From Lang, F. *et al.* (1970). *Comparative Biochemistry and Physiology*, **32,** 615–28.)

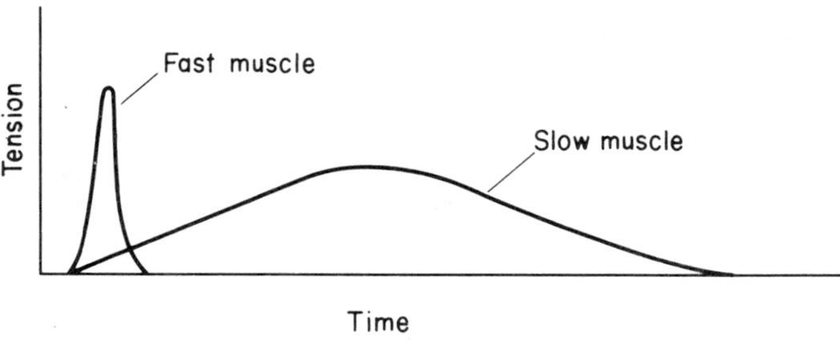


**Fig. 7.12** The development of tension in fast and slow muscles following stimulation of their motor nerves.

contraction is just repressed remains constant over quite a wide range of stimulation frequencies.

As with nerve cells (see p. 37), an increase in the external concentration of potassium ions lowers the membrane potential of muscle cells (i.e. depolarizes them). In addition, above a certain

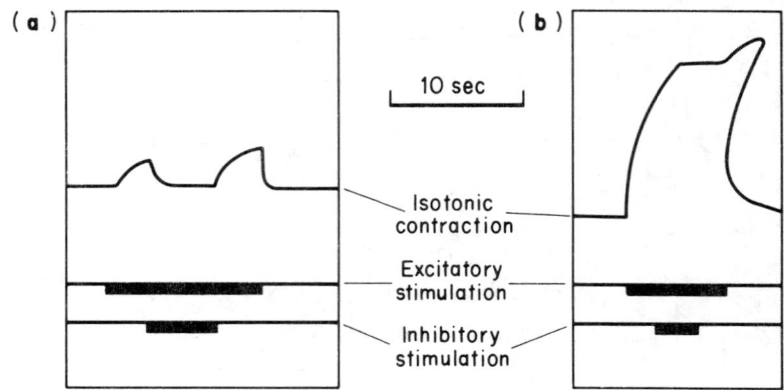


**Fig. 7.13** Kymograph records of (**a**) slow and (**b**) fast contractions of a limb muscle (bender of the propodite) of the crayfish *Procambarus* to show that inhibitory stimulation is more effective on the slow excitatory system. (From van Harreveld, A. and Wiersma, C. A. G. (1937). *Journal of Experimental Biology*, **14**, 448–61.)

threshold level of external potassium a prolonged contraction (a contracture) occurs. Further increase in external potassium concentration causes the strength of the contracture to increase rapidly. The rate of increase then slows down and ultimately a maximum is reached (Fig. 7.14). This contracture tension is reduced at low external calcium ion concentrations and, in the absence of calcium, the contractures ultimately fail.

**Excitation-contraction coupling**

It is known that the T-system tubules are involved in carrying the excitation of the surface membrane to the contractile mechanism, since local depolarizing currents applied adjacent to them—for example at the Z-lines in frog skeletal muscle and at the A–I boundary in relaxed crab muscles—elicit a local contraction.

In cross-striated muscle the depolarization of the excited muscle fibre membrane spreads inwards along the T tubules to the dyads and triads (see p. 13). In vertebrate skeletal muscle there is evidence of a regenerative mechanism (i.e. an action potential) in the T-system, involving an increase in sodium conductance. However, in those muscles whose surface membrane does not support an action potential, such as the multiterminally innervated skeletal muscles of arthropods, a tubular action potential does not occur. In these muscles the inward spread of depolarization is possibly electrotonic

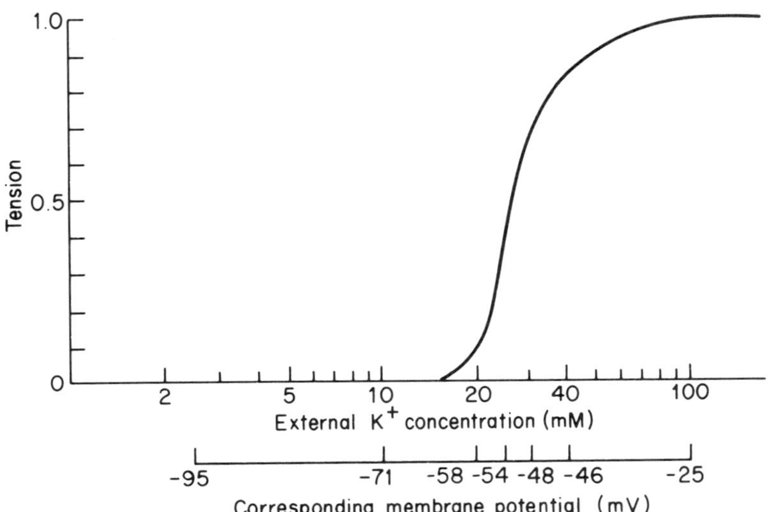


**Fig. 7.14** Relationship between peak tension and external potassium concentration or membrane potential in frog muscle fibres. (After Hodgkin, A. L. and Horowicz, P. (1960). *Journal of Physiology*, **153,** 386–403.)

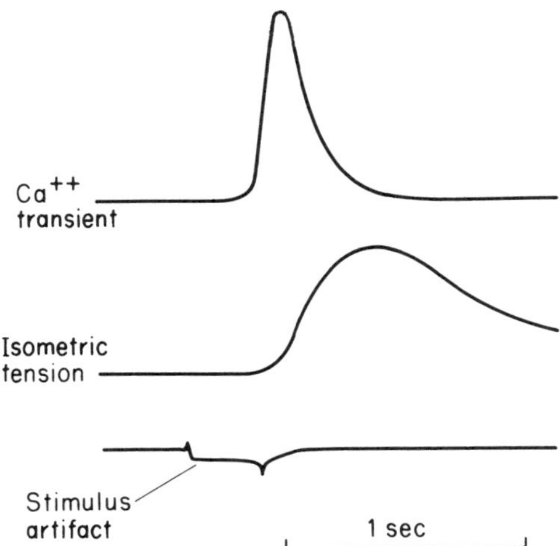


**Fig. 7.15** Relationship between the mobilization of calcium and the development of tension in a resting muscle fibre of a barnacle following a depolarization. The calcium transient is determined by measuring the light production from the cell following injection of the muscle fibre with the calcium bioluminescent protein aquorin (a sensitive calcium indicator which emits light in response to changes in the intracellular calcium ion concentration). (From Ridgeway, E. B. and Gordon, A. M. (1975). *Science*, **189,** 881–3. Copyright 1975 by the American Association for the Advancement of Science.)

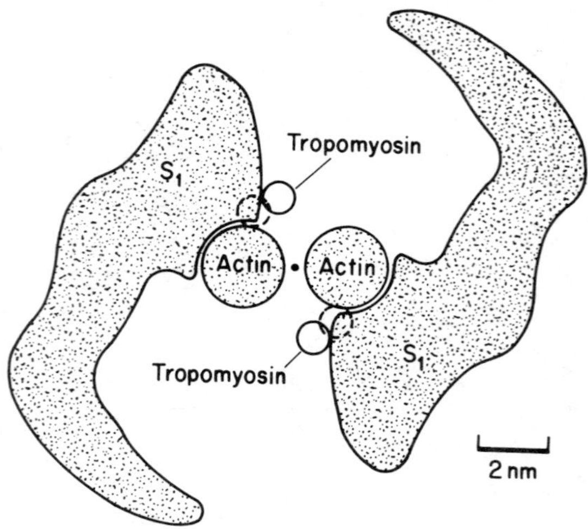


**Fig. 7.16** Model showing the possible role of tropomyosin in the formation of cross-bridges between the $S_1$ head of the myosin molecule and the actin filament. ◌, inhibitory position of the tropomyosin (i.e. the $S_1$ head of the myosin molecule cannot bind with the actin); ○, position taken up by the tropomyosin in the presence of calcium. (From Wakabayashi, T., Huxley, H. E., Amos, L. A. and Klug, A. (1975). *Journal of Molecular Biology*, **93,** 477–97.)

and the transfer of the signal to the intracellular components of the excitation–contraction coupling mechanism may simply involve depolarization of the dyads and triads. An alternative hypothesis, the 'channelled current' hypothesis, suggests that the current flow is channelled through the core of the tubules to a region of high chloride permeability in the tubular membrane at the dyads, and that specific ions transport a current across the latter.

Calcium, magnesium and ATP are all required in appropriate concentrations for a contraction to be elicited. While the last two occur in the right sort of concentration, the calcium ions are held at a below-threshold concentration level in the muscle cytoplasm (sarcoplasm) by a calcium pump in the sarcoplasmic reticulum membrane. In consequence, in resting muscle there is a high concentration of calcium in the sarcoplasmic reticulum. Depolarization of the dyads or triads elicits a movement of calcium ions into the cytoplasm, presumably by inhibiting the calcium pump. The relationship between the time course of the release of calcium into the sarcoplasm and the development of tension in the muscle fibres of a barnacle (Crustacea) is shown in Fig. 7.15.

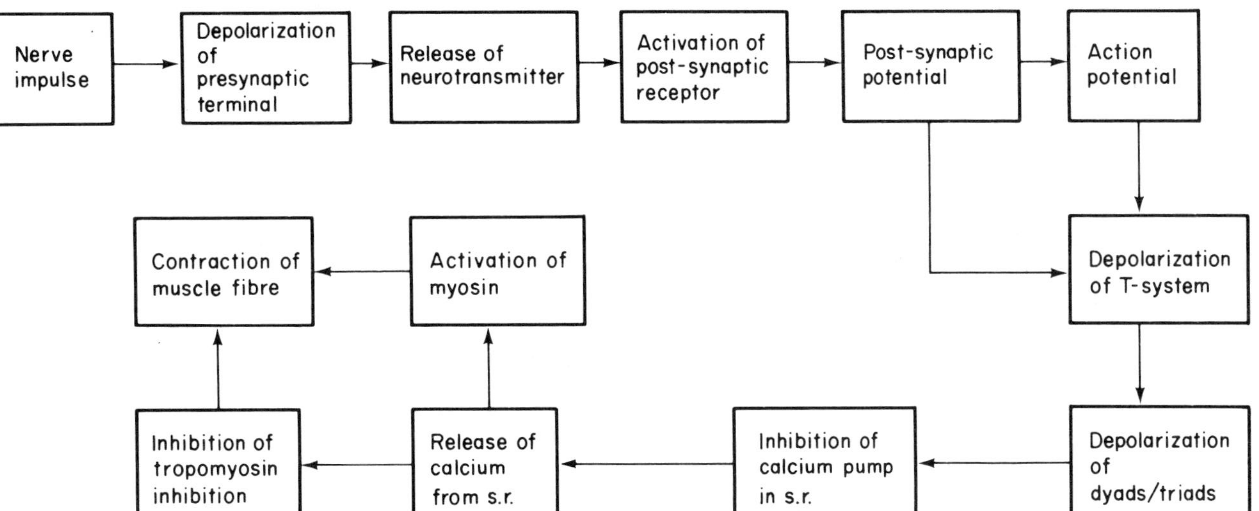


**Fig. 7.17** Flow diagram to show the sequence of events between the initiation of a nerve impulse in a motor axon and the contraction of the muscle fibre which it innervates.

There is evidence that the way in which calcium activates the contraction mechanism differs in different groups of animals. In vertebrates, decapod crustaceans and some sipunculids the effect of calcium is on the actin filaments. It is suggested that, in relaxed muscle, the position of the tropomyosin prevents cross-bridge formation. When calcium is released into the sarcoplasm it binds to the C subunit of the troponin complex and so causes movement of the tropomyosin, thereby releasing the inhibition (Fig. 7.16). This is supported by X-ray diffraction studies, which indicate that tropomyosin does indeed alter its position in response to an increase in sarcoplasmic calcium. This is referred to as I-filament control.

Alternatively, in molluscs, echiuroids, brachiopods, nemertines and holothurians there is A-filament control, mediated by the part of the myosin molecule containing the calcium-binding site. In annelids, nematodes, most arthropods and most sipunculids both mechanisms occur.

A summary of the sequence of events between motor nerve activation and contraction of a muscle is shown in Fig. 7.17. After excitation has ceased, the calcium is pumped back into the sarcoplasmic reticulum.

# 8

# *Sense Organs: Introduction and Mechanoreceptors*

## INTRODUCTION

Irrespective of the sensory modality to which they respond, receptors are generally divided into those which provide information on change in the environment (***phasic receptors***) and those which primarily indicate the *status quo* (***tonic receptors***), although there are many which combine both roles. The nature of the receptor potential induced by a stimulus and the basic relationship between the stimulus and the sensory nerve response have been described in Chapter 4 (Figs 4.1–4.7). In this and the following chapter, examples are given to illustrate the types of receptor which mediate the various sensory modalities.

## MECHANORECEPTION

There is a very wide range of receptors which provide the animal with mechanoreceptive information. Broadly speaking, most mechanoreceptors can be categorized into one of the three main groups—tactile receptors, proprioceptors and auditory receptors—although a certain amount of 'blurring' occurs at the edges of the groups.

### Tactile receptors

The tactile (touch) receptors are located exclusively in the epidermal or dermal layers of the body.

In soft-bodied invertebrates such as annelids the sensory cells bear cilia with a 9 + 2 arrangement of tubules. These cilia pass through the cuticle and hence project outwards from the animal.

Many of the sensory cells are grouped together into discrete sense organs. In *Lumbricus* there are two types of sensory cells with projecting cilia (Fig. 8.1). It is, at present, uncertain which of these (if either) responds to touch and which to chemical stimulation; and whether the sensory cells are primary sensory cells with an axon

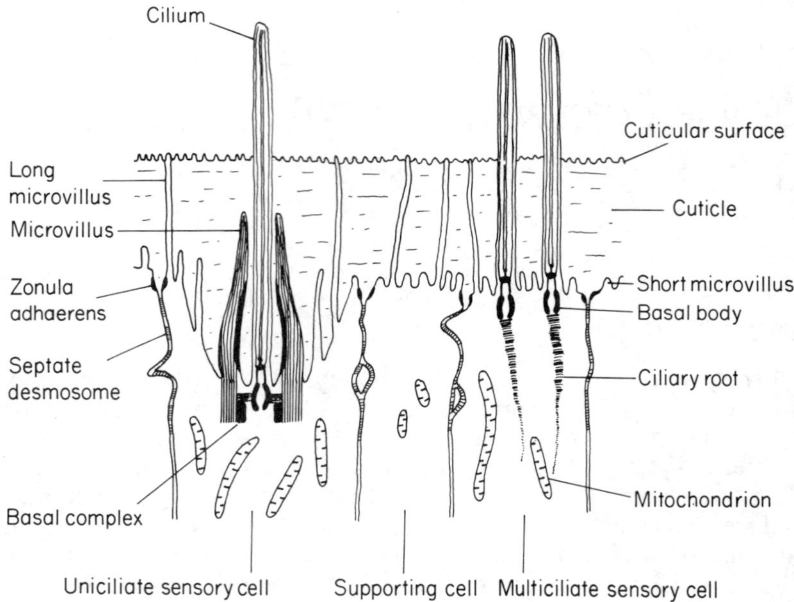


**Fig. 8.1** Diagram of a longitudinal section through a uniciliate and a multiciliate sensory cell and supporting cells of an earthworm epidermal sense organ. (From Mill, P. J. (1978). In *Physiology of Annelids*, (Mill, P. J., ed.), pp. 63–114. Academic Press, London; after Knapp, M. F. and Mill, P. J. (1971). *Tissue and Cell*, **3**, 623–36.)

passing to the central nervous system or whether they are secondary receptor cells with which a sensory neuron makes synaptic contact.

Tactile sensitivity is probably also mediated by unspecialized dendritic endings at or close to the surface of the body. Certainly oligochaetes and leeches have a few sensory cells which are touch receptors (T cells), and which have their cell bodies in the central nervous system and their dendritic terminations probably ending freely in the periphery.

In arthropods the tactile sensory cells are clearly primary sensory cells with an axon and a dendrite, the latter giving rise distally to a modified ciliary structure. This usually possesses a recognizable basal body, immediately distal to which the dendrite narrows abruptly and contains a 9 + 0 arrangement of double tubules. This 'ciliary region' is typically very short and gives way to a 'paraciliary region', characterized by the presence of single tubules. At its extreme distal end the modified cilium becomes dilated and packed to a varying extent with microtubules and often some electron-dense material. This region, called the 'tubular body', makes contact with the base of a hair (sensillum trichodeum) (Fig. 8.2). The receptor potential is

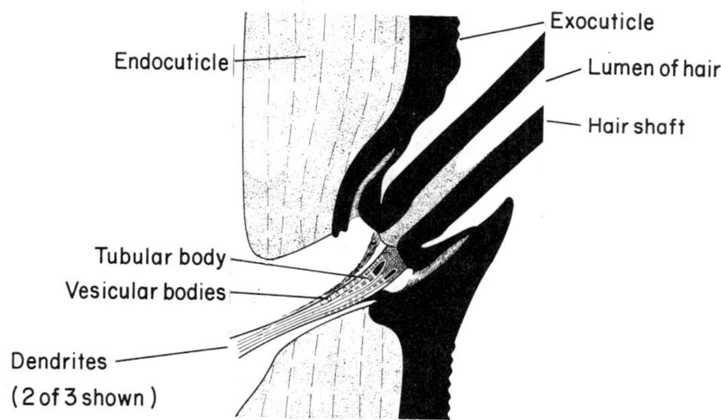


**Fig. 8.2** Diagram of a longitudinal section through the base of a tactile hair from the leg of a spider to show its innervation (From Harris, D. J. and Mill, P. J. (1977). *Journal of Comparative Physiology, A*, **119**, 37–54.)

probably produced as a result of compression of this tubular body. Other sensilla trichodea are chemoreceptors (see p. 185). The modified cilium lies in an extracellular space and is surrounded by a tube of extracellular material, the dendritic sheath. Three of the epidermal cells have become modified for specific functions associated with the sensillum. One of these 'enveloping cells' is thought to secrete the dendritic sheath; the other two secrete, respectively, the socket (tormogen cell) and the hair (trichogen cell).

Insect and most crustacean tactile hairs are each innervated by a single sensory cell. However, some tactile receptors on the thorax of lobsters are dually innervated, each sensory cell signalling a different direction of movement. In arachnids, the tactile sensilla are innervated typically by three sensory cells enclosed in a common dendritic sheath. Apart from the dually-innervated lobster sensilla there is no marked directional sensitivity associated with tactile hairs, although they do respond maximally to depression of the hair.

In mammals the skin consists of an outer epidermis, and an underlying dermis in which all the various 'skin' receptors are located. Thus touch, for example, is relayed to the receptors via deformation of the epidermis and the outer part of the dermis overlying the receptors. The 'skin' receptors include the Krause end bulbs, the Ruffini cylinders and the Meissner and Pacinian corpuscles, as well as free nerve endings.

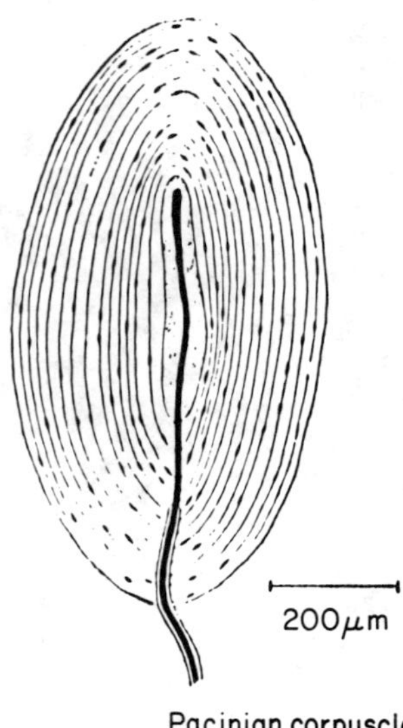


**Fig. 8.3** Diagram of a Pacinian corpuscle. (From Matthews, P. B. C. (1972). *Mammalian Muscle Receptors and their Central Actions.* Edward Arnold, London.)

The Pacinian corpuscles (Fig. 8.3) are sensitive exclusively to touch, but the functions of the other dermal sense organs are somewhat problematical. The Meissner corpuscles are generally considered to be touch receptors, and the Krause end bulbs and Ruffini cylinders sensitive to cold and warmth respectively. However, the so-called 'Law of Specific Nerve Energies', which states that however any one type of receptor is stimulated the sensation will always be the same, does not always hold for the dermal receptors and there is evidence that the Meissner corpuscles, Krause end bulbs and Ruffini cylinders can signal different sensory modalities apart from the one to which they are apparently mainly sensitive. Furthermore, experiments on the cornea, which only contains free nerve endings, have shown that this region is sensitive to touch, cold, warmth and pain.

The sensation of touch adapts fairly rapidly. This is, in part, a result of the elasticity of the skin overlying the receptor, which will tend to return to its original shape, but is due primarily to the phasic properties of the receptor potential. In the case of the Pacinian corpuscle this is partly a function of the dendrite itself, but the rate of adaptation is markedly enhanced by the presence of the capsule of connective tissue (see p. 49).

**Proprioception**

Proprioceptors have been defined by Lissmann (1950; see p. 259) as 'Sense organs capable of registering continuously deformation (changes in length) and stress (tensions, decompressions) in the body, which can arise from the animal's own movements or may be due to its weight or other external mechanical forces'. Thus all mechanoreceptors which provide the animal with information regarding the position, movement and orientation of the whole animal or its parts within its environment are included as proprioceptors. This is a very wide definition and indeed covers the majority of mechanoreceptors.

*Flow receptors*

Most flow receptors are concerned primarily with registering changes in the flow of the medium over the surface of the body. However, they are also important in the orientation of the body relative to the medium and as such can be considered to be proprioceptors.

Among terrestrial animals, structures which fall into this category include the hairs on the front of the head of the locust, which are directionally sensitive to wind direction and are fairly slowly adapting, and the hairs on the anal cerci of cockroaches. The former are associated with the initiation of, and adjustments to, flight; the latter, when stimulated, initiate an escape reflex. The trichobothria of spiders (Fig. 8.4) are exceptionally sensitive flow receptors, monitoring the slightest movements of the air. Trichobothria occur in longitudinal rows on the legs, and each is innervated by four sensory cells. Their structure is very similar to that of tactile hairs, except that there is an additional 'helmet-shaped' extracellular structure associated with the insertion of the dendrites at the base of the socket. The sensory cells innervating them are phasic and both directionally and positionally sensitive; different sensory cells covering different parts of the range of movement (Fig. 8.5).

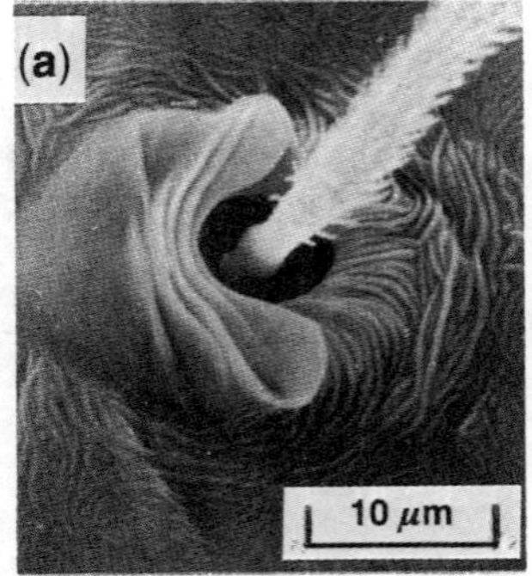


**Fig. 8.4** The base of a trichobothrium from the leg of a spider. (**a**) (*left*) Scanning electron micrograph; (**b**) (*below*) diagram of a longitudinal section to show the innervation. (From Harris, D. J. and Mill, P. J. (1977). *Journal of Comparative Physiology, A,* **119,** 37–54.)

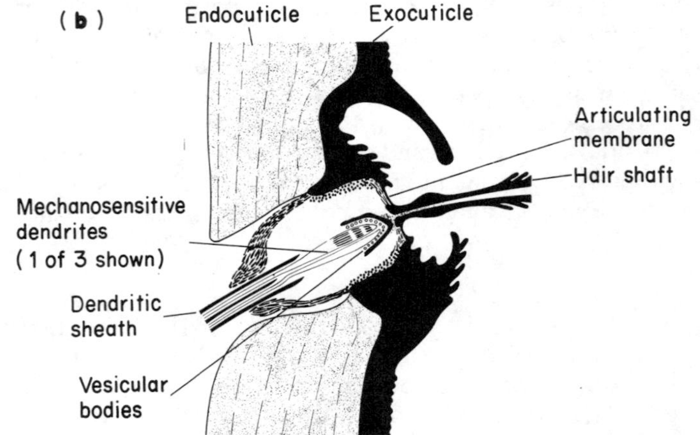


Flow receptors are also found in animals inhabiting an aquatic environment. Examples are the hair fans (Fig. 8.6a) and hair pegs found on the legs, claws and carapace of lobsters and the two rows of plumose hairs (Fig. 8.6b) found on the antennae of the rock-lobster, all of which are sensitive to water currents. These receptors are each innervated by at least two sensory cells, and at least the hair fans and hair pegs possess directional sensitivity. The posteriorly-directed spines on the abdomen of dragonfly larvae are possibly flow receptors, but differ from the above structures in that they are each innervated by a single sensory cell.

Elasmobranch and teleost fish, larval amphibians and the adults of aquatic amphibians such as *Xenopus* possess groups of sensory hair cells (neuromasts) lying in pits or grooves on the head and body (Fig. 8.7a). This is referred to generally as the 'lateral line system',

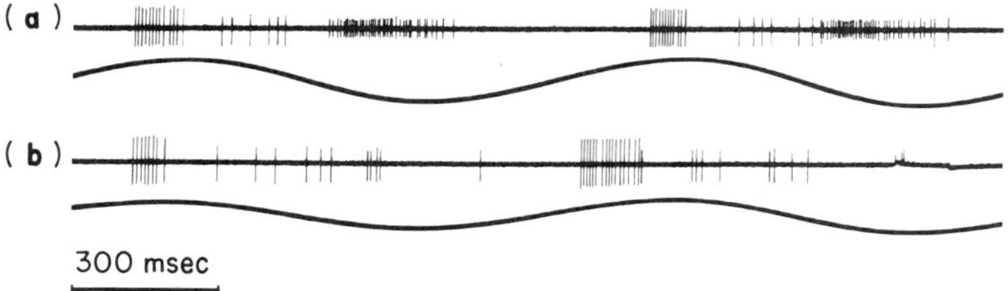


**Fig. 8.5** Extracellular recording of the response of a trichobothrium from the leg of a spider to movement (**a**) at right angles to the leg (down on the monitor trace corresponds to posterior movement) and (**b**) along the leg (down on the monitor trace corresponds to movement towards the body). The lower line in (**a**) and (**b**) is the monitor trace. Note the presence of three units, which are clearly distinguishable in (**a**) by the three different sizes of spikes, and their discrete response ranges. (From Harris, D. J. and Mill, P. J. (1977). *Journal of Comparative Physiology, A,* **119,** 37–54.)

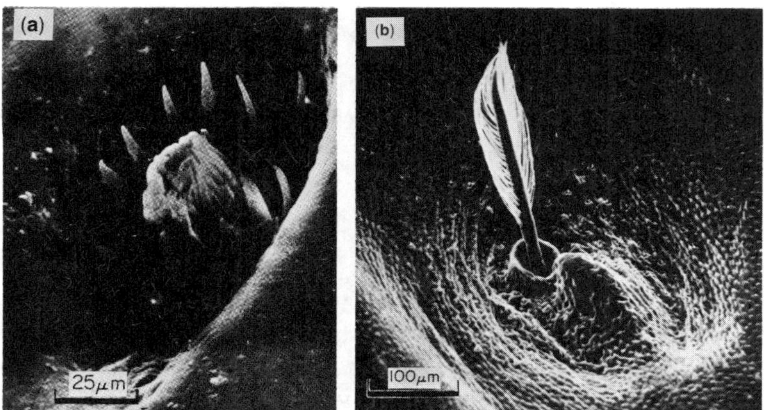


**Fig. 8.6** Scanning electron micrographs of (**a**) a hair fan from the carapace of a lobster and (**b**) a plumose hair from the antennal hydrodynamic organ of a rock-lobster. ((**a**) From Shelton, R. G. J. and Laverack, M. S. (1970). *Journal of Experimental Marine Biology and Ecology*, **4,** 201–10; (**b**) from Laverack, M. S. (1976) (photograph by Clarac, F., Vedel, J. P. & Moulins, M.). In *Structure and Function of Proprioceptors in the Invertebrates.* (Mill, P. J., ed.) Chapman and Hall, London.)

although only the row of pits down either side of the body are the 'lateral lines' in the strict anatomical sense.

In the Agnatha (jawless fishes) the pits are open and lie in somewhat irregular rows. In fishes there is a single row along either side of the body, lying in a canal which may be open, or roofed over with just a few openings to the surface. In teleosts there are also several rows on the head and the hairs of each neuromast are

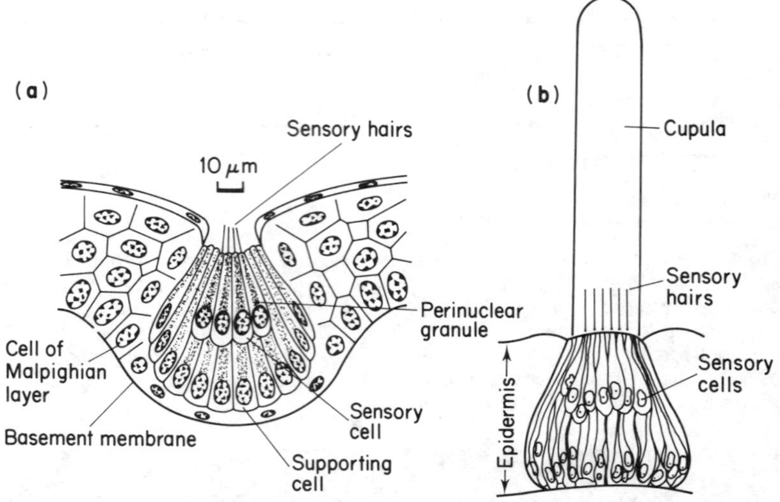


**Fig. 8.7** Diagrams of (**a**) a single lateralis organ from the epidermis of *Xenopus*, (**b**) a neuromast of a teleost with the hair cells embedded in a cupula. ((**a**) From Murray, R. W. (1955). *Quarterly Journal of Microscopical Science*, **96,** 351–61; (**b**) from Dijkgraaf, S. (1952). *Experientia*, **8,** 205–16.)

embedded in a gelatinous cupula (Fig. 8.7b). In aquatic amphibians there are several rows of pits both on the head and on the body, while in elasmobranchs and the southeast Asian catfish *Plotosus* the organs on the head lie at the end of long mucus-filled canals and are called the Ampullae of Lorenzini.

Each hair cell bears a number of hairs, one of which has a ciliary structure and is referred to as a kinocilium. The kinocilium lies to one side of the other hairs, the stereocilia, (Fig. 8.8) and is important in determining the directional sensitivity of the cell. In any one group of hair cells the orientation of the kinocilia is the same in each cell and the hairs of each group of hair cells are embedded in a gelatinous cupula. These organs are sensitive to water flow. In the lateral line some groups of cells have their kinocilia orientated in one direction, in others they are orientated in the opposite direction. Thus water flow in one direction excites some receptors and inhibits others, while water flow in the opposite direction has the reverse effect.

In teleosts the lateral line organs can detect a moving object some distance away, presumably by monitoring changes in pressure. This has been referred to as the 'distant touch' sense and is extremely well-developed in blind cave fish, which use it to avoid obstacles. In addition to the detection of flow and pressure, the Ampullae of Lorenzini in elasmobranchs are sensitive to other stimuli such as temperature and electrical fields.

*Peripheral stress detectors*

Peripheral stress detectors are receptors, mainly located in the periphery, which signal tensions and decompressions of the body surface.

In oligochaetes and leeches there are sensory cells with their cell bodies in the central nervous system, morphologically similar to the large touch (T) cells mentioned above (p. 116). These are, however, associated with stronger mechanical stimulation of the body surface and are called pressure or P cells. In leeches, at least, still stronger stimulation elicits a response in the so-called nociceptive (N) or pain cells. Hence, in these animals, touch, pressure and pain sensitivity are separated on the basis that different degrees of deformation of the body wall elicit responses in different groups of specific sensory cells, identified both by the location of their cell bodies within the central nervous system and by their physiological properties (Fig. 8.9). In earthworms there are also ciliated cells, with cilia running horizontally below the cuticle but above the epidermis, which are ideally situated to act as pressure detectors.

In mammals also, the difference between touch and pressure is often a question of the degree of deformation of the surface. Indeed, it would seem that, in animals without a hard exoskeleton, touch could be included within the definition of proprioception, in so far as it does involve some (minimal) deformation of the body surface. Furthermore, in mammals pressure is probably monitored by the touch sensitive Pacinian corpuscles. However, touch is clearly definable in humans as a sensation and is normally dealt with separately from proprioception, as in this chapter.

Stress in the hard exoskeleton of insects and crustaceans is detected by campaniform sensilla. In insects these sensilla are each innervated by a single sensory neuron, and are similar to tactile hairs in all respects except that the hair has become replaced by a domed, cuticular cap, which bears a thickened ridge. The sensilla are found in groups, as on the legs of cockroaches (Fig. 8.10a), or singly near the bases of tactile spines. When in groups they are usually arranged so that their thickened ridges are all aligned in the same direction—that in which cuticular stress is likely to be experienced. In crustaceans the appearance of the campaniform sensilla is rather different (Fig. 8.10b). Each sensillum is innervated by two sensory neurons and they occur in small groups at the ends of limbs and near the bases of some

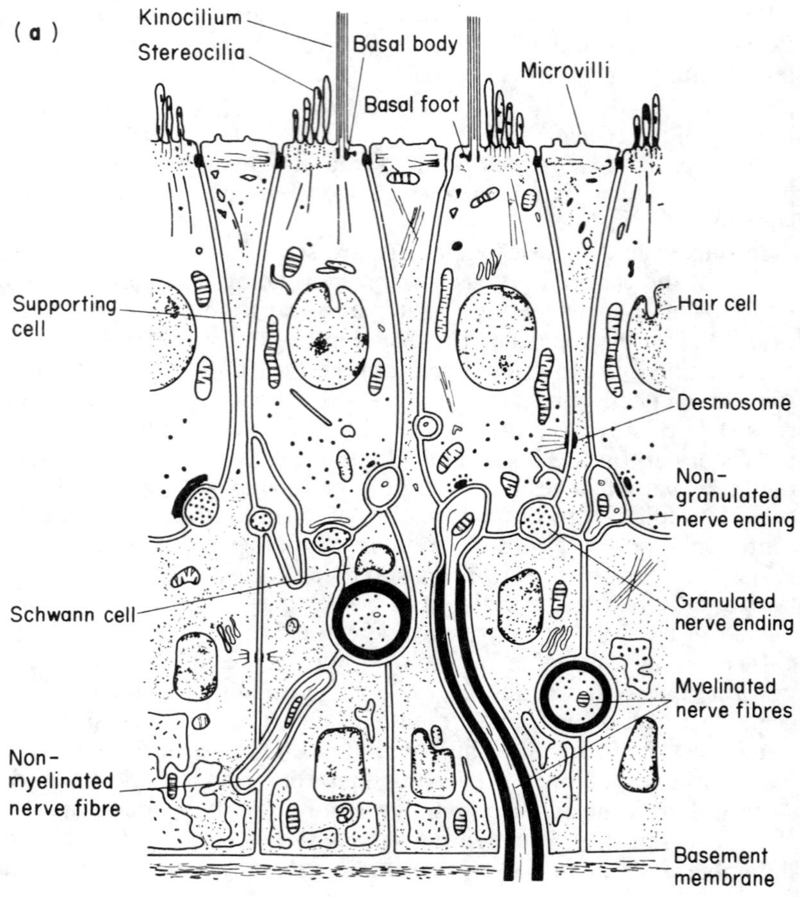


tactile hairs. Campaniform sensilla are also found on the antennae of both insects and crustaceans.

In spiders and scorpions the campaniform sensilla are replaced by slit sensilla and lyriform organs. Slit sensilla, as the name implies, appear externally as short slits or grooves in the cuticle (Fig. 8.10c) and are found scattered over the limbs and body. Lyriform organs are composed of several slits oriented in the same direction as one another (Fig. 8.10d) and occur on the limbs, often close to the joints. Each slit is dually innervated. Both slit sensilla and lyriform organs measure stress applied at right angles to the slit(s).

Decapod crustaceans are able to shed their limbs at a special

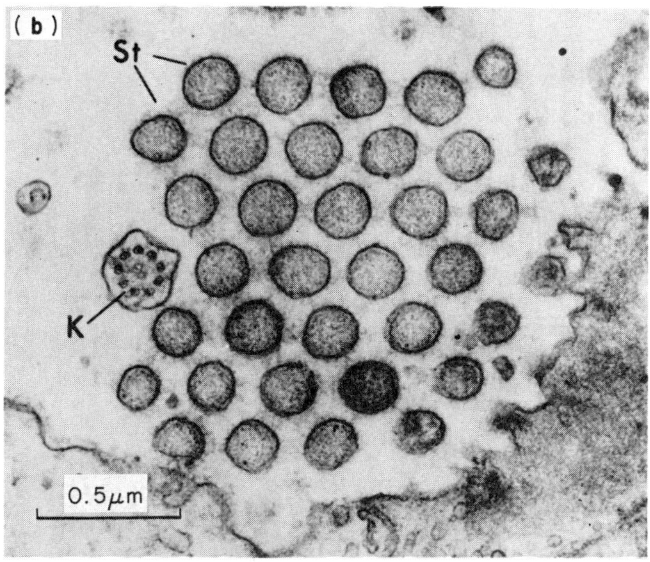


**Fig. 8.8** (**a**) (left) Diagram of the structure of the sensory cells of a lateral line canal neuromast in the teleost fish *Lota vulgaris*. (**b**) (above) Electron micrograph of a transverse section through the sensory hair bundle of a lateral line organ to show the hexagonal arrangement of stereocilia (St) behind the kinocilium (K). (From Flock, Å. (1965). *Cold Spring Harbor Symposia on Quantitative Biology*, **30**, 133–44.)

autotomy plane. This capability is particularly well-developed in the brachyurans (crabs), where the autotomy plane occurs in one of the basal segments (the basi-ischiopodite). Two chordotonal organs (p. 140) are associated with the cuticle of this region—CSD (cuticular stress detector)1 and CSD2—both of which insert on to areas of comparatively thin cuticle and are able to detect stress in this region. There is evidence that CSD1 is involved in initiating the autotomy (leg-shedding) reflex in response to cuticular stress.

*Muscle stress receptors*

The Golgi tendon organs and the apodeme tension receptors are found in the muscle tendons of vertebrates and crustaceans respectively. Their dendrites are directly associated with the tendons and hence these sense organs are in series with the muscle. They respond to increase in tension in the tendon, which may be brought about either by active contraction or by passive stretch of the muscle. In vertebrates the arrangement of the insertion of the muscle fibres on

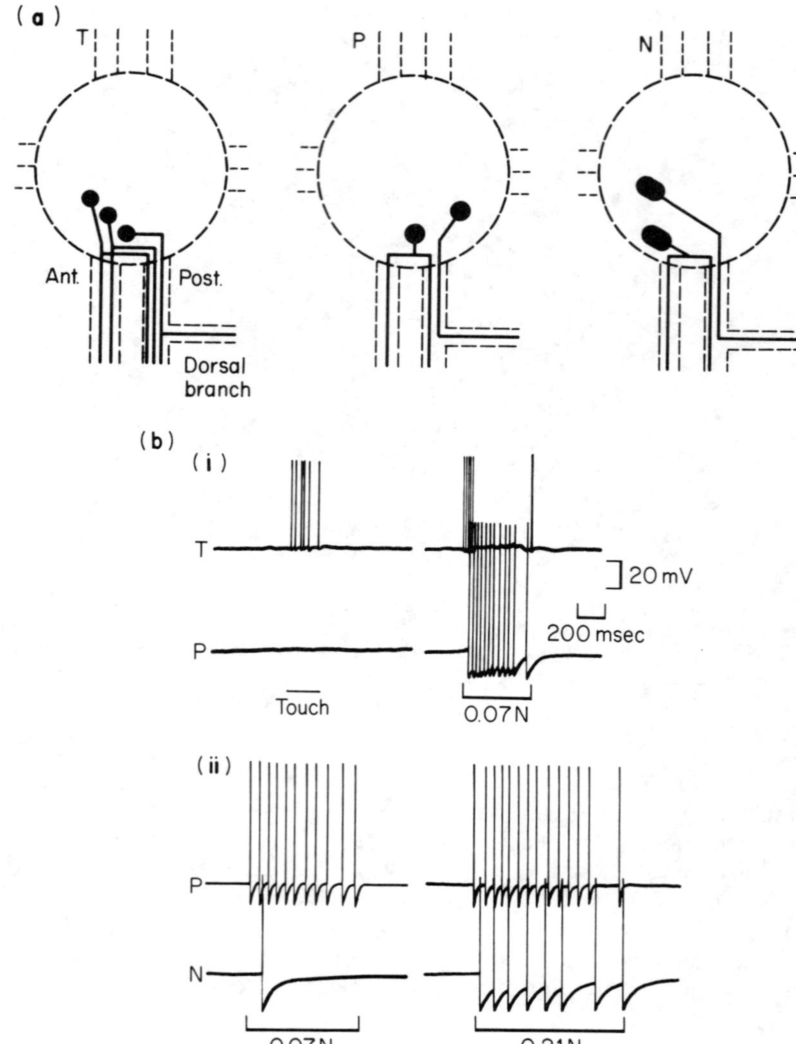


**Fig. 8.9** (**a**) Diagram showing the position of the T (touch), P (pressure) and N (nociceptive) sensory cells in a ganglion of a leech, and the arrangement of their axons in the segmental nerves. (**b**) Intracellular recordings from the T, P and N cells to show the effect of different strengths of stimulation; (**i**) the responses of T and P cells to light touch and slight indentation of the body wall (0.07 Newtons); (**ii**) the responses of P and N cells to slight (0.07 Newtons) and marked (0.21 Newtons) indentations of the body wall. (From Nicholls, J. G. and Baylor, D. A. (1968). *Journal of Neurophysiology*, **31,** 740–56.)

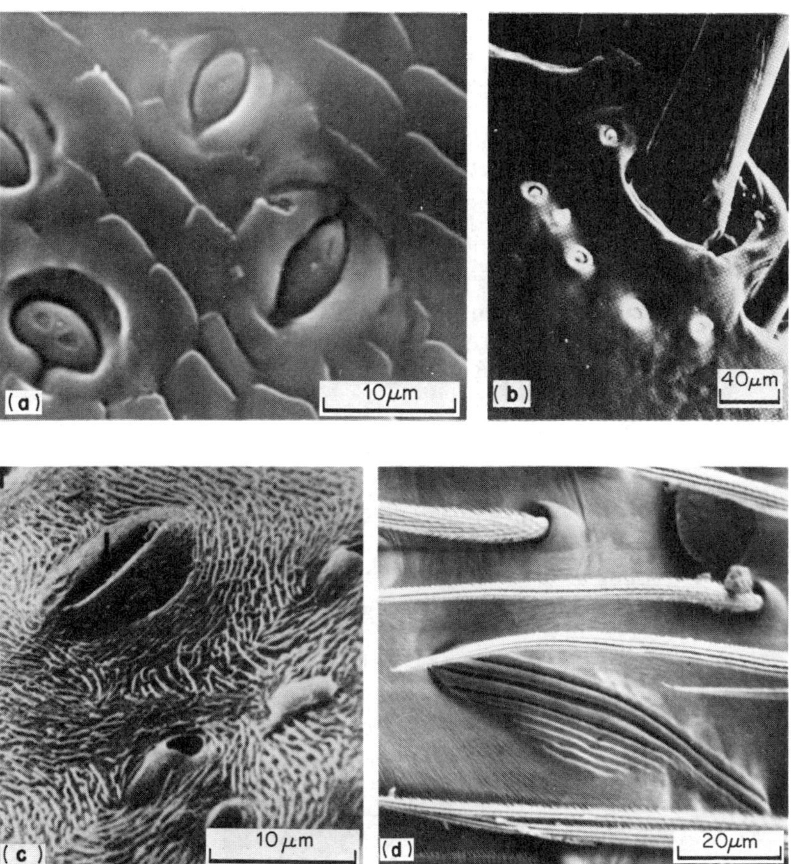


**Fig. 8.10** Scanning electron micrographs of (**a**) insect campaniform sensilla from the leg of a cockroach; (**b**) campaniform sensilla from the antennule of a lobster; (**c**) a slit sensillum from the leg of a spider (arrow indicates site of dendrite attachment; and (**d**) a lyriform organ from the leg of a spider. ((**a**) Photograph by courtesy of S. Rankin, Department of Pure and Applied Zoology, University of Leeds; (**b**) from Laverack, M. S. (1976). In *Structure and Function of Proprioceptors in the Invertebrates*. (Mill, P. J., ed.) Chapman and Hall, London; (**c**) from Barth, F. G. (1981). In *Sense Organs* (Laverack, M. S. and Cosens, D. J., Eds), pp. 112–41. Blackie.

the tendon and the pattern of innervation are such that the response of any given sensory cell varies according to which muscle motor units are activated. The Golgi tendon organs have a low threshold (although the tension produced by passive stretch of the muscle may be partly dissipated mechanically by the sheath surrounding the muscle) and both they and the apodeme tension receptors adapt slowly to a maintained tension.

*Movement and position receptors*

This category covers a very wide range of receptor types. There are some, in arthropods, which are located externally, but the majority are found internally.

External receptors

The best known external receptors are the hair plates of various insects (Fig. 8.11a), located, for example, at the bases of the legs, on the antennae and mouthparts, and in the neck region. They have not been found in crustaceans, although some decapods have organs called CAPs (cuticular articulated pegs) associated with certain leg joints (Fig. 8.11b). On the antennae, the hair plates may be associated with an internal mechanoreceptor (Johnston's organ) which is sensitive to vibrations. The CAPs are always associated with internal chordotonal organs (p. 140).

The hair plates are positioned such that movement of the joint causes a deflection of the hairs. While the hairs composing the plate have a structure similar to that of individual hair sensilla (p. 116), their response is fairly tonic, with increase in displacement causing an increase in the firing frequency of the sensory cells. They thus have a unidirectional sensitivity and provide the central nervous system with information on position.

Internal receptors

Any categorization of internal receptor types is somewhat arbitrary, but it does help to separate stretch receptors from joint receptors in discussing the plethora of mechanoreceptors which fall within this group. The stretch receptors generally lie parallel to, and are often associated with, muscles. As the name implies, joint receptors are associated with the joints of the appendages.

*Stretch receptors* Stretch receptors range in complexity from simple connective tissue strands with an associated sensory cell, as found in many insects, to the complex muscle receptor organs of decapod crustaceans and muscle spindles of vertebrates.

In most insects there is a pair of stretch receptors oriented longitudinally above the dorsal musculature in the majority of abdominal segments and, in some cases, in the thorax as well. In some, a second, vertically oriented pair, is also present.

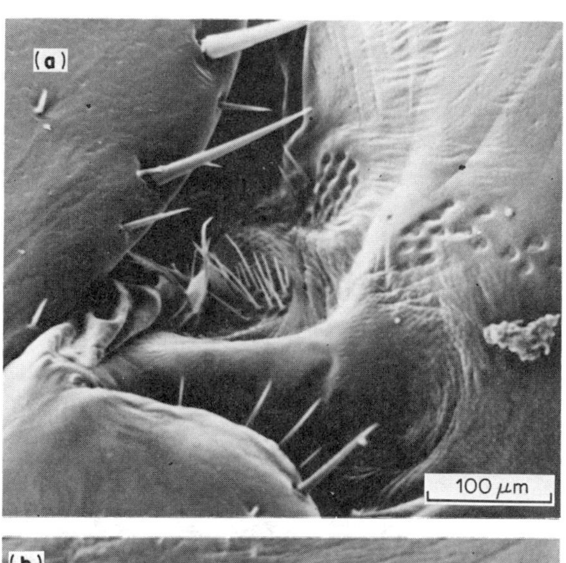


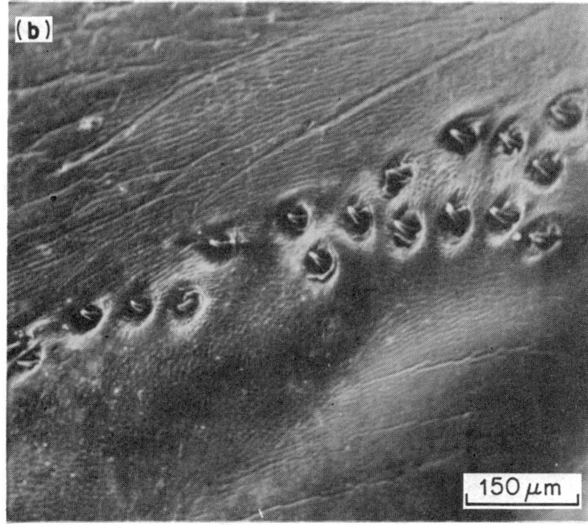


**Fig. 8.11** Scanning electron micrographs of (**a**) a hair plate from a cockroach leg; (**b**) a CAP (cuticular articulated peg) organ from a walking leg of lobster. ((**a**) Photograph by S. Rankin, Department of Pure and Applied Zoology, University of Leeds; (**b**) photograph by P. Lund, Department of Pure and Applied Zoology, University of Leeds.)

The receptor may consist either of a strand of connective tissue, which generally runs more or less parallel with the longitudinal muscles (Fig. 8.12a), or of a strand of connective tissue closely associated with a single muscle fibre which receives motor innervation (Fig. 8.12b). The latter structure is referred to as an MRO

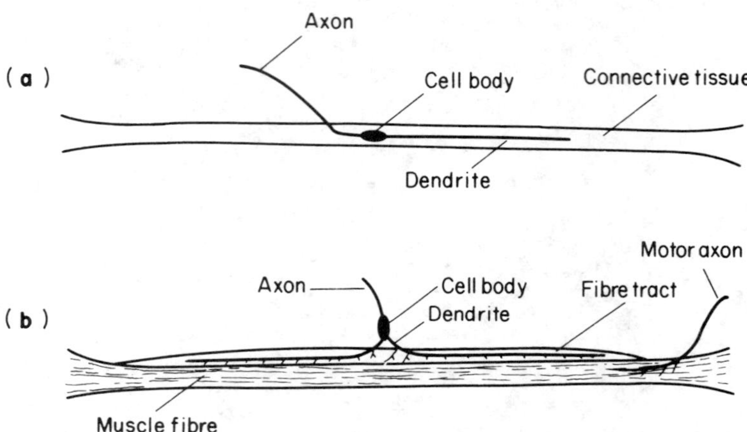


**Fig. 8.12** Diagrams showing the morphology of abdominal stretch receptors from (**a**) a dragonfly larva and (**b**) a lepidopteran. The latter includes a muscle fibre and hence is a muscle receptor organ (MRO).

(muscle receptor organ). In both cases the dendrites of the single sensory cell are embedded in the connective tissue strand. Where the strand is not directly associated with a muscle fibre the endings are simple. In the MROs of Lepidoptera (the peak of complexity among insect stretch receptors) the dendrites send side branches into longitudinally oriented bundles of connective tissue, and the central region of the muscle fibre contains less contractile material than the ends.

All of these receptors give information on both movement and position. Providing that there is a certain minimum tension on the receptor, the sensory cell fires with a steady (tonic) discharge which is faster the greater the receptor length. A sudden increase in length produces a rapid increase in the firing frequency which then adapts rapidly (phasic response) to the new steady level. The reverse occurs on shortening the receptor (Fig. 8.13a).

The response of the MRO of the lepidopteran caterpillar has been studied in most detail and this shows acceleration and deceleration responses, in addition to the movement (phasic) and position (tonic) responses. These are illustrated in Fig. 8.13b. Here the application of a stretch which increases slowly at constant velocity and is then maintained, results in an initial rapid increase in firing frequency, followed by some adaptation; then a steady increase while the stretch continues. At the end of the period of stretching there is a rapid decrease in firing frequency, followed by some recovery before slow adaptation to the new tonic level. The dashed line in the figure

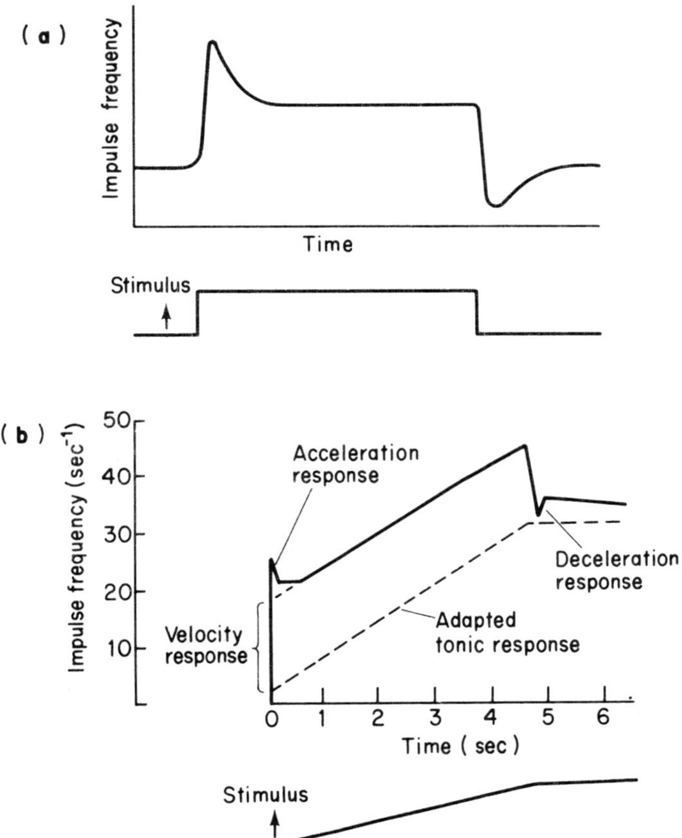


**Fig. 8.13** Relationship between the frequency of action potentials (impulses) and stretch in abdominal stretch receptors of (**a**) a dragonfly larva and (**b**) a lepidopteran. In (**a**) the stimulus is in the form of a step function; (**b**) the stimulus is applied as a ramp in order to differentiate the velocity and acceleration (and deceleration) responses. ((**b**) After Weevers, R. de G. (1966). *Journal of Experimental Biology*, **44,** 177–94.)

indicates the adapted tonic response to the applied stretch. The difference between the two lines is the velocity response, while the overshoot at the onset of stretch and the undershoot at the cessation of stretch are responses to acceleration and deceleration respectively. Thus the information provided by this receptor is quite complex.

In crustaceans, the stretch receptors are mainly MROs. Their positioning is similar to that in insects, but there are nearly always two pairs of receptors in each abdominal segment, with a division of labour between the members of a pair. One (MRO1) has a tonic response; the other (MRO2) has a phasic response. Each receptor consists of a muscle fibre (the receptor muscle, RM) and a sensory neuron (SN). The dendrites of the sensory neuron end in a region near the centre of the muscle fibre, which contains connective tissue and little or no contractile material (Fig. 8.14). Each receptor muscle

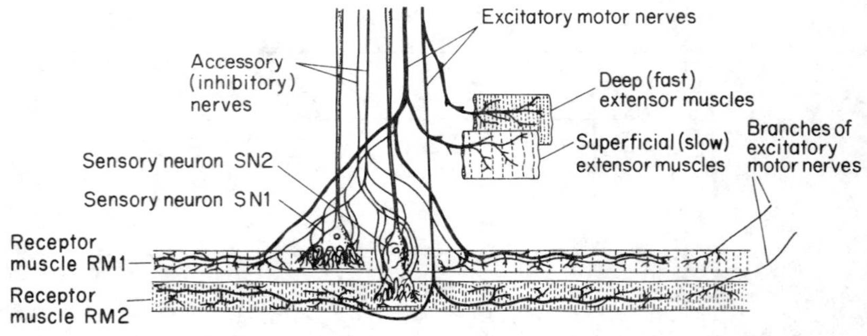


**Fig. 8.14** Diagram of the slow (RM1/SN1) and fast (RM2/SN2) MROs (muscle receptor organs) of the lobster. (From Alexandrowicz, J. S. (1967). *Biological Reviews*, **42**, 288–326.)

is innervated by its own excitatory motor fibre. Two or three inhibitory motor fibres are common to both receptors. Of these, one innervates the receptor muscle and the sensory dendritic endings while another innervates just the sensory dendritic endings. The receptor muscles also receive branches of excitatory motor fibres innervating adjacent muscles.

In response to a maintained stretch the rhythmic firing frequency of the tonic receptor (MRO1) has been recorded for up to $3\frac{1}{2}$ hours; the phasic burst of the other receptor (MRO2) is usually less than 60 seconds in duration. The threshold for MRO1 is lower than that for MRO2. Their rates of adaptation and thresholds are properties of the neurons themselves, not of the elastic properties of the 'in series' muscle fibres. In MRO1 there is a linear relationship between the firing frequency of the sensory neuron and the length of the receptor (p. 51).

Since the dendritic and contractile regions are in series, stimulation of the receptors can be achieved either by passive stretch of the receptor muscles or by their isometric contraction (p. 101). In both cases there is an increase in tension in the central connective tissue region of the receptor and it increases in length. The resultant deformation of the dendritic endings produces a receptor potential with subsequent production of spikes at the spike-initiating zone. Even a single action potential in the excitatory motor axon innervating RM1 may produce a long-lasting discharge in SN1 and this effect becomes greater as the initial length of the receptor is increased (Fig. 8.15). Similarly, the higher the impulse frequency in the excitatory motor neuron, the greater the contraction of the receptor muscle and hence the higher the frequency of action potentials in SN1. MRO2 is most sensitive to fast stretch or twitch contractions of RM2. The tonic firing of SN1 can be blocked by stimulating the large inhibitory motor neuron to the receptors (Fig. 8.16). The inhibitory junction potentials (IJPs) produced by this stimulation are larger the greater the depolarization (Fig. 8.16, see also Fig. 4.10).

A somewhat different type of MRO is found at the bases of the limbs in decapod crustaceans. These thoracic-coxal MROs each consist of a muscle fibre with a non-contractile region at its proximal end which is innervated by a sensory neuron (T fibre). In astacurans (lobsters and crayfish) and palinurans (rock-lobsters) a second sensory fibre (S fibre) innervates the proximal region of the receptor muscle distal to the non-contractile region. In brachyurans (crabs) the S fibre enters two connective tissue strands which flank the receptor muscle at its base and, more distally, merge into the connective tissue sheath surrounding the receptor muscle (Fig. 8.17). In some cases a third, small sensory neuron (P fibre) is also present. The dendrites of all three sensory neurons terminate in vacuolated connective tissue strands and the arrangement is such that the T fibre endings are in series with the receptor muscle while the S fibre endings are in parallel with it. The receptor muscle also receives efferent innervation.

The cell bodies of the sensory neurons lie within the central nervous system and transmission of information along the axons is by graded potential and not by action potentials, and is therefore decremental (i.e. the size of the potential diminishes as it travels further from the sensory endings). The responses of the T and S fibres to a steady increase in length of the receptor muscle, followed

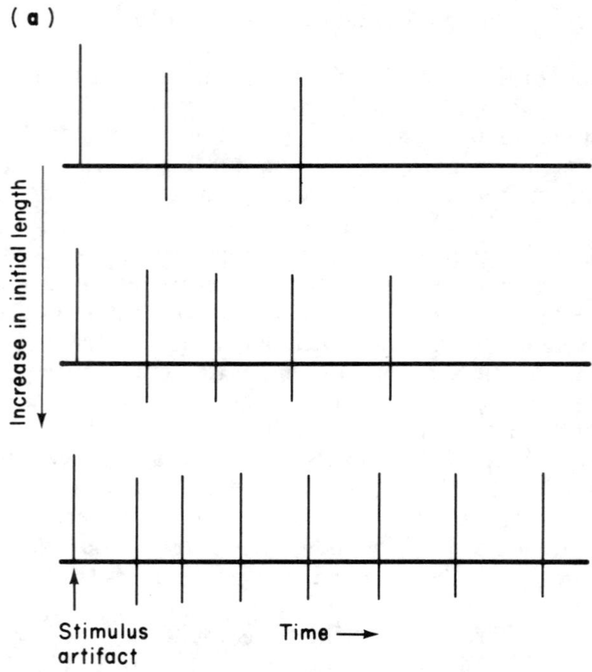


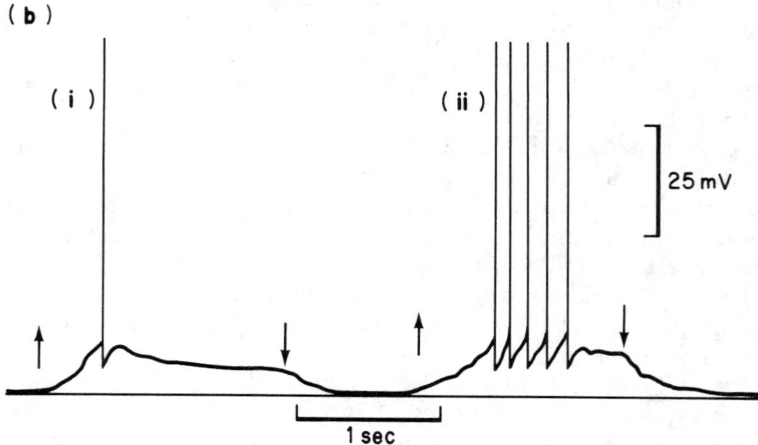


**Fig. 8.15** Recordings from the sensory neuron of the crustacean tonic MRO. (**a**) Extracellular recordings to show the reponse to a single stimulus to the excitatory motor neuron at three different initial lengths of the receptor muscle; (**b**) intracellular

by maintenance of the new length and then return to its original length, are shown in Fig. 8.18. It can be seen that the responses of both of these sensory neurons have phasic and tonic components. Furthermore, in each case the phasic component contains both velocity and acceleration responses. The acceleration response of the T fibre is marked; that of the S fibre is much smaller. (Note the similarities between the response of the S fibre and that of the lepidopteran MRO shown in Fig. 8.13b.)

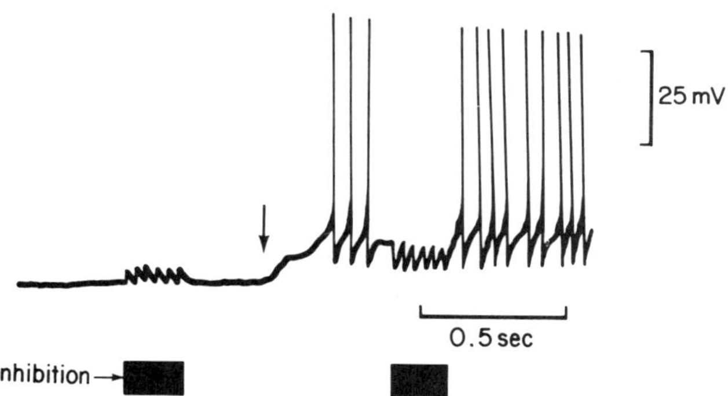


**Fig. 8.16** Intracellular recording from the sensory neuron of the tonic MRO of a lobster. The inhibitory motor neuron was stimulated twice at 30 Hz. During the first period the receptor muscle was relaxed and the inhibitory potentials were depolarizing. The receptor was then stretched sufficiently to elicit continuous firing (↓). Inhibitory stimulation now produced hyperpolarizing potentials and interrupted the receptor discharge. (From Kuffler, S. W. and Eyzaguirre, C. (1955). *Journal of General Physiology*, **39,** 155–84.)

*Muscle spindles* The corresponding receptors in vertebrates are the muscle spindles (Fig. 8.19), several of which are found in most vertebrate muscles. Each muscle spindle consists of several muscle fibres (intrafusal fibres), each with a non-contractile central (equatorial) region. These fibres are several millimetres long and about 100$\mu$m wide in their equatorial region, tapering towards their ends. There are two types of intrafusal fibres—nuclear bag fibres and

---

recording to show the effect of two stretches, (**i**) just above threshold, producing a single action potential, and (**ii**) a somewhat greater stretch, producing a larger generator potential and a discharge of five action potentials. ↑, start of stretch; ↓, end of stretch. ((**a**) After Kuffler, S. W. (1954). *Journal of Neurophysiology*, **17,** 558–74; (**b**) from Eyzaguirre, C. and Kuffler, S. W. (1955). *Journal of General Physiology*, **39,** 87–119.)

nuclear chain fibres. In their equatorial region the nuclear bag fibres have a cluster of nuclei lying two or three deep transversely across the fibre, while the nuclei in the nuclear chain fibres lie in single file. Other differences between them are somewhat variable. However, the nuclear bag fibres are often thicker than the nuclear chain fibres and are usually rather longer. Furthermore, the nuclear chain fibres

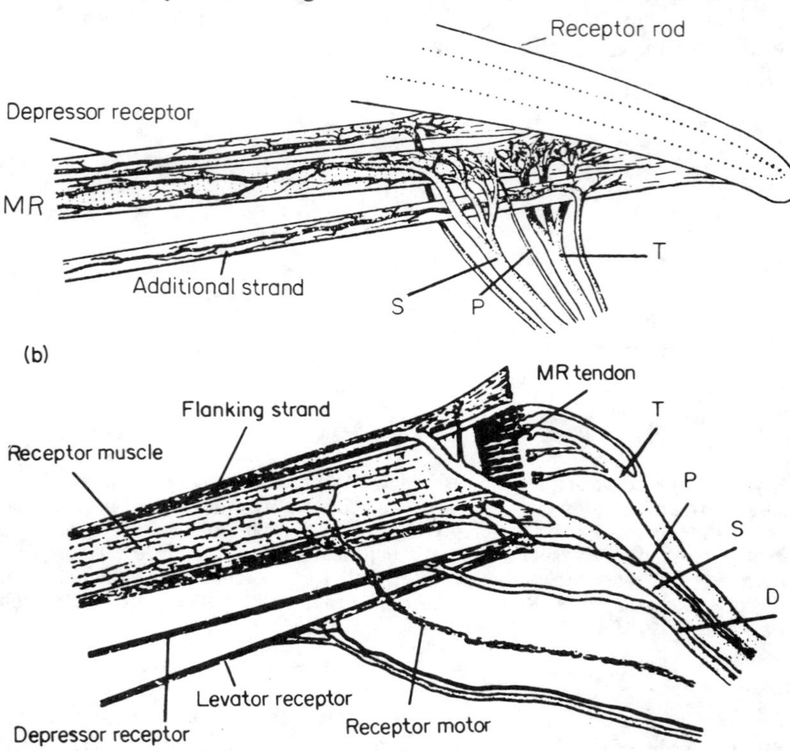


**Fig. 8.17** Diagrams of thoracic–coxal (TC) MROs in (**a**) the lobster *Palinurus vulgaris* and (**b**) the crab *Carcinus maenas*. ((**a**) from Alexandrowicz, J. S. (1967). *Journal of the Marine Biological Association, U.K.*, **47,** 415–32; (**b**) from Alexandrowicz, J. S. and Whitear, M. (1957). *Journal of the Marine Biological Association, U.K.*, **36,** 603–28.)

have a less regular array of myofibrils and contain more sarcoplasm, mitochondria and myofibrillar ATPase. The M-line and H-zone are present in the nuclear chain fibres but in the nuclear bag fibres the M-line is absent and the H-zone is only poorly developed.

There are two sensory fibres associated with each muscle spindle (Fig. 8.19). One is referred to as a primary or group I afferent, the

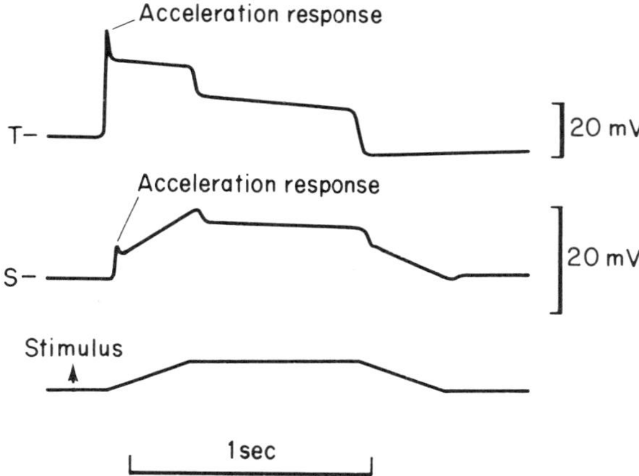


**Fig. 8.18** Intracellular recordings of receptor potentials from the T and S sensory neurons of the thoracic–coxal MRO of the crab *Carcinus*, elicited by stretching the receptor. (After Bush, B. M. H. (1976). In *Structure and Function of Proprioceptors in the Invertebrates*. (Mill, P. J., ed.) Chapman and Hall, London. (By Bush, B. M. H. and Cannone, A. J.))

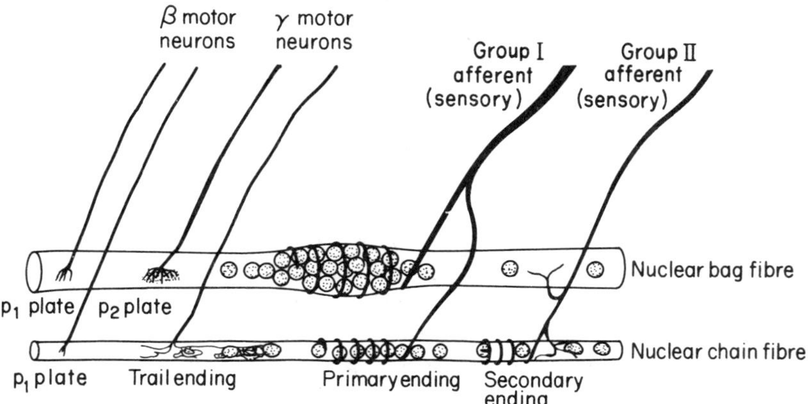


**Fig. 8.19** Simplified diagram of the central region of a vertebrate muscle spindle to show the sensory and motor innervation of the nuclear bag and nuclear chain fibres: There are in fact two types of nuclear bag fibres: dynamic ($bag_1$) fibres and static ($bag_2$) fibres, controlled respectively by 'dynamic' and 'static' $\gamma$ (and, in some spindles, $\beta$) motor neurons. (After Boyd, I. (1961). *Journal of Physiology*, **159,** 7P–9P; and Jansen, J. K. S. and Matthews, P. B. C. (1962). *Journal of Physiology*, **161,** 357–78.)

other as a secondary or group II afferent (p. 30; Table 1.1). The primary afferent has a similar, spirally-organized ending on both types of intrafusal fibre in the equatorial region. In contrast, the secondary afferent has spiral endings only on the nuclear chain fibres. In some cases the secondary afferent has no ending on the nuclear bag fibres, but when it does the endings are simple. The secondary endings lie on either side of the equatorial region.

The motor innervation of the muscle spindles of mammals is by both $\beta$ and $\gamma$ motor neurons (p. 28; Table 1.1). The synapses of the $\beta$ motor neurons, the $p_1$ plates, are similar to normal motor end-plates, and at least some of the $\beta$ neurons which innervate the muscle spindles also innervate the ordinary (extrafusal) muscle fibres. Some

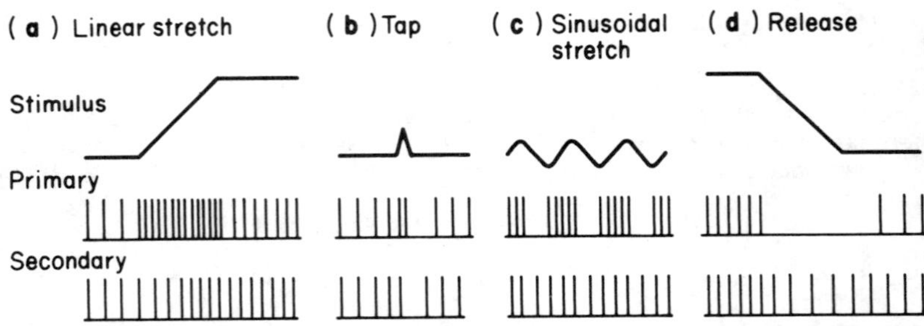


**Fig. 8.20** Diagrams showing the typical responses of the primary and secondary sensory endings in a muscle spindle to large stretches applied in the absence of motor activity. (From Matthews, P. B. C. (1964). *Physiological Reviews*, **44**, 219–88.)

of the $\gamma$ motor neurons also terminate in end-plates, but these $p_2$ plates are about twice as long as the $p_1$ plates and the subsynaptic membrane is less folded. Other $\gamma$ motor neurons have trail endings similar to those on the slow muscle fibres of frogs. There is a tendency for the plate endings to occur on the nuclear bag fibres and the trail endings on the nuclear chain fibres (Fig. 8.19).

As with the MROs of crustaceans, the sensory endings can be stretched, and hence excited, both by passive stretch of the muscle and by active contraction of the receptor muscle (intrafusal) fibres. Conversely, contraction of the muscle reduces the excitation by shortening the muscle spindles.

The axons of the primary afferents are of larger diameter and conduct at greater velocities than those of the secondary afferents (see Table 1.1), although there is some overlap. Both types of afferent have phasic and tonic components but, while their tonic components are of similar sensitivity, the phasic component is much more marked in the primary afferents (Fig. 8.20). The primary afferents also have acceleration and deceleration responses (Fig. 8.21a). These are particularly noticeable when the efferent innerva-

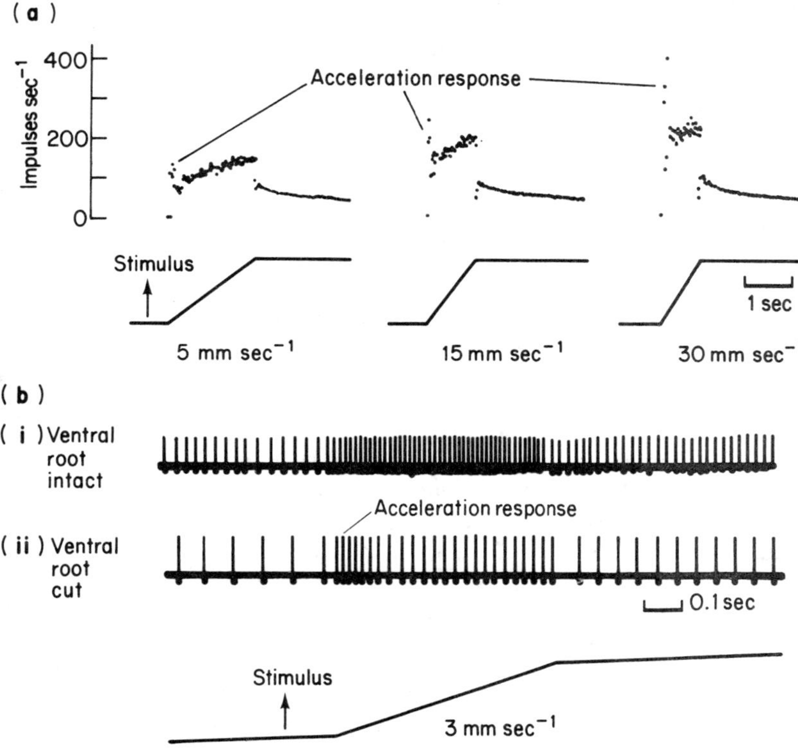


**Fig. 8.21** Extracellular recordings from a primary sensory ending of a mammalian muscle spindle. (**a**) Instantaneous frequency plots resulting from three different rates of stretch of the muscle spindle. (**b**) The effect of a slow stretch applied (**i**) during steady motor excitation of the muscle spindle and (**ii**) to a de-efferented muscle spindle (i.e. no motor innervation). Note that in (**b**) the acceleration response is absent in the presence of steady motor excitation of the muscle spindle. (**a**) From Matthews, P. B. C. (1972). *Mammalian Muscle Receptors and their Central Actions*. Edward Arnold, London; after Matthews, P. B. C. (1963). *Journal of Physiology*, **168,** 660–78. (**b**) From Jansen, J. K. S. and Matthews, P. B. C. (1962). *Journal of Physiology*, **161,** 357–78.)

tion is abolished, and may be virtually absent when the tone of the spindle is maintained by its efferent nerve supply (Fig. 8.21b).

The primary endings, because of their greater phasic sensitivity, show a response to brief stretches, as elicited, for example, by tapping the tendon, when there is little effect on the secondary endings (Fig. 8.20b). Similarly, the primary endings show a much greater sensitivity to repetitive, sinusoidal stretching and relaxing of the spindle (Fig. 8.20c). Both types of ending show a linear response to low amplitudes of sinusoidal stretch, i.e. a doubling of the amplitude of the stimulus doubles the amplitude of the response.

The $\gamma$ (fusimotor) neurons are of two functionally distinct types—static and dynamic fusimotor neurons. Stimulation of either increases the tonic activity of the primary endings at constant muscle length. However, they have different effects on the phasic (dynamic) response to stretching. Thus stimulation of a static neuron causes a reduction in the phasic response, whereas stimulation of a dynamic neuron produces a marked increase in the phasic response. (The phasic response is generally measured by the so-called 'dynamic index'; this is the fall in firing frequency which occurs during the first 0.5 sec after completion of a ramp stretch.) Static neurons have a similar effect on the secondary endings as on the primary endings, but dynamic neurons have no apparent effect on the secondary endings.

*Joint receptors* In arthropod limbs the joint receptors are each composed of a number of sensory cells associated with a receptor strand containing cells and connective tissue. The receptor strand may or may not span the joint, but it is always arranged so that joint movement alters its length. Each joint has either one or two of these receptors associated with it (Fig. 8.22). In arachnids the dendrites are thought to end fairly simply within the receptor strand; but in insects and crustaceans the dendrites end in a modified ciliary structure and there is considerable modification of the surrounding cells. This latter type is referred to as a chordotonal organ and the terminal region of the dendrite, together with its surrounding structures, is referred to as a scolopidium. In some cases there are two dendrites per scolopidium. The number of sensory cells in a single chordotonal organ varies from a few (e.g. the abdominal chordotonal organs of anisopteran dragonfly larvae) up to about a hundred (e.g. some of the limb chordotonal organs of decapod crustaceans). In the limbs of decapod crustaceans there are one or two chordotonal organs which are directly associated with a small 'accessory flexor' muscle in one of the central joints of the legs. These are called myochordotonal organs (Fig. 8.22).

Typically, each sensory cell in a chordotonal organ bears a single dendrite. This contains a ciliary root (or axial filament) which ends distally in a basal body. At this point the dendrite narrows abruptly and gives rise to a modified cilium, usually called a centriolar

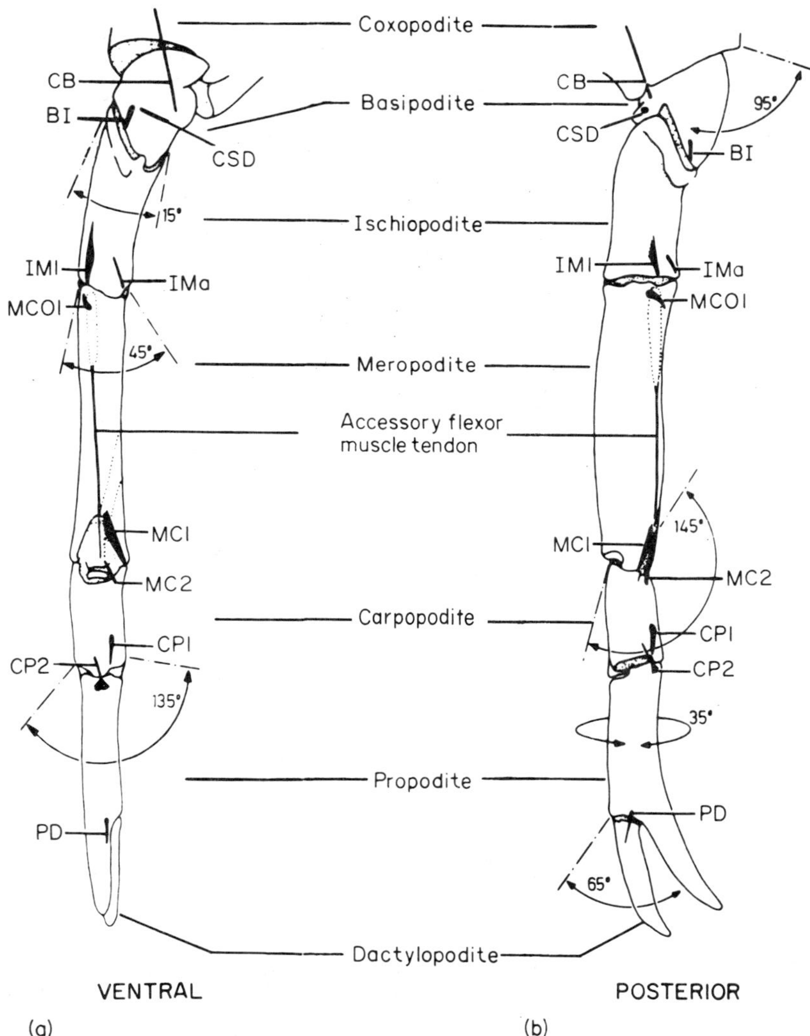


**Fig. 8.22** (**a**) Ventral and (**b**) posterior views showing the positions of the joint chordotonal organs, the myochordotonal organ (MCO1) and the cuticular stress detector (CSD) in a left walking leg of the lobster *Homarus gammarus*. Where two chordotonal organs monitor one joint they are differentiated by suffixes, i.e. CP1 and CP2; MC1 and MC2; IM1 and IMa. Each chordotonal organ is named after the joint which it monitors, for example the PD organ monitors the propodite-dactylopodite joint. (After Wales, W., Clarac, F., Dando, M. R. and Laverack, M. S. (1970). *Zeitschrift für vergleichende Physiologie*, **68,** 345–84.)

derivative. There are two types of centriolar derivative (Fig. 8.23). In one (type 1, Fig. 8.23a) there is a $9+0$ arrangement of double microtubules (one of each pair has an electron-dense core and a pair of arms) forming an axoneme, which extends the full length of the cilium. Just before the tip there is a ciliary dilation which contains, in

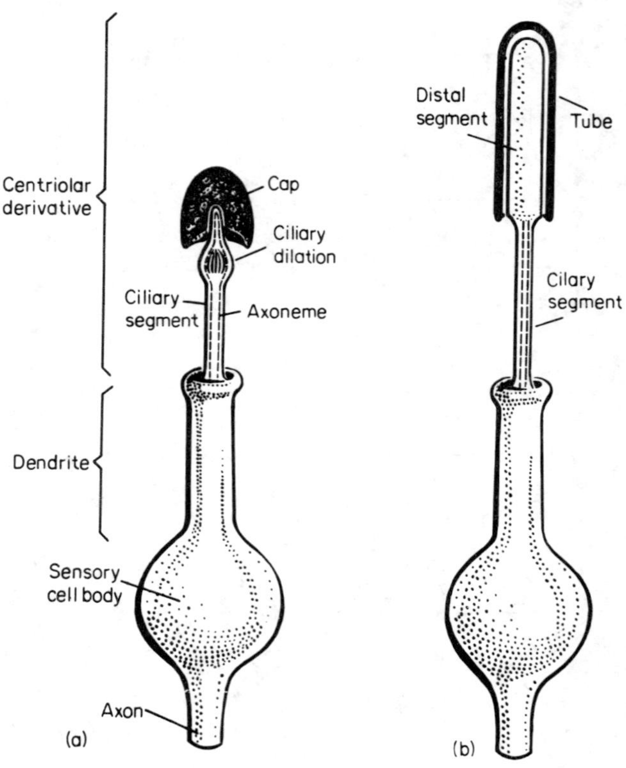


**Fig. 8.23** Diagrams showing the sensory cells of scolopidia. (**a**) Type 1 (centriolar derivative without a distal segment) and (**b**) type 2 (centriolar derivative with a distal segment). (From Moulins, M. (1976). In *Structure and Function of Proprioceptors in the Invertebrates.* (Mill, P. J., ed.) Chapman and Hall, London.)

addition to the axoneme, an electron-dense material laid down around a matrix of longitudinally oriented microtubules. This type is found in, for example, the abdomen and legs of insects. In the other type (type 2, Fig. 8.23b) the cilium is separable into two zones, a basal ciliary segment containing the axoneme and a distal segment containing a number of single, longitudinally oriented microtubules.

In many cases the ciliary segment can be subdivided into a ciliary region, containing only the axoneme, and a paraciliary region, containing the axoneme plus additional microtubules. This type is found in, for example, decapod crustacean limbs.

The distal region of the dendrite and the cilium are enclosed by a scolopale cell containing an electron-dense structure, the scolopale. The dendrite is anchored closely to the scolopale by desmosomes, and the cilium lies in a large extracellular 'scolopale' space. Distal to the scolopale cell, and often interdigitating with it, there is an electron-dense extracellular structure (Fig. 8.23). In cells with a type 1 centriolar derivative this forms a cap over the end of the dendrite and the scolopale space, while in those with a type 2 centriolar derivative it is elongated into a tube which surrounds the distal segment and there is usually an enveloping cell surrounding the scolopale cell and tube. In most scolopidia there is an attachment cell which is juxtaposed either to the cap or, where there is an enveloping cell, to the distal region of the latter (Fig. 8.24) and the attachment and enveloping cells are surrounded mainly by a cellular matrix (strand cells). However, in some scolopidia with a type 2 centriolar derivative, there is no attachment cell and the enveloping cell is in direct contact with collagen fibres.

The most complex chordotonal organs are probably those found in the limbs of decapod crustaceans where, within any one receptor, there is a clear structural and physiological differentiation, both between phasic and tonic sensory cells and between phasic cells responding to the two opposite directions of joint movement. The arrangement of the major cell types in the chordotonal organ which spans the most distal limb joint of a crab (called the PD organ after the initial letters of the names of the two adjacent segments—the propodite and the dactylopodite (Fig. 8.22)) is shown in Fig. 8.25. The proximal end of this receptor is attached to the tendon of the dactylopodite flexor muscle while the distal end inserts on the cuticle of the dactylopodite. The larger, proximal sensory cells have a purely phasic response (movement sensitive) (Fig. 8.26a) while the distal row of smaller cells have predominantly tonic responses (position sensitive). The movement sensitive cells can be divided into those which insert into the sides of the receptor strand and respond to elongation of the strand (produced by joint flexion) and those which insert dorsally into the strand and respond to relaxation or shortening of the strand (produced by joint extension). The scolopidia of the flexion (elongation) sensitive cells have an attachment cell and are embedded in a cellular region of the receptor strand; those of the extension (relaxation) sensitive cells lack an attachment cell and are

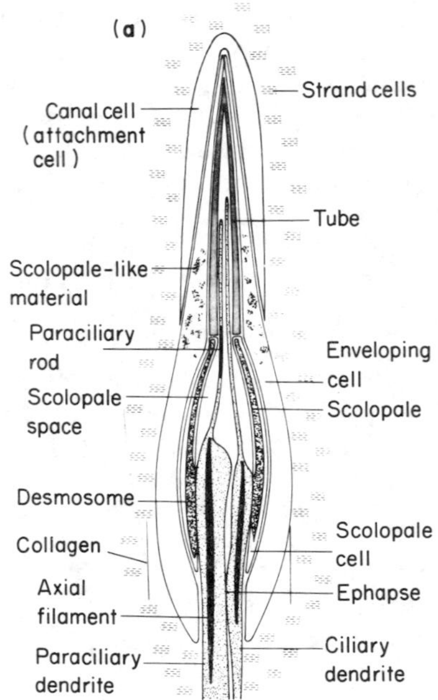


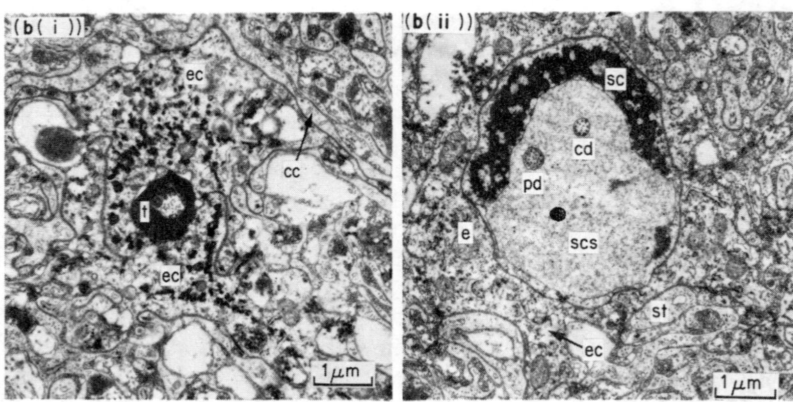


**Fig. 8.24** A scolopidium containing elongation sensitive sensory cells from the PD joint chordotonal organ of the crab *Cancer pagurus*. (**a**) Diagram of a longitudinal section; (**b**) electron micrographs of transverse sections through (**i**) the tube region and (**ii**) the scolopale region. cc, canal cell; cd, ciliary dendrite; e, ephapse; ec, enveloping cell; pd, paraciliary dendrite; sc, scolopale; scs, scolopale space; st, strand cell; t, tube. (From Mill, P. J. and Lowe, D. A. (1973). *Proceedings of the Royal Society, B,* **184,** 179–97.)

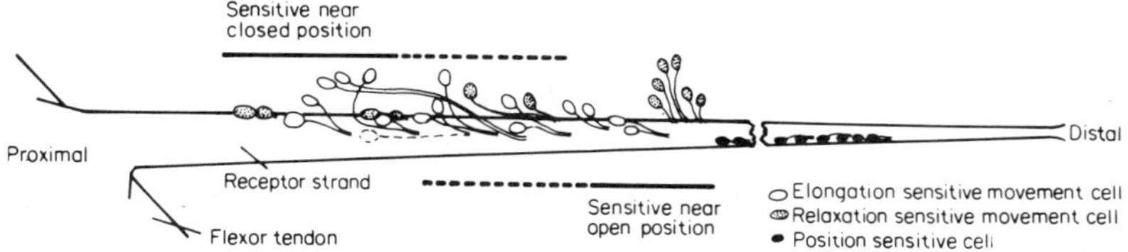


**Fig. 8.25** Diagram from the anterior side to show the organization of the sensory cells in the PD joint chordotonal organ of the crab *Cancer*. The horizontal lines refer to the movement sensitive cells, the dashed parts indicating cells which are equally sensitive in any position. The axons are not shown. (After Hartman, H. B. and Boettiger, E. G. (1967). *Comparative Biochemistry and Physiology*, **22**, 651–63.)

largely surrounded by longitudinally oriented collagen fibres. In the PD organ there are two dendrites in each scolopidium and there is evidence that these differ in their threshold level (Fig. 8.26b).

In the PD organ some phasic cells respond to velocity; others are almost pure movement cells, showing velocity sensitivity only at very low rates of movement (Fig. 8.26a). The firing frequency of some velocity sensitive cells also depends on the position of the joint. Thus, those lying proximally on the receptor strand tend to be more sensitive in flexed joint positions, while those lying distally tend to be more sensitive in extended joint positions; irrespective of whether they are flexion-sensitive or extension-sensitive cells. The tonic cells generally respond maximally towards one or other of the extremes of the movement range (flexed or extended) and they have an asymmetric response in that their firing frequency for a given position is higher if that position is achieved by movement of the joint in the direction towards which the sensory cell is maximally active (Fig. 8.27).

In mammals there are several types of joint receptor: Golgi endings in the ligaments, Ruffini endings and Paciniform corpuscles (which look like smaller versions of Pacinian corpuscles). The Golgi endings are position sensitive, whereas the Paciniform corpuscles respond to movement. The Ruffini endings provide information both on position and on the velocity of angular movement.

**Vibration**

Vibrations may be received through the substrate or as pressure waves in the medium and are differentiated from sound waves on the basis of their lower frequencies. A number of the more highly sensitive mechanoreceptors respond to vibrational stimuli and indeed most, if not all, vibration receptors respond to other forms of mechanical stimulation.

The hair fans and hair pegs of lobsters and the plumose hairs on the antennae of rock-lobsters detect water-borne vibrations, the former two with a synchronous response up to about 100 Hz; while stimulation of certain abdominal hairs in the water-bug *Notonecta* elicits an orientation response towards vibrations.

Phasic mechanoreceptors in the limbs are ideally situated to monitor substrate-borne vibrations. The most sensitive pure movement cells in the PD organ of decapod crustaceans (p. 145) are capable of responding to vibrations, and one of the myochordotonal organs in *Cancer* (p. 140) responds up to a frequency of about 150 Hz. The myochordotonal organs in the terrestrial crab *Ocypode* are likewise sensitive to high frequency vibrations and also respond to air-borne sound. The primary endings of mammalian muscle spindles respond to vibrations up to 500 Hz and are sensitive to displacements of as little as 50 $\mu$m.

The thread hairs and the free-hook hairs in the statocysts of crabs (p. 157) are sensitive to vibrations of the antennules, and hairs in all three crista systems of the statocysts of *Octopus* (p. 157) have a high vibration sensitivity.

**Gravity receptors**

Many invertebrates have evolved specialized receptors, called statocysts, for the detection of linear accelerations, such as result from gravity. Essentially a statocyst comprises a group of sensory hair cells, the hairs of which support a structure called a statolith. Movement of the statolith tangential to the surface of the sensory cells, caused by a change in body position, results in a shearing force on the loaded hairs, thereby stimulating the sensory cells.

Statocysts are found in many coelenterates, notably the Leptomedusae and Scyphozoa in which they are suspended near the margin of the bell. Each statocyst contains one or more calcareous statoliths which are secreted by the surrounding cells (lithocytes), and the structure is surrounded by a layer of mesoglea and ectoderm (Fig. 8.28a). The sensory cells may surround the base of the statocyst or be borne on the statocyst itself. In the latter case the statocyst is partially or completely enclosed in a vesicle. Each sensory cell bears one

---

**Fig. 8.26** Extracellular recordings from the PD joint chordotonal organ of the crab *Cancer* to show the response of elongation sensitive movement cells (ESMCs) to different rates of elongation of the receptor strand. (**a**) Details of the response of a single cell. Arrows indicate the beginning and end of stretch. (**b**) The response of a pair of sensory cells to show that both members of a pair are sensitive to the same direction of movement. (Spikes retouched.) Downward movement of the stimulus traces indicates elongation of the receptor strand. ((**a**) From Mill, P. J. and Lowe, D. A. (1972). *Journal of Experimental Biology*, **56,** 509–25; (**b**) after Hartman, H. B. and Boettiger, E. G. (1967). *Comparative Biochemistry and Physiology*, **22,** 651–63.)

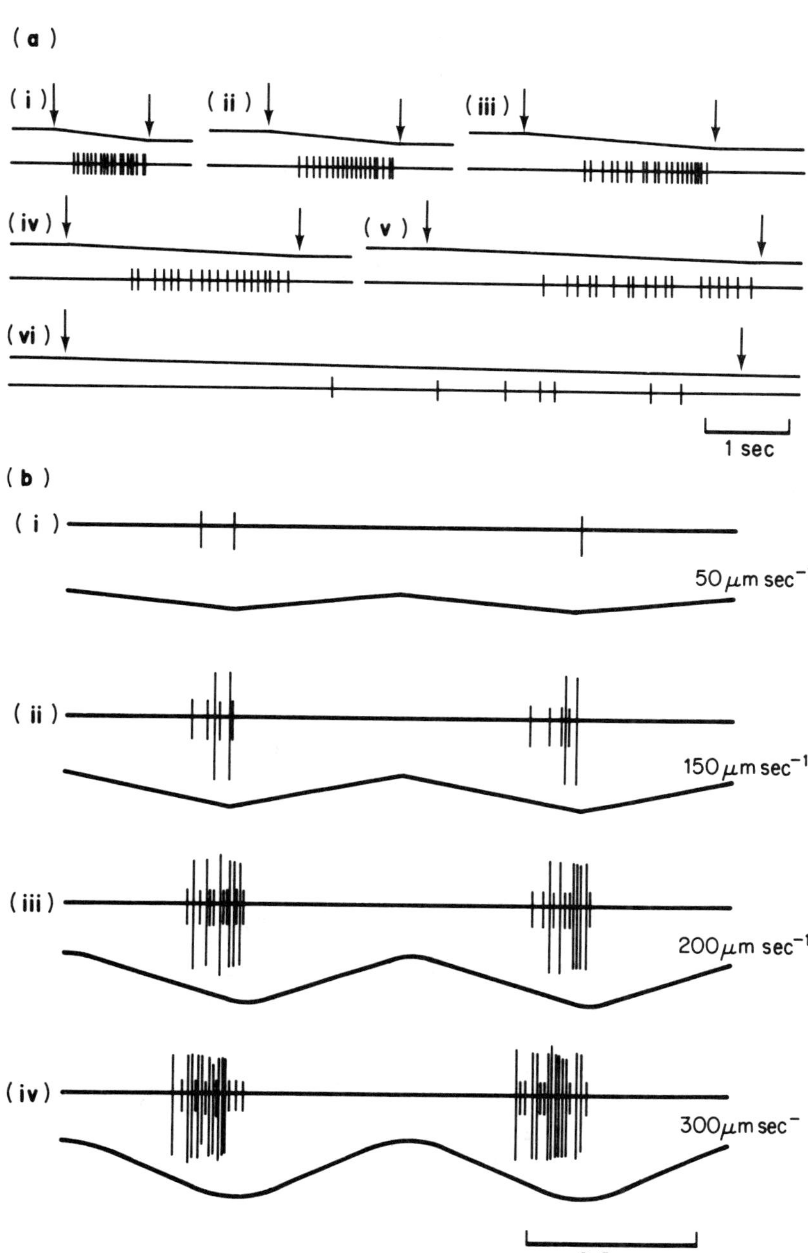
(a)
(i)
(ii)
(iii)
(iv)
(v)
(vi)
1 sec
(b)
(i)
50 μm sec⁻¹
(ii)
150 μm sec⁻¹
(iii)
200 μm sec⁻¹
(iv)
300 μm sec⁻
0.5 sec

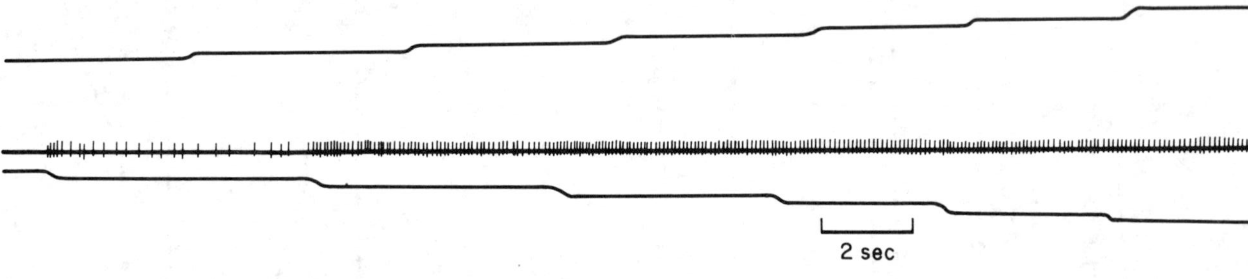


**Fig. 8.27** Extracellular recording from the PD joint chordotonal organ of the lobster *Homarus* to show the response of an asymmetric relaxation sensitive position cell (RSPC) to different lengths of the receptor strand. The recordings are continuous. Upward movement of the stimulus trace indicates elongation; downward movement relaxation of the receptor strand. (From Mill, P. J. and Lowe, D. A. (1972) *Journal of Experimental Biology*, **56,** 509–25.)

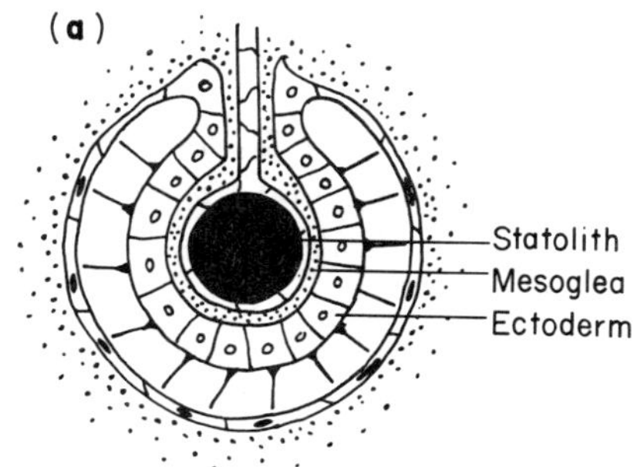


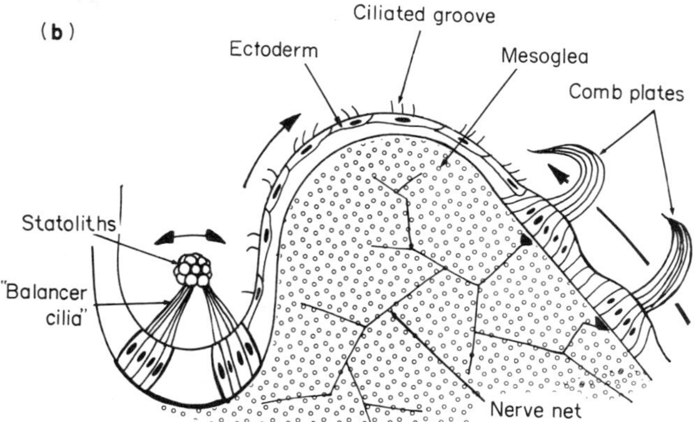


**Fig. 8.28** Diagrams of the statocysts of (**a**) a coelenterate and (**b**) a ctenophore. (From Dorsett, D. A. (1976). In *Structure and Function of Proprioceptors in the Invertebrates* (Mill, P. J., ed.). Chapman and Hall, London; after Horridge, G. A. (1969). *Tissue and Cell*, **1**, 341–53.)

kinocilium (p. 122) surrounded by numerous sterocilia and, in the Scyphozoa, the latter are fused into a ridged collar. In ctenophores the statocyst lies in a depression and comprises a group of statoliths supported by four groups of balancer cilia (Fig. 8.28b), each cilium having a $9 + 2$ ciliary structure. Statocysts are also found in many sedentary polychaetes, where there are from one to approximately twenty pairs at the anterior end of the animal. In *Scoloplos* each statocyst consists of an open groove (statocrypt), but in the majority of animals they are in the form of a vesicle which may or may not be connected to the surface. Sand grains are, in some cases, used as statoliths. In *Arenicola marina* the receptor cells each bear five or six kinocilia, but no stereocilia.

In general, terrestrial arthropods do not possess statocysts. Although they are not often found in insects, insects do orientate with respect to gravity, relying on information from a variety of receptors. Proprioceptive information from the limbs may be utilized, as in the stick insect *Carausius*, and other insects, for example the ant *Formica polyctena*, rely to a considerable extent on hair plates located at various body joints and at the bases of the legs. A

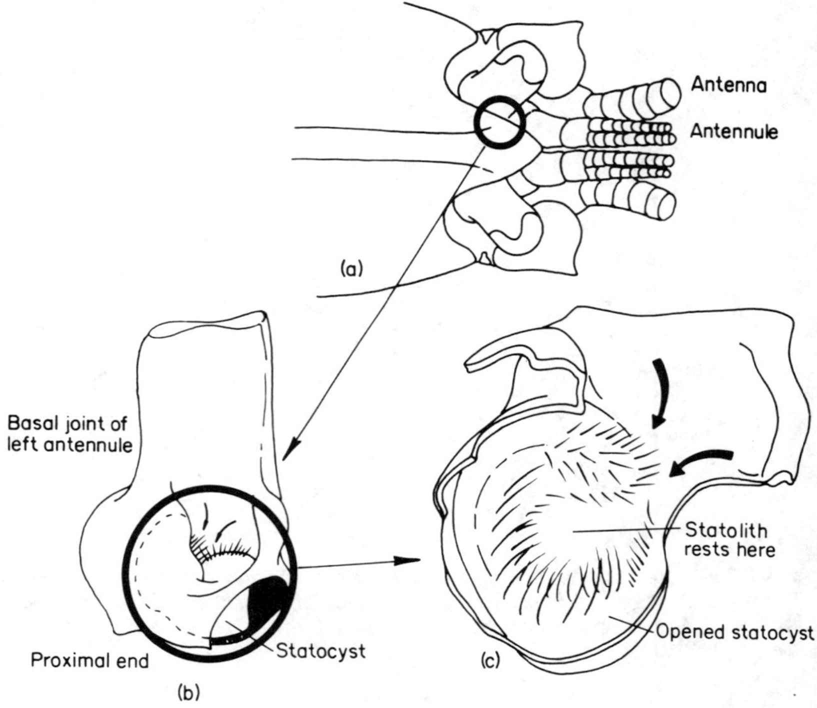


**Fig. 8.29** Diagrams illustrating the position of the statocysts of the crayfish *Cherax destructor*. The statocysts are contained within the basal joints of the antennules (**a**, **b**). The sensory hairs, (**c**), have their tips directed inwards to enclose the statolith, which is composed of sand particles. (From Sandeman, D. C. (1976). In *Structure and Function of Proprioceptors in the Invertebrates.* (Mill, P. J., ed.) Chapman and Hall, London.)

compound chordotonal organ (Johnston's organ), lying in the second joint of each antenna of insects, monitors movements of the more distal joints and, in many insects, this is used as a gravity receptor. Johnston's organ may also be used in the control of flight and as a hearing organ.

In contrast to insects, most crustaceans are aquatic, and statocysts

(**a**)

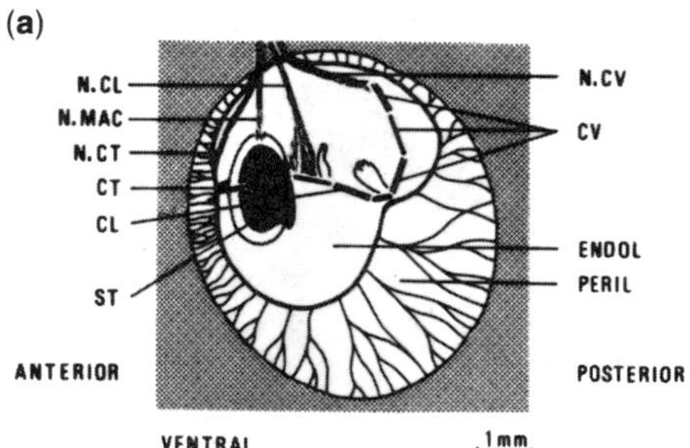


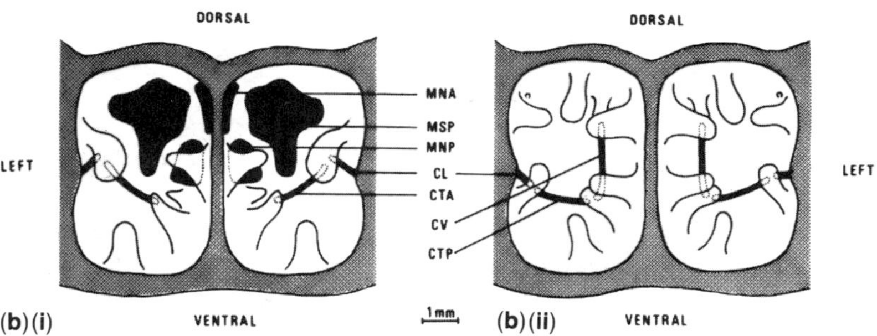


(**b**)(**i**) (**b**)(**ii**)

**Fig. 8.30** Diagrams of (**a**) a lateral view of the left statocyst of the octopus *Octopus vulgaris* and (**b**) anterior (**i**) and posterior (**ii**) views of a transverse section through the statocyst of the squid *Sepia officinalis*. CL, crista longitudinalis; CT, crista transversalis; CTA, crista transversalis anterior; CTP crista transversalis posterior; CV, crista verticalis; ENDOL, endolymph; MNA, macula neglecta anterior with statoconial layer; MNP, macula neglecta posterior with statoconial layer; MSP, macula statica princeps with statolith; N.CL, nerve of crista longitudinalis; N.CT, nerve of crista transversalis; N.CV, nerve of crista verticalis; N.MAC, nerve of macula; PERIL, perilymph; ST, statolith. (From Budelmann, B.-U. (1976). In *Structure and Function of Proprioceptors in the Invertebrates.* (Mill, P. J., ed.) Chapman and Hall, London.)

occur quite commonly in this group. In decapod crustaceans a statocyst is found typically in the basal joint of each antennule. In the crayfish it is a relatively simple structure, consisting of an invagination lined with a crescent of sensory hairs surrounding a statolith (Fig. 8.29). Each sensory hair is innervated by a chordotonal organ comprising three sensory cells. There is no connective tissue strand and the extracellular tube is replaced by a long 'chorda' which inserts at the base of the hair. One apparent problem is that the statocyst is located in an appendage which is itself moveable with respect to the body, but it has been demonstrated that, in the lobster, movements of the atennules alone do not have any effect on orientation because

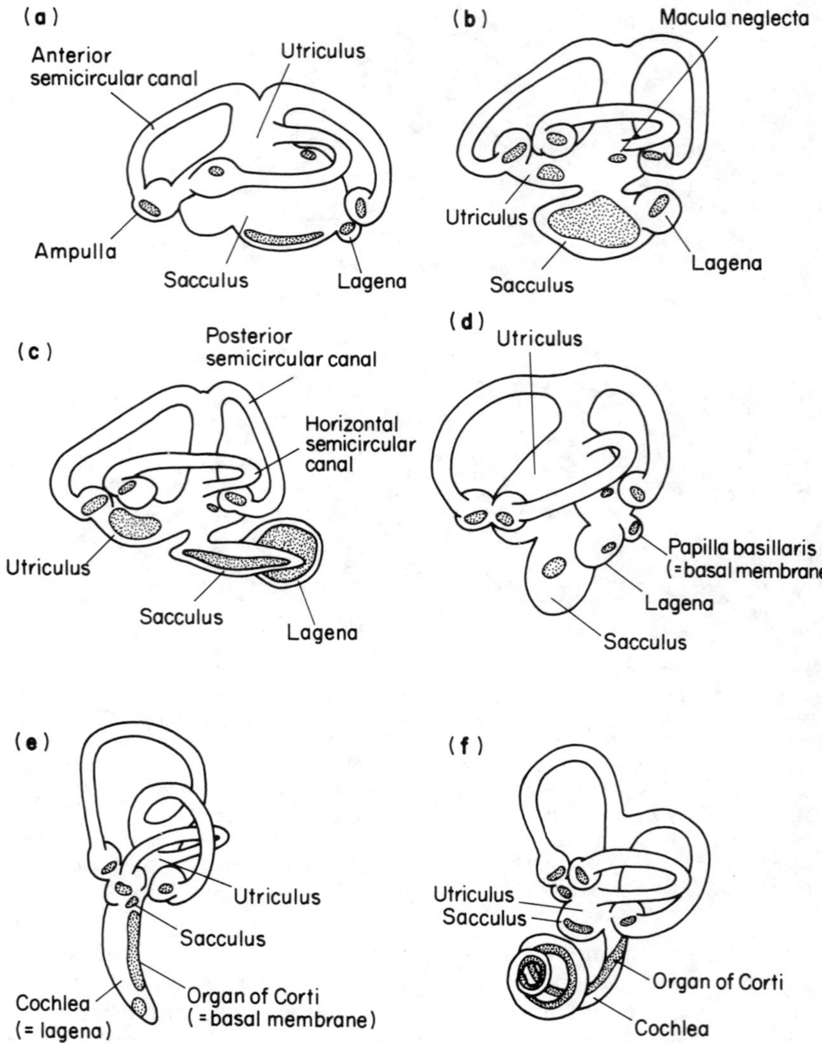


**Fig. 8.31** Diagrams of the inner ear of various vertebrates: (**a**) elasmobranch (*Raja*); (**b**) teleost fish (*Salmo*); (**c**) teleost fish (*Phoxinus*); (**d**) frog (*Rana*); (**e**) bird (*Columba*); and (**f**) mammal (*Cavia*). The positions of sensory hair patches (maculae), which are internal, are indicated by dots. ((**a**), (**d**) After Retzius, G. (1881). *Das Gehörorgan der Wirbelthier. I Das Gehörorgan der Fische und Amphibien*; (**b**), (**c**) after von Frisch, K. (1935). *Biological Reviews*, **11,** 210–46; (**e**), (**f**) after Retzius, G. (1884). *Das Gehörorgan der Wirbelthiere. II Das Gehörorgan der Reptilien, der Vögel und der Säugethiere.*)

the input from the statocysts is apparently counteracted by input from other antennal proprioceptors.

Statocysts are also found in molluscs. They consist of a fluid-filled sac lying in or near the central nervous system, and the cavity is often connected to the exterior by a canal. In some there is a single statolith (Fig. 8.30a), in others a group of small structures called statoconia. The sensory cells bear numerous kinocilia and microvilli but there are no stereocilia. In gastropods and bivalves the structure of the statocysts is simple but in cephalopods it is more complex with two main sensory systems, one a gravity receptor system, the other for the detection of angular accelerations. In octopods (e.g. *Octopus vulgaris*) the former comprises an oval-shaped plate of sensory and

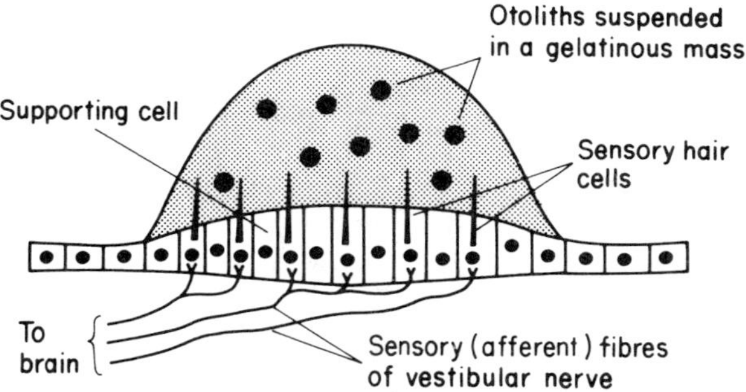


**Fig. 8.32** Diagram to show the sensory cells of the macula (sensory pad) of a mammalian utriculus or sacculus. (From Usherwood, P. N. R. (1973). *Nervous Systems*. Studies in Biology, no. 36. Edward Arnold, London.)

supporting cells (called a macula), the hairs of the sensory cells supporting a statolith (Fig. 8.30a). In decapods (e.g. *Sepia* and *Loligo*) there are three maculae arranged at almost right angles to one another (two vertical and one horizontal) (Fig. 8.30b). One of the vertical maculae supports a statolith; the other two are covered by a layer of statoconia.

The complexity in decapod cephalopods is comparable with that in vertebrates, in which group the gravity receptors are located in the membranous labyrinth of the inner ear, which has developed from part of the anterior lateral-line system (p. 120). In all vertebrates there are two chambers, the utriculus and the sacculus, concerned with the detection of linear accelerations such as gravity; while in agnathans, elasmobranchs, teleosts and amphibians a third chamber, the lagena, is also involved (Fig. 8.31). There is usually more than one macula in each chamber. In place of a statolith, the sensory hairs are embedded in a gelatinous structure containing dense particles (otoliths) (Fig. 8.32).

Individual sensory cells are excited by movement of their hairs in the direction of their basal feet and inhibited by the reverse movement. The basal feet of the hairs of a single sensory cell may be oriented in different directions. This occurs in pulmonate gastropods. Figure 8.33 shows the response from a single sensory cell in the pulmonate *Arion empiricorum* to rotation around the longitudinal axis of the body. In accord with the arrangement of the basal feet, it responds to rotation in either direction. This particular cell is

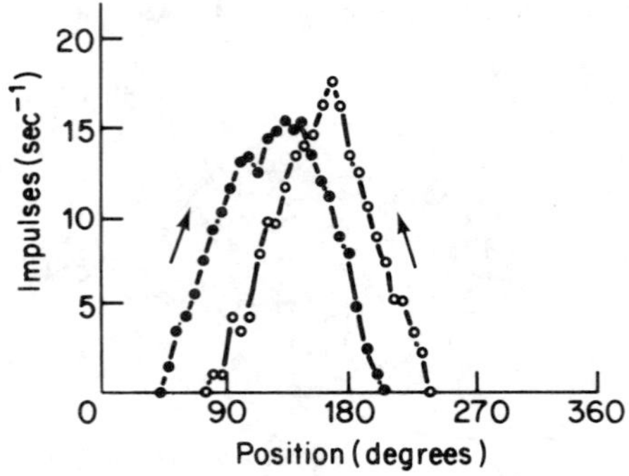


**Fig. 8.33** The frequency of sensory impulses in a single axon in the nerve from the right statocyst of the slug *Arion empiricorum* during complete rotation of the animal around its longitudinal axis at a velocity of 1.67 rpm. Arrows indicate the direction of tilt; ●, rotation to the left; ○, rotation to the right. (From Budelmann, B.-U. (1976). In *Structure and Function of Proprioceptors in the Invertebrates* (Mill, P. J., ed.). Chapman and Hall, London; after Wolff, H. G. (1973). *Fortschritte der Zoologie*, **21**, 80–99.)

maximally active close to the upside-down position (180°) of the animal. (Peak activity varies slightly, depending on the direction of rotation.) In the sensory cells of cephalopods the basal feet are all oriented in the same direction, but those of different cells in a macula are oriented in different directions (Fig. 8.34). The orientation of the basal feet in the maculae of an elasmobranch fish is shown in Fig. 8.35.

In general, while different cells do vary in the position of the body at which their response is maximal, the overall input from a statocyst is minimal when the animal is in its normal, horizontal rest position (i.e. when the shearing force exerted on the supporting sensory hairs by the statolith is minimal) and increases with the degree of tilt (either roll or pitch) of the animal.

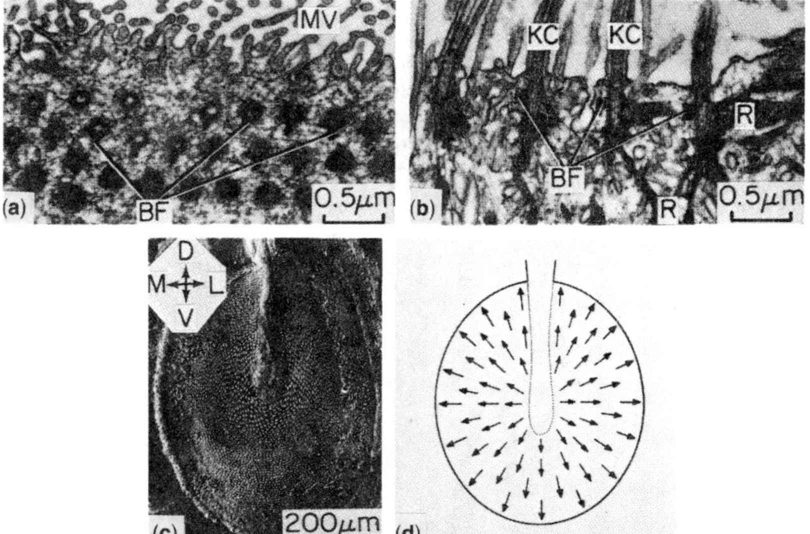


**Fig. 8.34** Structure of the statocyst of the octopus *Octopus vulgaris*. (**a**) Transverse section through the basal body region of the sensory cells; (**b**) longitudinal section through the bases of four kinocilia KC; (**c**) surface view of the macula to show the arrangement of the groups of cilia (D, dorsal; L, lateral; M, medial; V, ventral); and (**d**) polarization pattern of the macula, the arrows indicating the direction in which the basal feet point. BF, basal foot; MV, microvilli; R, ciliary root. ((**a**), (**b**), (**d**) From Budelmann, B.-U.(1976). In *Structure and Function of Proprioceptors in the Invertebrates.* (Mill, P. J., ed.) Chapman and Hall, London; (**c**) from Budelman, B.-U. *et al.* (1973). *Brain Research*, **56,** 25–41.)

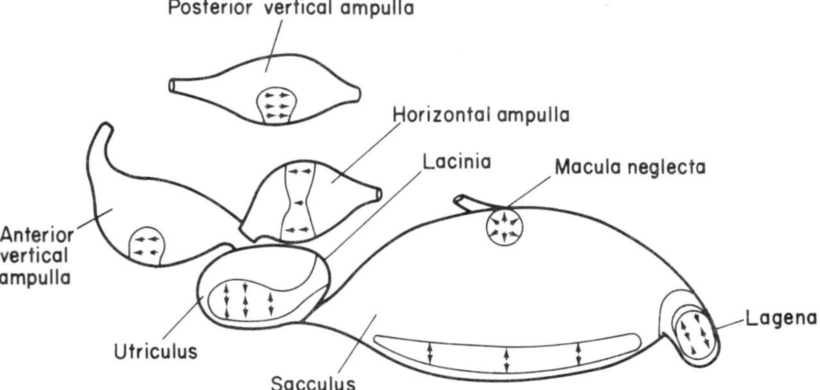


**Fig. 8.35** Diagram to show the orientation of the sensory hair bundles in the cristae and maculae of the left labyrinth of the ray. The arrows indicate the position of the kinocilium with respect to the stereocilia. (After Lowenstein, O. *et al.* (1964). *Proceedings of the Royal Society, B,* **160,** 1–12.)

## Angular acceleration detectors

There are indications that a number of invertebrates use general proprioceptive inputs for obtaining information on angular accelerations. However, some have evolved specialized receptors for this purpose. In decapod crustaceans and cephalopod molluscs part of the statocyst has taken on this function; in vertebrates the corresponding receptors are located in the semicircular canals of the membranous labyrinth of the inner ear (p. 158). In dipteran insects the role is

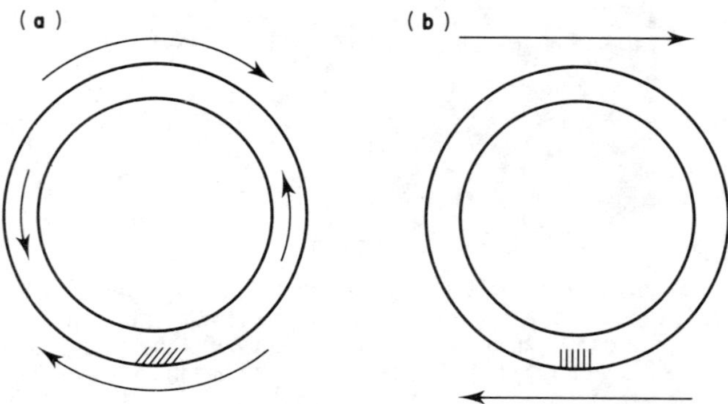


**Fig. 8.36** Diagrams illustrating the effect of (**a**) angular and (**b**) linear accelerations on the displacement of fluid in a hollow, circular canal. Note that only angular acceleration has an effect on the fluid and hence on any sensory hairs in the canal, and that the latter are bent in the opposite direction to the imposed movement. (After Sandeman, D. C. (1976). In *Structure and Function of Proprioceptors in the Invertebrates*. (Mill, P. J., ed.) Chapman and Hall, London.)

fulfilled by sense organs called halteres, which are modified hindwings.

If sensory cells in a fluid-filled system, such as a statocyst, are to detect angular, as opposed to linear, accelerations, their hairs should ideally protrude into a canal so that they can detect fluid movements in the latter. The effects of angular and linear accelerations on such a system are shown in Fig. 8.36. The presence of a canal will impose directionality on the system in that the sensory hairs will be deflected maximally by angular movements in the plane of the canal (Fig. 8.36a) and will be unaffected by movements at right angles to the canal (Fig. 8.36b).

In the lobster statocyst long 'thread' hairs, which are not associated with the statolith, lie in a simple canal. In crabs there are two canals (horizontal and vertical) (Fig. 8.37) arranged so that movement in the three primary planes can be detected. One group of thread hairs lies in that part of the canal system which is common to both canals, and a second group lies towards the bottom of the vertical canal. There are also some short bent hairs, the free-hook hairs, in the posterior part of the vertical canal. Each thread hair is associated with a pair of sensory cells, to which it is attached by

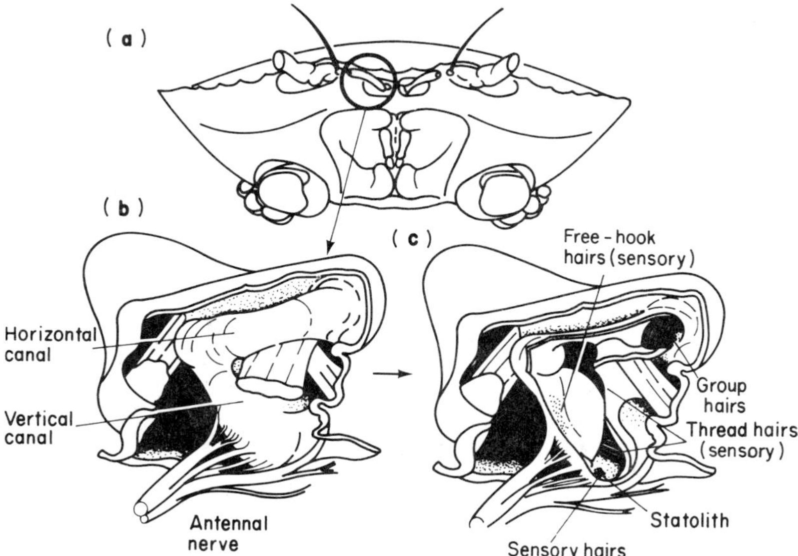


**Fig. 8.37** Diagrams illustrating the position of the statocysts of a crab. (**a**) Statocysts contained within the basal joints of the antennules; (**b**) and (**c**) the basal joint of the right antennule as seen from behind. In (**b**) the exoskeleton has been removed to show the two canals at right angles to each other. In (**c**) the canals have been opened to show the positions of the receptor hairs, the statolith and the group hairs. (From Sandeman, D. C. (1976). In *Structure and Function of Proprioceptors in the Invertebrates.* (Mill, P. J., ed.) Chapman and Hall, London.)

scolopale organs. The sensory cells associated with both types of hair respond unidirectionally.

In cephalopod molluscs the sensory hair cells lie on ridges called cristae, which are divided into sections, each section supporting a sail-like cupula. The sensory 'hairs' are all kinocilia and their basal feet are oriented at right angles to the line of the crista in which they lie. In octopods there are three cristae (longitudinal, vertical and transverse), each of which is subdivided into three sections (Fig.

8.30a). The central section of each crista bears a single row of sensory cells; the outer sections bear two rows. In decapods there are four cristae (longitudinal, vertical and two transverse) (Fig. 8.30b), each with four main rows of sensory hair cells.

The longitudinal crista is most sensitive to angular accelerations around the longitudinal axis of the animal, the vertical crista to those around the vertical axis and the transverse crista(e) to those around the transverse axis. In addition to this form of directionality, the sensory cells, in *Octopus* at least, are themselves directionally sensitive, being excited by movement of their hairs in one direction and inhibited by their movement in the opposite direction. In the

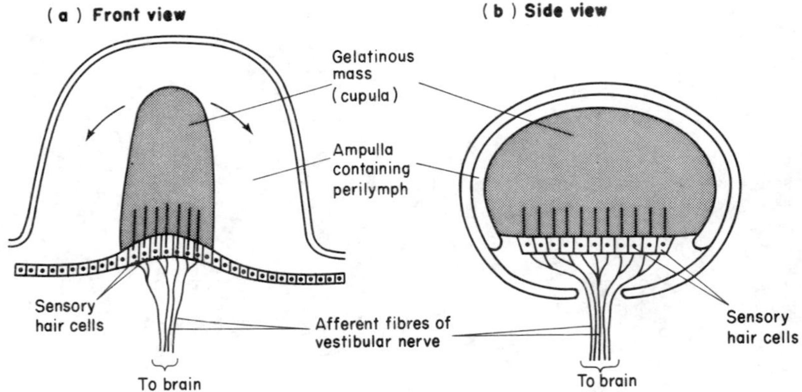


**Fig. 8.38** Diagrams of the ampulla of a mammalian semicircular canal to show the sensory cells. (**a**) Front and (**b**) side view. The arrows in (**a**) indicate the direction of movement. ((**a**) From Usherwood, P. N. R. (1973). *Nervous Systems.* Studies in Biology, no. 36. Edward Arnold, London.)

longitudinal and vertical cristae all of the sensory cells are oriented in the same way. Hence rotation of the animal in one direction causes excitation and inhibition during acceleration and deceleration respectively, while rotation in the reverse direction has the opposite effect. In the transverse crista some cells are excited and others are inhibited by each direction of rotation.

In the Agnatha there are one (in hagfishes) or two (in lampreys) vertical semicircular canals in the membranous labyrinth of the inner ear; in all other vertebrates there are three (two vertical and one horizontal) semicircular canals (Fig. 8.31), all lying at right angles to one another and each bearing an ampulla containing a single crista. Each crista consists of several rows of sensory hair cells whose cilia (hairs) are embedded in a single gelatinous cupula (Fig. 8.38). Each hair cell has a single kinocilium and a number of stereocilia, as in the maculae of the vertebrate gravity detection system. The kinocilia of each crista are all oriented in the same direction and the sensory cells, as with the similar cells in the gravity detection system,

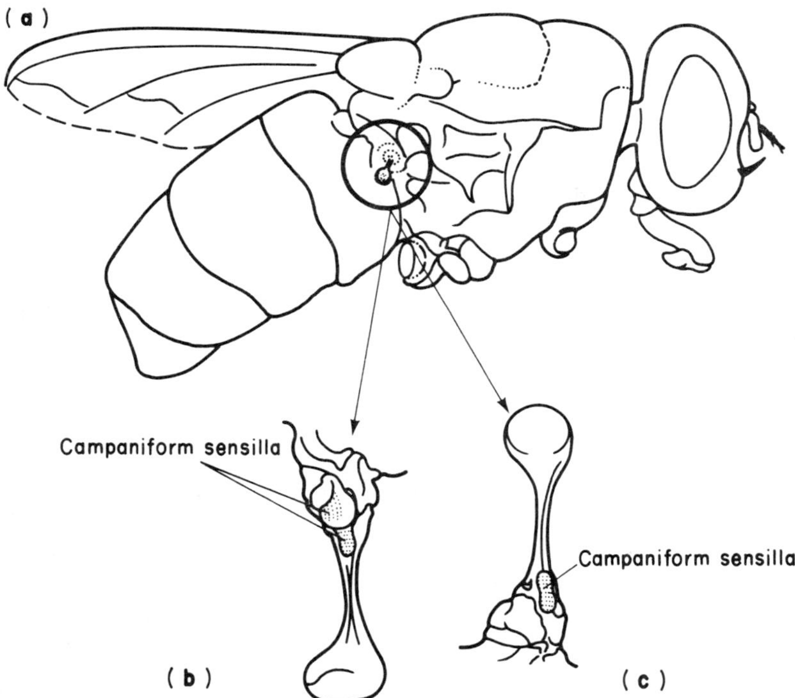


**Fig. 8.39** Diagrams illustrating the halteres of the fly *Lucilia cuprina*. (**a**) The right haltere; (**b**) dorsal and (**c**) ventral views of a right haltere to show the campaniform sensilla which are sensitive to the distortion of the cuticle at the base of the haltere. (From Sandeman, D. C. (1976). In *Structure and Function of Proprioceptors in the Invertebrates.* (Mill, P. J. ed.) Chapman and Hall, London.)

are excited by bending of their kinocilium in the direction of its basal body. Hence, not only are the individual sensory cells direction sensitive, but so is each crista.

The halteres of flies are club-shaped structures (Fig. 8.39a), which are oscillated during flight at the same frequency as the wings but in antiphase with them, and behave effectively like gyroscopes. Groups of campaniform sensilla (p. 123) are located at the base of each haltere (Fig. 8.39b) and are ideally sited to detect alterations in the plane of oscillation of the latter, brought about by angular accelerations imposed on the animal, notably those in the yaw plane.

In *Octopus* the angular acceleration receptor system is also sensitive to gravity, in that the magnitude of the resting discharge depends on the animal's position, and the magnitude of the response to rotation of the animal depends on the range of the movement arc covered. This is not the case in vertebrates.

**Hearing**

Hearing is the detection of non-substrate borne vibrations, and auditory receptors are particularly well-developed in terrestrial animals. In air, sound consists of a displacement wave, which is very directional, and a pressure wave, effective in all directions. To detect displacement requires an easily moveable diaphragm (tympanum), as is found in the insect tympanal organs. Conversely, pressure detection needs a very stiff diaphragm which only moves a very small amount, as in the mammalian ear.

The tympanal organs of insects are found on the legs, thorax, abdomen or antennae. The tympanum consists of a thin, taut membrane to which a chordotonal organ is attached (Fig. 8.40). The number of sensory neurons varies from two (noctuid moths) to as many as 80 (*Locusta migratoria*). Movements of the tympanum stretch the dendrites of the sensory cells and so activate them. The frequency range of noctuid moths extends as high as 60 kHz and hence they can detect the sonar of bats, but most insects probably have a lower limit than this. There is little or no frequency discrimination in insects, but there is often intensity discrimination. However, in *Locusta migratoria* there are four groups of sensory cells associated with the tympanum and the frequency to which each group is maximally sensitive differs.

Among crustaceans hearing is unusual. However, in the land crab *Ocypode*, the cuticle overlying the myochordotonal organ in each walking leg is very thin and serves as a tympanum and the dendrites of the myochordotonal organ anchor in this region. The crab can only hear when a leg is extended because of the arrangement of the muscle associated with the myochordontal organ.

Most fish have no tympanum and hence a very limited hearing capability and they respond only up to a frequency of about 1 kHz. In elasmobranchs, the sacculus and utriculus function as auditory receptors as well as gravity receptors. The sacculus has the same function in teleosts. In addition, in teleosts auditory receptors are found in another region of the inner ear, the lagena (Fig. 8.31b, c). In some teleosts (cyprinoids and siluroids) the range of hearing is extended by a coupling device, consisting of a chain of ossicles derived from processes of several vertebrae (the Weberian ossicles), between the swim bladder and the sacculus (Fig. 8.41). This enables the swim bladder to act as a tympanum and detect water-borne sound.

In anuran amphibians (frogs and toads) there is an external tympanum on each side of the head. Each tympanum is separated from the inner ear by a chamber, the middle ear, which is in

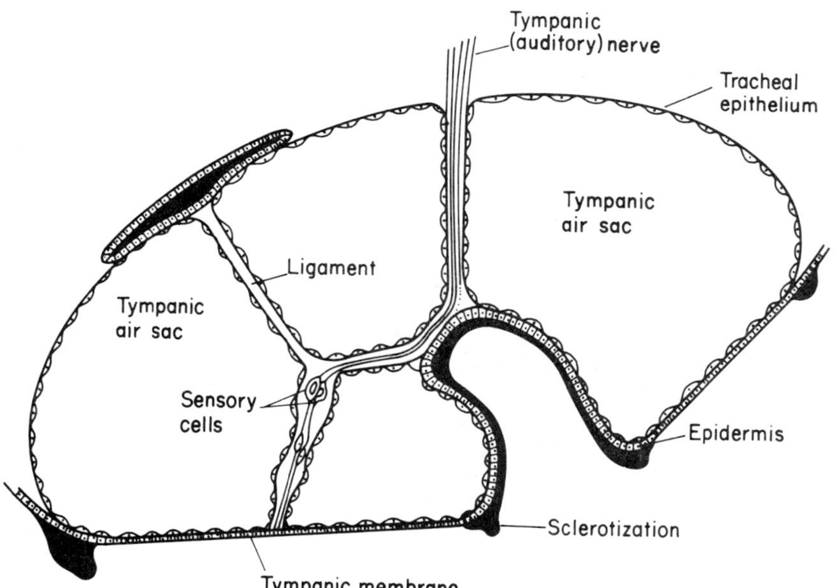


**Fig. 8.40** Diagram of a section through the left tympanic organ of a noctuid moth. The displacement wave moves the tympanic membrane and hence the dendrites of the two sensory cells. (From Roeder, K. D. and Treat, A. E. (1957). *Journal of Experimental Zoology*, **134,** 127–57; after Eggers, F. (1919). *Zoologisches Jahrbuch, Anatomie*, **41,** 273–376.)

communication with the pharynx via the eustachian tube. Movements of the tympanum are transmitted across the middle ear by two ossicles (columella and stapes) to a thin oval area, the oval window (fenestra ovalis). The subsequent fluid movements in the sacculus and lagena stimulate the sensory cells and so, as in teleosts, the sacculus serves two functions. The lagena contains a tectorial membrane which overlies some of the sensory cells, and there is a rudimentary basilar membrane (see below).

In reptiles the sacculus only serves as a gravity receptor and sound reception is the function solely of the lagena. In some reptiles (e.g. crocodiles) this contains a basilar membrane. Geckos probably have the highest frequency response; about 10 kHz.

In birds and in cetaceans (whales) and pinnipedes (seals, etc.) the

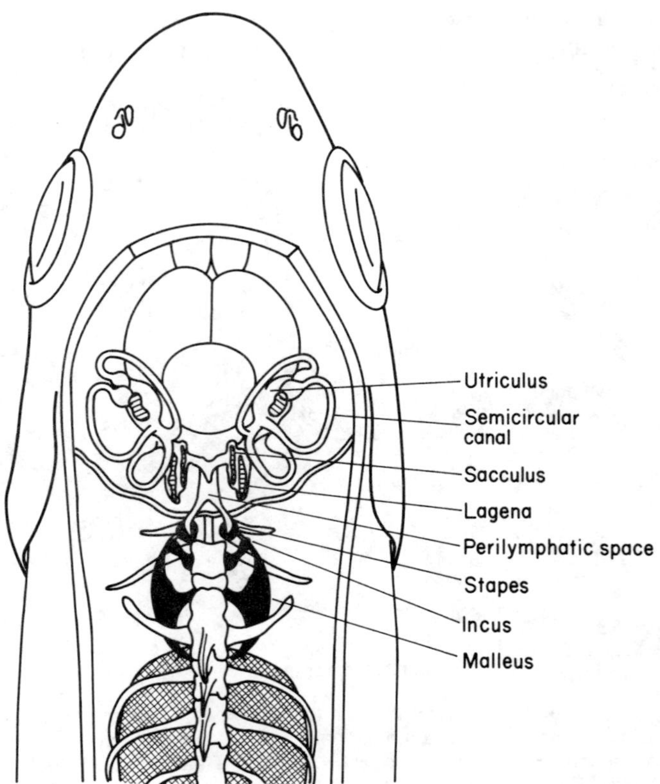


**Fig. 8.41** Diagram to illustrate the relationship between the inner ear and the Weberian ossicles (shown in black) in Ostariophysi. (From Frisch, K. von (1936). *Biological Reviews*, **11**, 210–46.)

tympanum is on the surface of the head, but in most mammals it lies at the base of a depression (the outer ear) associated with which there is a flap (pinna) which helps to impose directionality on sound detection. Movement of the tympanum is transmitted across the middle ear to the oval window, with little or no change in amplitude, by a single ossicle (columella) in birds and by three ossicles (malleus, incus and stapes) in mammals. Since the surface area of the oval window is considerably less than that of the tympanum, the force exerted on the former is effectively amplified. This is necessary because of the much greater density, and hence resistance (impedence) to movement, of fluids (the cochlear is filled with fluid) than of air. The transformation ratio of this impedence matching device is about 25:1. In mammals the ossicles in the middle ear buckle when they are subjected to excessive vibrations caused by very loud sounds and they thus protect the inner ear. Also, during talking, muscular contraction reduces the sensitivity of the middle ear.

In both birds and mammals a cochlea has developed from the lagena. In birds it is rather short and almost straight and the macula of the lagena is still present at its apex; in mammals the macula of the lagena is absent and the cochlea is very long and coiled. Many birds and mammals have a frequency range up to about 25 kHz, but bats and cetaceans, which use acoustic signals for echolocation, have ranges up to about 200 kHz.

In mammals the cochlea is divided longitudinally into three canals, a central scala media containing endolymph, and the scala vestibuli and scala tympani containing perilymph (Fig. 8.42a). The scala vestibuli is juxtaposed to the middle ear at the oval window, while the scala tympani is similarly juxtaposed to the middle ear at a second membranous region, the round window (fenestra rotunda). These two outer canals are interconnected by a gap, the helicotrema, at the apex of the cochlea, and the function of the round window is to equilibrate the pressure in the inner ear. The scala media is separated from the scala vestibuli by a thin membrane called Reissner's membrane, and from the scala tympani by the basilar membrane, which contains the sensory cells. There are four rows of sensory cells: an inner row separated by the rods and tunnel of Corti from three outer rows (Fig. 8.42). These cells possess only stereocilia, which are embedded in the tectorial membrane overlying the sensory epithelium. The basilar membrane undergoes a four-fold increase in breadth between the base and the apex of the cochlea. The tectorial and basilar membranes (including the sensory cells) are known collectively as the Organ of Corti.

In birds the structure of the cochlea is similar to that of mammals in many respects. However, Reissner's membrane is heavily vascularized, the scala vestibuli is narrower, there is no helicotrema, there are 30–50 rows of sensory cells and the increase in width of the basilar membrane from the base to the apex of the cochlea is much less marked.

Individual sensory cells are directionally sensitive and respond to displacement, but they are not velocity sensitive. The basilar membrane vibrates in response to sounds and the sensory cells are stimulated by the shearing force on their hairs caused by the relative movement of the basilar membrane with respect to the tectorial

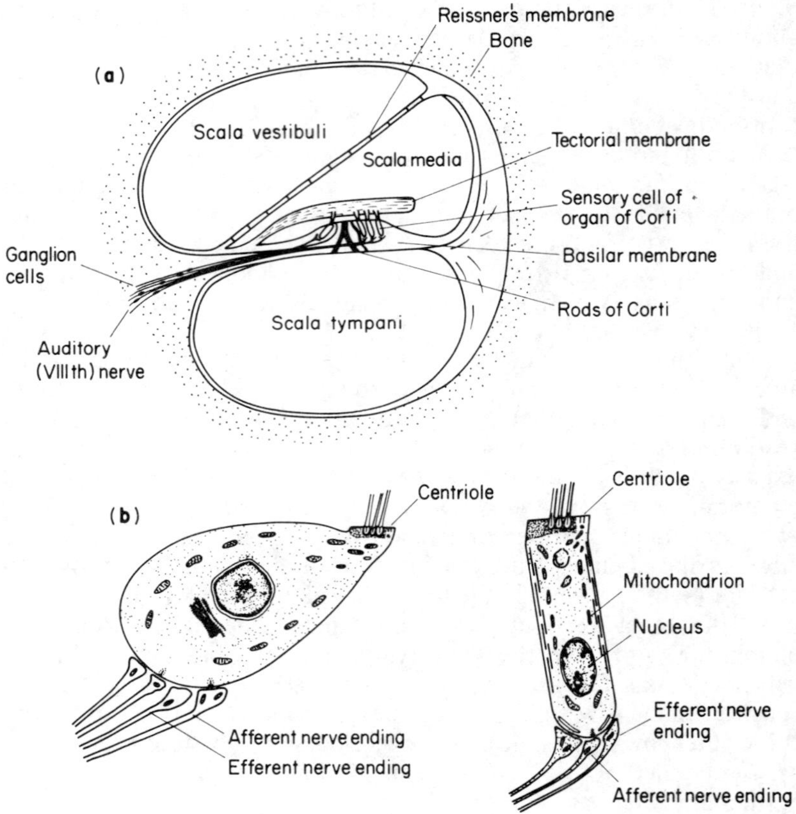


**Fig. 8.42** (**a**) Diagram of a transverse section through the cochlea of the mammalian ear. (**b**) Diagrams of an inner and an outer hair cell in the organ of Corti. ((**b**) After Wersäll, J., Flock, A. and Lundquist, P.-G. (1965). In *Cold Spring Harbor Symposia on Quantitative Biology*, Vol. 30. *Sensory Receptors*, (Frisch, L., ed.), pp. 115–32.)

membrane. In mammals, at low frequencies (i.e. below about 50 Hz) the basilar membrane vibrates synchronously along its length with the compressions of the perilymph in the outer canals, and certainly up to this frequency the individual neurons can follow the stimulus synchronously. However, the structure of the basilar membrane is such that, above 50 Hz, a travelling wave passes along it from the base of the cochlea to the apex, with a maximum displacement in a region of the membrane which varies with the frequency of the stimulus. High frequencies produce maximum displacements near the base (stapes end), low frequencies near the apex. This provides for frequency discrimination. In birds the system probably operates in a similar manner, while the macula of the lagena (which is at the apex of the cochlea—Fig. 8.31e) may be used to detect very low frequencies.

# 9

# *Photoreceptors, Chemoreceptors, Thermoreceptors and Electroreceptors*

## PHOTORECEPTION

Photoreceptors are activated by electromagnetic energy of wavelengths between 300 nm and 1000 nm, although individual receptor cells are only sensitive to part of this range, and indeed the receptors of most animals do not cover the entire range. There are many different types of photoreceptor, ranging from single cells to the complex eyes of vertebrates. A plethora of names has been used for these but, in this chapter, they have been grouped under six headings to obtain some degree of order—single-celled photoreceptors, simple ocelli, ocelli, eyespots, compound eyes and eyes.

### *Single-celled photoreceptors*

Many invertebrates and some fishes and amphibians have a general, so-called 'dermal', light sensitivity. In annelids this is the result of numerous single-celled photoreceptors scattered throughout the epidermis, particularly at the anterior end of the body, and along the length of some of the main nerves. The receptor cells contain a vacuole surrounded by a border of microvilli. The vacuole may be simple, as in the leech *Hirudo*, or have an irregular outline, as, for example, in *Lumbricus* (Fig. 9.1a).

### *Simple ocelli*

Simple ocelli are composed of one or more photoreceptor cells enclosed in a common pigment cup. The latter presumably increases the efficiency of the receptors by improving their light gathering capacity. In *Hirudo* the sensitive cells are of the same structure as the

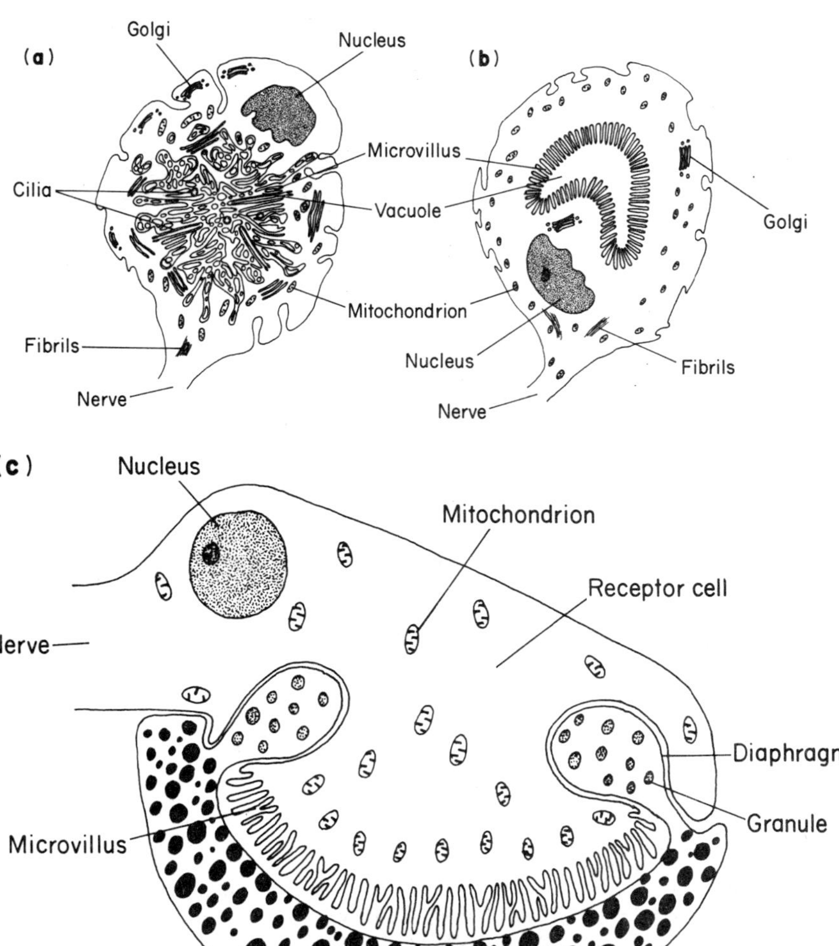


**Fig. 9.1** Diagrams of (**a**) a single-celled photoreceptor cell of the earthworm *Lumbricus terrestris*; (**b**) a photoreceptor cell from a simple ocellus of the leech *Hirudo medicinalis* and (**c**) a simple ocellus of the polychaete *Armandia brevis*. (From Mill, P. J. (1978). In *Physiology of Annelids*. (Mill, P. J., ed.) Academic Press, London. (**a**) After Röhlich, P., Aros, B. and Virágh, S. (1970). *Zeitschrift für Zellforschung and mikroscopische Anatomie*, **104,** 345–57; (**b**) after Röhlich, P. and Török, L. J. (1964), *Zeitschrift für Zellforschung und mikroscopische Anatomie*, **63,** 618–35; (**c**) after Hermans C. O. and Cloney, R. A. (1966). *Zeitschrift für Zellforschung und mikroscopische Anatomie*, **72,** 583–96.)

single-celled photoreceptors (Fig. 9.1b), but in the polychaete *Armandia* it is the distal border of the cell which bears the microvilli and this lies adjacent to the pigment cup (Fig. 9.1c).

*Ocelli*

Ocelli include all those photoreceptors in which a group of sensory cells shares a common pigment cup and a common lens, but in which

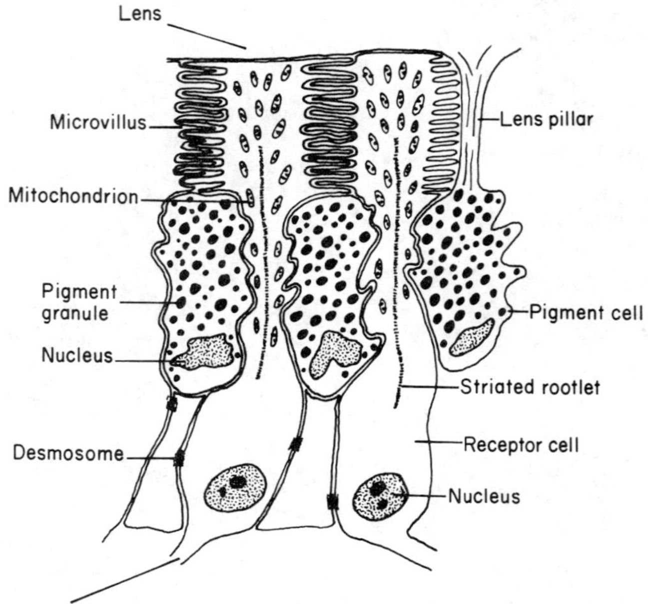


**Fig. 9.2** Diagram of a section through the retina of the ocellus (eye) of the polychaete *Nereis virens*. (From Mill, P. J. (1978). In *Physiology of Annelids*. (Mill, P. J., ed.) Academic Press, London; after Dorsett, D. A. and Hyde, R. (1968). *Zeitschrift für Zellforschung und mikroscopische Anatomie*, **85,** 243–55.)

there is no mechanism for altering the focal length of the optical system. In invertebrates other than arthropods, ocelli are often called eyes. Such 'eyes' are found in errant polychaetes, where the lens lies below a cornea of cuticle and epidermal cells. In most cases the lens consists of highly interfolded, membrane-bound processes and is derived from the pigment cells, to which it often remains connected (Fig. 9.2). However, in *Vanadis* the lens is a secreted structure consisting of membrane-bound droplets. The retina comprises photoreceptor and pigment cells and in some cases the former also contain pigment granules. The arrangement is such that there is an effective pigment cup. The photoreceptor cells are prolonged distally into the cup and the lateral borders of these prolongations bear microvilli (Fig. 9.2). Although the presence of a striated rootlet suggests a ciliary origin for the photoreceptor cells, the microvilli develop from the sides of the cell below the cilium.

A rather similar type of photoreceptor is found on the tentacles of gastropod molluscs such as *Agriolimax* and *Helix*. However, in *Agriolimax* the microvilli are arranged radially around the end of the receptor cells, while in *Helix* they arise mainly from the distal ends of the receptor cells and hence are almost parallel to the incident light (rather than at right angles to it as in annelids). The pallial eyes of lamellibranch molluscs such as *Pecten* are rather different, with an inverted retina consisting of two layers of receptor cells, below which there is a reflective layer (the argentea) composed of guanine crystals (Fig. 9.3). The proximal receptor cells bear microvilli, the distal ones numerous modified cilia.

In *Pecten* the microvillous receptor cells respond to increase in, and maintenance of, illumination. These are also the only types of response recorded in the optic nerves of the gastropod *Otala*, which has exclusively microvillous receptor cells in its retina. On the other hand, the ciliate receptor cells of *Pecten* respond only to decrease in illumination. In consequence of this and behavioural evidence, it has been suggested that photoreceptor cells bearing microvilli are concerned with orientation responses, whilst those bearing cilia are concerned with shadow responses. This is supported by the ciliary structure of the eyespots in sabellid polychaetes (see below), which mediate the marked withdrawal (escape) response of these animals to shadow stimuli.

### *Eyespots*

Eyespots are found on the tentacles of sabellid polychaetes and may occur singly (e.g. *Dasychone*) or be grouped together to form compound eyespots (e.g. *Branchiomma*). Each photoreceptor cell contains a transversely-oriented membranous structure, which is thought to be the photosensitive region of the cell. The membranes are of ciliary origin and hence eyespots are unlike the vast majority of invertebrate eyes. Each photoreceptor cell is surrounded by a pigment cell and has a lens lying distal to it (Fig. 9.4).

### *Compound eyes*

Compound eyes are exclusive to the arthropods. In surface view the compound eye appears as an array of, usually, hexagonal facets,

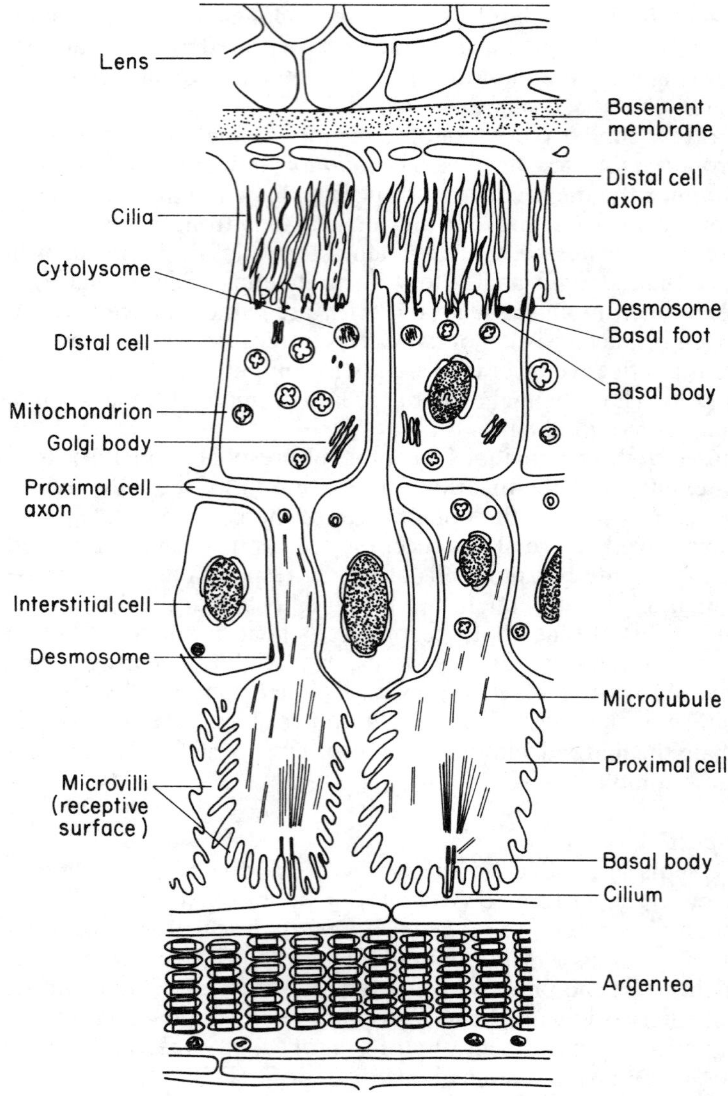


**Fig. 9.3** Diagram of a section through the retina of the mollusc *Pecten maximus*. A single layer of cells (the cornea) bearing microvilli on their distal borders lies peripheral to the lens. (After Barber, V. C., Evans, E. M. and Lund, M. F. (1967) *Zeitschrift für Zellforschung und mikroskopische Anatomie*, **76,** 295–312.)

each facet representing the outer surface of a single visual unit called an ommatidium (Fig. 9.5c). The number of ommatidia varies from a few (some ants) up to over 2000 (some anisopteran dragonflies). Each ommatidium comprises a group of sensory (retinula) cells, distal to which is a structure called the crystalline cone and a corneal lens (Fig. 9.5a,b), the cone and lens functioning together as a lens of fixed focal length.

In some eyes there are four retinula cells in each ommatidium (e.g. *Aeshna* and *Daphnia*), in others seven (e.g. *Drosophila*) and in

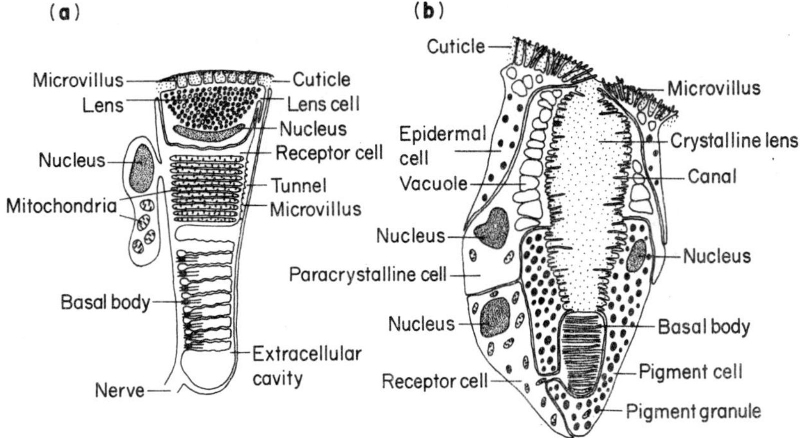


**Fig. 9.4** Diagrams of (**a**) a single unit from an eyespot from a tentacle of the polychaete annelid *Branchiomma pulvonina* and (**b**) a simple eyespot from a branchial tentacle of the polychaete annelid *Dasychone bombyx*. (From Mill, P. J. (1978). In *Physiology of Annelids*. (Mill, P. J. ed.) Academic Press, London; (**a**) after Krasne, F. B. and Lawrence, P. A. (1966). *Journal of Cell Science*, **1**, 239–48; (**b**) after Kerneis, A. (1968). *Zeitschrift für Zellforschung und mikroskopische Anatomie*, **86**, 280–92.)

*Limulus* 10–15. The retinula cells are elongated perpendicular to the surface of the eye and those of each ommatidium form a circular array (Fig. 9.5d). The medial border of each cell consists of numerous, transversely-oriented microvilli, which appear as lamellae in transverse sections through the cells and as densely packed tubules in appropriate longitudinal sections (Fig. 9.6a). This structure, known as a rhabdomere, corresponds functionally to the outer segment of the rod and cone cells of the vertebrate retina (see below). The rhabdomeres of a single ommatidium constitute a rhabdom. In some cases the rhabdomeres of a rhabdom are not in close apposition and this 'open' type of rhabdom is found, for example, in the Diptera (Fig. 9.6b). In other arthropods (e.g. Odonata, Dictyoptera, Orthoptera and Lepidoptera) the rhabdomeres are juxtaposed to one

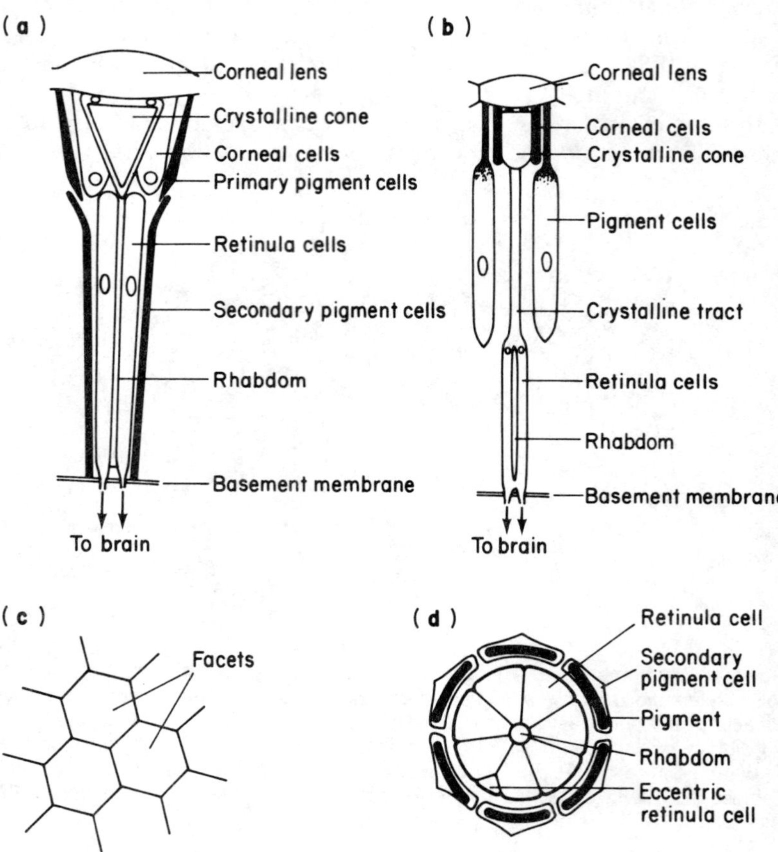


**Fig. 9.5** Diagrams of ommatidia from (**a**) an apposition eye and (**b**) a superposition eye. (**c**) Hexagonal arrangement of ommatidia seen from the surface of the eye. (**d**) Transverse section of (**a**) at the level of the retinula cells. (From Usherwood, P. N. R. (1973). *Nervous Systems.* Studies in Biology, no. 36. Edward Arnold, London, after Wigglesworth, V. B. (1965). *The Principles of Insect Physiology.* Methuen, London.)

another to form a 'closed' rhabdom (Fig. 9.6c). In closed rhabdoms the rhabdomeres constitute a greater proportion of the retinula cells than in the open type. The retinula cells are primary sensory cells, each with an axon running to the optic lamina. In most arthropods,

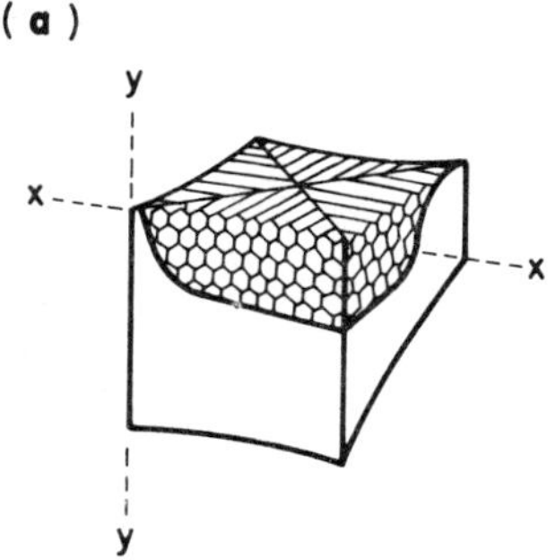


**Fig. 9.6** (**a**) Diagram of an example of a rhabdom of an arthropod ommatidium to show the arrangement of the microtubules in the rhabdomeres. This is the closed or fused type. X-X indicates the transverse plane, Y-Y indicates the longitudinal plane. (**b**) and (**c**) electron micrographs of transverse sections of (**b**) the open type of rhabdom (*Drosophila melanogaster*) and (**c**) the closed type of rhabdom (the crustacean *Leptodora kindtii*). R, rhabdomeres. (From Wolken, J. J. (1968). In *Symposium of the Zoological Society of London*, **23** (Invertebrate Receptors) (Carthy, J. D. and Newell, G. E., eds), pp. 113–33. Academic Press, London.)

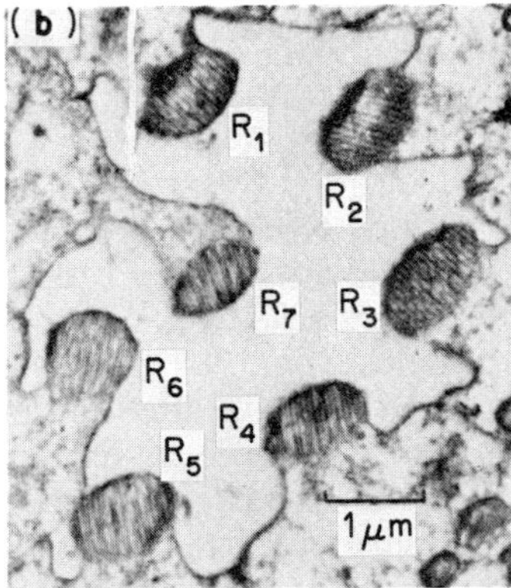


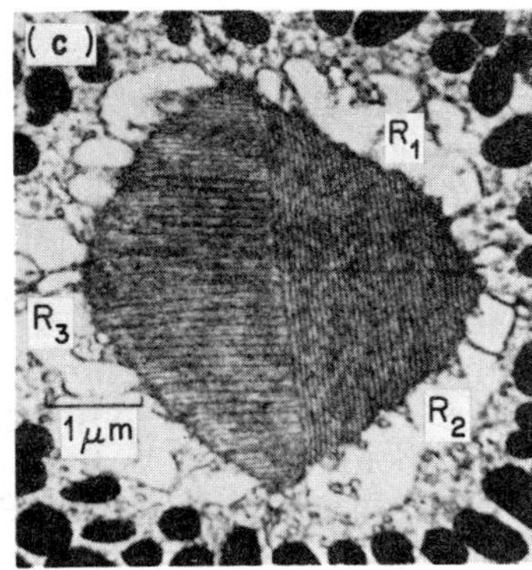


each retinula cell, when activated, elicits a response in its axon. However, in *Limulus* these axons appear to be non-functional and the retinula cells of each ommatidium excite a single eccentric cell, which does have a functional axon.

There are two anatomically distinct types of compound eye—apposition eyes and superposition eyes. In apposition eyes the rhabdomeres abut against the crystalline cone (Fig. 9.5a), but in superposition eyes the receptor cells lie well below the crystalline cone and the rhabdom is connected to the latter by a crystalline tract (Fig. 9.5b).

Each ommatidium is separated from its neighbours by pigment cells, and the disposition of these differs in the two types of eye. In apposition eyes each ommatidium is completely surrounded by pigment and so its rhabdom only receives light falling directly on its own lens and within about 10° of the perpendicular. In light-adapted superposition eyes the arrangement of the pigment is similar to that in apposition eyes, but in dark-adapted superposition eyes the pigment becomes concentrated around the crystalline cones, thereby allowing lateral penetration of light from that falling on adjacent ommatidia.

It has been suggested that apposition and superposition eyes are characteristic, respectively, of species which are active in high light intensities and those which are active in low light intensities. However, superposition eyes are found in diurnal as well as in nocturnal animals.

Arthropods with a closed rhabdom, with the exception of the Odonta, possess a 'slow' type eye, in which there is a monophasic, negative electroretinogram (ERG), the magnitude of which is dependent upon the level of dark adaptation. Conversely, insects with an open rhabdom possess a 'fast' type eye in which the ERG is diphasic and independent of the level of dark-adaptation.

*Eyes*

Included within this category are those photoreceptors in which there is a retina of sensory cells upon which a focused image can be formed by altering the position or shape of the lens. Eyes occur in both cephalopod molluscs and in vertebrates (Fig. 9.7). In the vertebrate eye not only the lens but also the cornea and the fluid in front of and behind the lens (aqueous and vitreous humour respectively) contribute to focusing, since they all have a refractive index greater than 1 (that of air). Indeed, in terrestrial animals the cornea is responsible for most of the focusing. Not only does it have a greater curvature than the lens, but the air-cornea interface is that of greatest change in refractive index. Conversely, in fish the cornea is usually fairly flat and has a refractive index similar to that of water, and hence plays little part in focusing.

Changes in focal length (accommodation) are brought about either by moving the lens (as in octopod molluscs, fishes, amphibians and snakes) or by altering the curvature of the lens by means of the ciliary muscle (as in reptiles other than snakes, birds and mammals). Birds and some lizards can also alter the shape of their cornea.

The retina in the cephalopod eye consists of photoreceptor cells and supporting pigment cells (Fig. 9.8). The distal (inner with respect to the eye) end of each photoreceptor cell is very elongated and is termed the rod region. In transverse section this region is slightly flattened, each of the long sides forming a rhabdomere composed of numerous microvilli lying at right angles to the rod. The rods are fairly regularly arranged so that four adjacent rhabdomeres form an

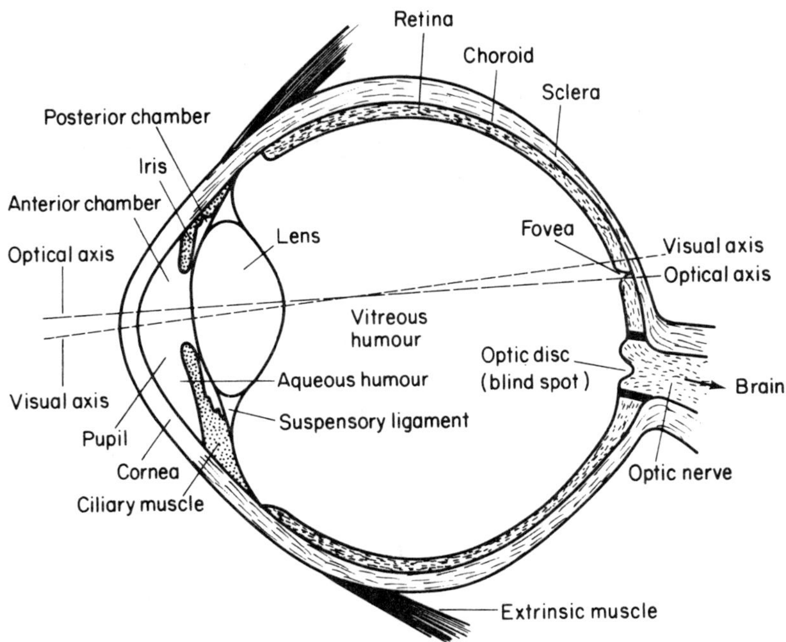


**Fig. 9.7** Diagram of a section through the human eye. (From Usherwood, P. N. R. (1973). *Nervous Systems.* Studies in Biology, no. 36. Edward Arnold, London; after Maximov, A. A. and Bloom, W. (1957). *Textbook of Histology.* W. B. Saunders, Philadelphia.)

open type of rhabdom. The rod region and the region immediately proximal to it contain pigment granules. These photoreceptor cells are primary sensory cells, each with an axon running to the appropriate optic lobe. The axons also have collaterals, which presumably synapse with each other and possibly also with efferent fibres from the optic lobes.

The retina of the vertebrate eye is a layered structure (Fig. 9.9a) which contains two types of photoreceptor cells (rods and cones), together with four other types of neuron: horizontal cells, bipolar cells, amacrine cells and ganglion cells. In contrast to the retina of cephalopods, the vertebrate retina is inverted so that the photoreceptor cells lie proximal to the other neurons and their photoreceptive processes point away from the cornea. Hence light has to travel through the retina to activate them.

The rod and cone cells differ in the shape of their distal region, this being longer and narrower in the rods than in the cones. However, in

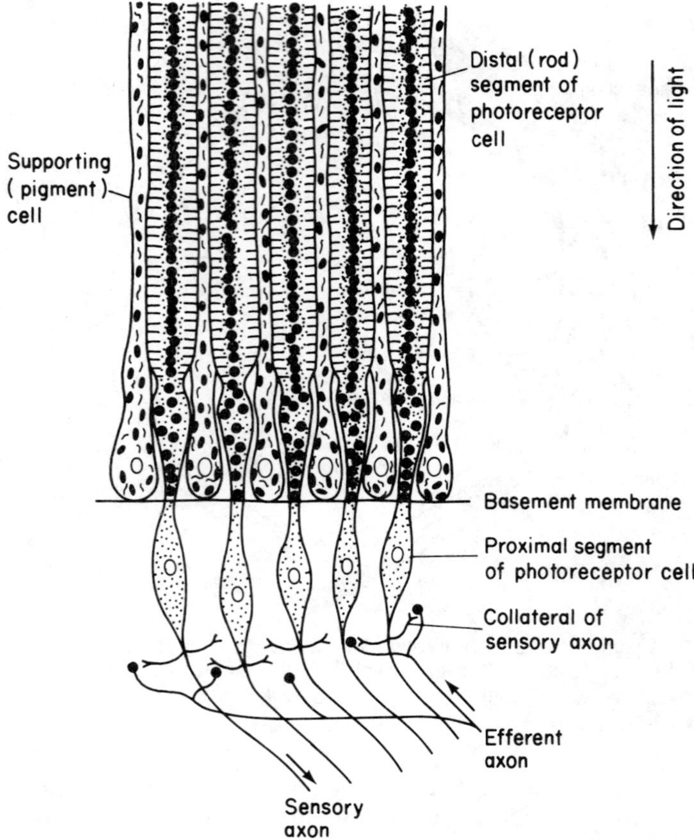


**Fig. 9.8** Diagram of the retina of the octopus eye. (After Young, J. Z. (1971). *The Anatomy of the Nervous System of Octopus vulgaris*. Oxford University Press, New York.)

both types of receptor cell this region is divisible into two parts. The inner segment (with respect to the eye) contains mitochondria (which are particularly numerous at its distal end in cone cells) and the double basal body of a short, ciliary structure. The outer segment is highly lamellate and contains the photosensitive pigment on or between the lamellae (Fig. 9.9b).

The rods are far more light sensitive than the cones, and indeed the latter are not activated in dim light. The retina of nocturnal animals thus usually contains a preponderance of rods and indeed in some (e.g. bats) consists entirely of rods. Cones, on the other hand, tend to predominate in the retinae of diurnal animals, and many birds have very few rods. Cones provide much greater image resolution (acuity) than rods, apparently because individual ganglion cells receive input from far fewer cones than rods. Thus animals with a rod-dominated retina have poor image resolution, but good vision in dim light; while those with a cone-dominated retina have good image resolution, but poor vision in dim light. Cones, in the majority of animals which possess them, are particularly abundant in a region in the centre of the retina called the fovea, and indeed rods may be absent from here. This is the region where images are normally focused and hence where it is particularly important to have good visual acuity. Many diurnal birds have an enlarged fovea.

Activation of the rods and cones involves bleaching of the photoreceptive or visual pigments (see below). In a mixed retina (i.e. with both rods and cones) much of the rod visual pigment becomes bleached in bright light and there is thus a shift (the Purkinje shift) from rod to cone vision. Subsequent transfer to very dim light results in a period of adaptation during which vision is gradually improved. This dark-adaptation of the cones only takes about 5 minutes. However, the rods, which are required for good vision in dim light, have had their pigment bleached, and their dark-adaptation takes 30–40 minutes.

**Photoreceptive pigments**

In animals with a single photoreceptive pigment, colour vision is not possible since any two monochromatic lights of appropriate sensitivities can elicit the same response from a photoreceptor cell. Two types of cell, each with its own photoreceptive pigment, confer limited colour vision but, although two monochromatic lights can be separated, a white light can still produce identical responses in the receptor cells to that elicited by some monochromatic lights. For full colour vision three types of cell, each with its own pigment, are necessary. Under such conditions all single monochromatic lights are distinguishable, not only from each other, but also from white light. Even so, pairs of monochromatic lights with complementary wavelengths (red-green, yellow-blue) do duplicate the response to white light. Colour vision occurs in comparatively few mammals (e.g. man) but is common in birds and many lower vertebrates.

The photosensitive pigments found in the retinal cells of many invertebrates and in the rods and cones of the vertebrate retina are composed of a colourless protein, opsin, and a yellow carotenoid (derived from vitamin A) called retinaldehyde (retinene).

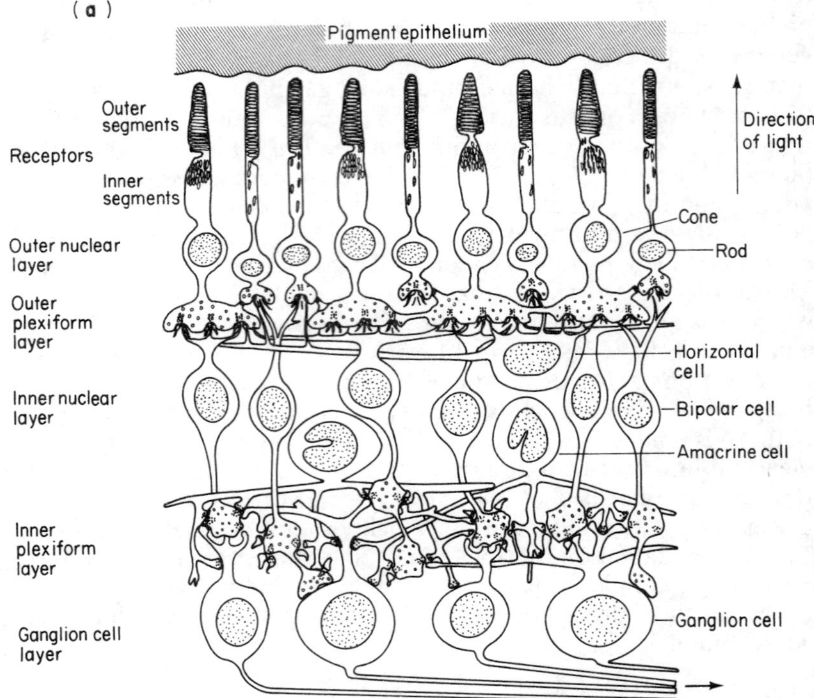


**Fig. 9.9** Diagrams of (**a**) the retina of the vertebrate eye and (**b**) part of a mammalian rod to show the junction between the outer and inner segments. ((**a**) From Dowling, J. E. and Boycott, B. B. (1966). *Proceedings of the Royal Society, B*, **166,** 80–111; (**b**) from de Robertis, E. (1960). *Journal of General Physiology*, **43** (Suppl. 2), 1–13.)

Most of our knowledge of the mechanism of action of these pigments comes from studies on the photosensitive pigment rhodopsin. The rods of the vertebrate retina contain a single pigment—rhodopsin (visual purple) in terrestrial and marine vertebrates, and the almost identical porphyropsin (visual red) in freshwater vertebrates. These are red pigments which absorb yellow-green light. Rhodopsin, which contains retinaldehyde$_1$, has a maximum absorption peak at 498 nm (Fig. 9.10a), while that of porphyropsin, which contains retinaldehyde$_2$, is at 522 nm. The presence of only a single rod pigment means that, in dim light, when only the rods are activated, vertebrates do not have colour vision. (That the absorption spectrum is an important step in the chain of reactions between

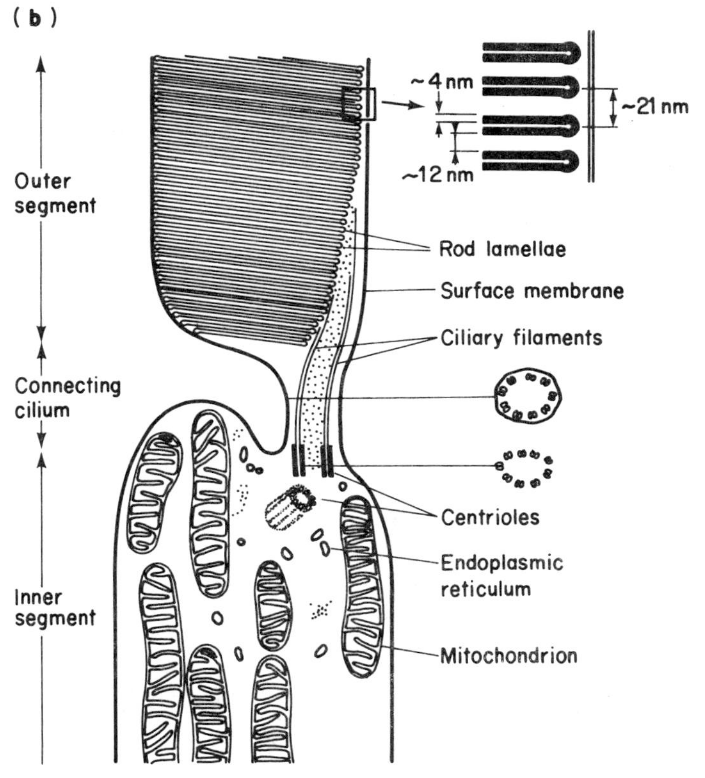


stimulus and response is shown by the close agreement between the absorption spectrum of rhodopsin and the relative sensitivity to light flashes at different wavelengths (Fig. 9.10b).)

There are three different cone pigments in vertebrates, located in different cone cells, with maximum absorption peaks at about 440 nm, 530 nm and 565 nm (Fig. 9.10b). This is the key to vertebrate colour vision. The differences in absorption spectra of these pigments are due both to the type of retinaldehyde and the type of opsin present. Thus the photoreceptive pigment iodopsin (found in chickens and pigeons) consists of a special cone opsin together with retinaldehyde$_1$, and a pigment isolated from freshwater fishes (cyanopsin) consists of cone opsin and retinaldehyde$_2$.

In all cases it seems that the retinaldehyde of photoreceptive pigments normally occurs in its 11-*cis* form. In rhodopsin at least it is converted by light to its all-*trans* form. It then goes through a series of

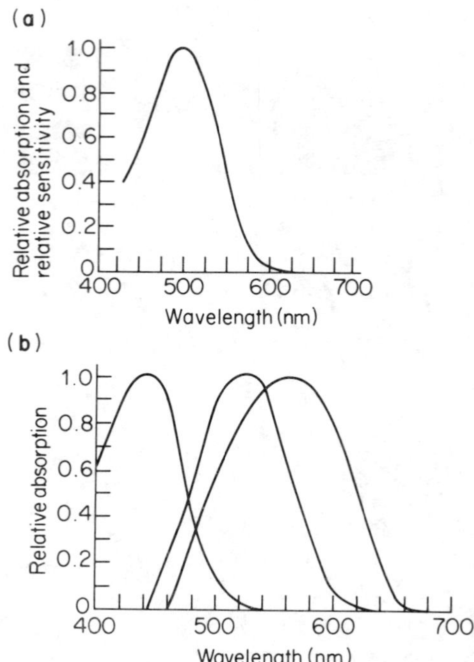


**Fig. 9.10** (**a**) The relative absorption of humal rhodopsin and the relative sensitivity of human rod vision plotted against wavelength. The two curves coincide precisely. (**b**) The relative absorption of the photopigments of three human cones plotted against wavelength. The maximum absorbances occur at 444 nm (blue sensitive), 530 nm (green sensitive) and 560 nm (red sensitive). ((**a**) After Wald, G. and Brown, K. (1958). *Science*, **127**, 222–6; (**b**) after Wald, G. and Brown, K. (1965). *Cold Spring Harbor Symposia on Quantitative Biology*, **30**, 345–61.)

reactions until the rhodopsin is finally split into opsin and retinaldehyde$_1$. This last stage is known as bleaching. The stages associated with activation of the rods are indicated in Fig. 9.11. There is evidence that one quantum of light activates a single rhodopsin molecule. Subsequently the photoreceptive pigment with its 11-*cis* form of retinaldehyde is reconstituted.

**Retinal potentials**

Small depolarizations, probably caused by an increased conductance to $Na^+$ and, possibly, $Ca^{++}$, can be seen in the retinula cells when a dark-adapted compound eye of *Limulus* is exposed to very low levels of illumination (Fig. 9.12). Each depolarization corres-

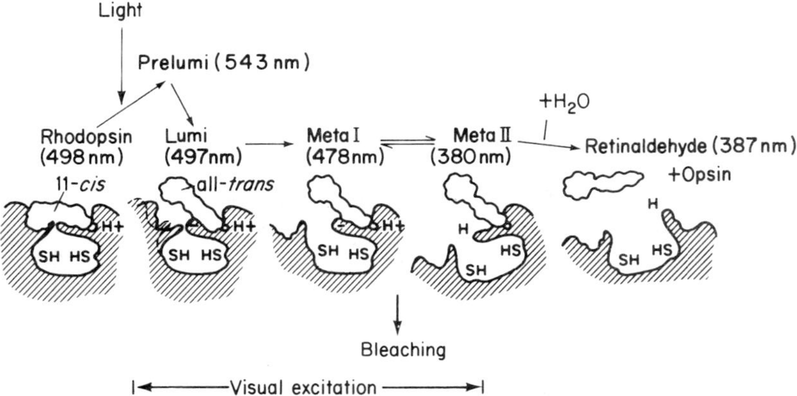


**Fig. 9.11** Sequence of bleaching of rhodopsin, with a theoretical scheme to explain the changes in configuration of retinaldehyde and opsin, and the exposure of optic groups. The figures indicate the wavelength of maximum absorption at each stage. Note the -SH groups and the $H^+$ binding group. Prelumi, Lumi, Meta I and Meta II are intermediate stages. (From Wald, G. and Brown, P. K. (1965). *Cold Spring Harbor Symposia of Quantitative Biology*, **30,** 345–59.)

ponds to the bleaching of a single rhodopsin molecule. At higher light intensities the depolarizations increase in frequency and sum to produce a smooth receptor potential (Fig. 9.12). Furthermore, the size of the individual depolarizations decreases with increase in light intensity such that the receptor potential is proportional to the logarithm of light intensity. The receptor potentials in the retinula cells of a single ommatidium produce a generator potential in the eccentric cell which, if it reaches the appropriate threshold level, activates the spike-initiating zone of that cell.

In contrast to *Limulus* and other invertebrates; the retinal potentials in, at least, the lower vertebrates, are slow hyperpolarizations of 10–20 mV amplitude which, in both rods and cones, increase with increase in light intensity. The probable mechanism is as follows. In the dark-adapted state the metabolic sodium pump is partially counteracted by sodium leaking in at one end of the cell. On exposure to illumination the $Na^+$ leak is blocked by a mechanism which may involve $Ca^{++}$, with a concomitant increase in internal negativity.

The photoreceptor cells are thought to release neurotransmitter continually in proportion to their level of depolarization. Thus the reduction in neurotransmitter release by the photoreceptor cells during a hyperpolarization probably explains why the horizontal cells

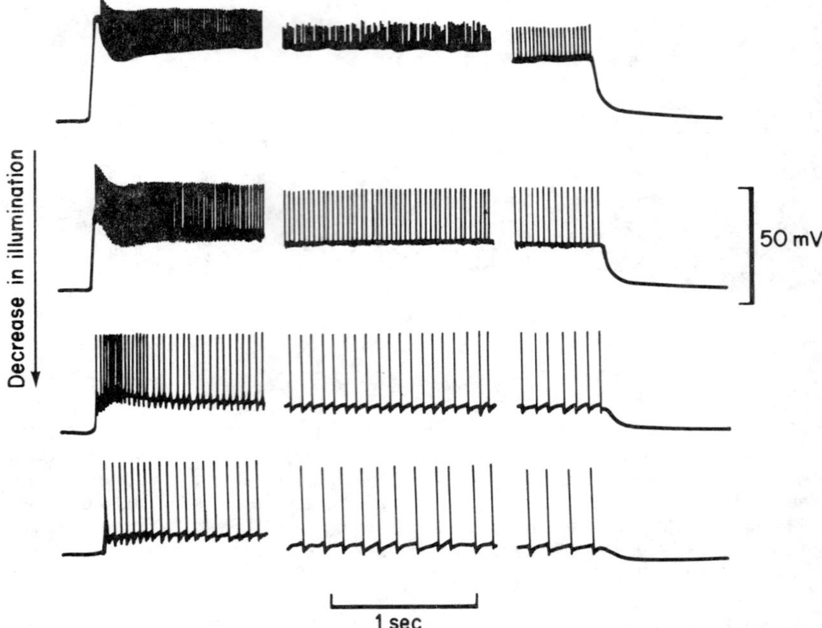


**Fig. 9.12** Intracellular records from an eccentric cell of *Limulus* eye at different levels of illumination. Steps of light lasted 20 seconds. Gaps between the three records in each row are 8.4 seconds each. (From Fuortes, M. G. F. and Poggio, G. T. (1963). *Journal of General Physiology*, **46**, 435–52.)

of the retina show a similar hyperpolarizing response. Some bipolar cells are also hyperpolarized by the photoreceptor cells, but are depolarized by the horizontal cells; others are affected in the reverse way. In all cases the hyperpolarizations and depolarizations increase in magnitude with increase in light intensity. However, those cells which are always hyperpolarized or always depolarized, irrespective of the wavelength of the light, cannot carry information on colour. This information can only be carried by those cells which are hyperpolarized by one wavelength, but depolarized by another. None of the above cell types produces action potentials.

Both the amacrine cells and the ganglion cells (whose axons pass to the central nervous system) show depolarizing potentials, giving rise, at least in the ganglion cells, to action potentials.

The ganglion cells are spontaneously active and have almost circular receptive fields of up to 4–8° (representing a retinal circle of 1–2 mm diameter). In mammals some ganglion cells are excited by

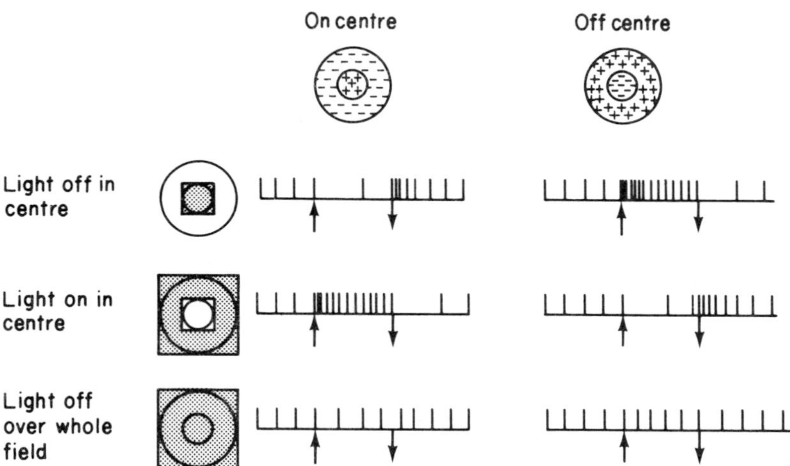


**Fig. 9.13** Diagrams of the receptive fields and response patterns of retinal ganglion cells. The centre of the field is either excitatory (on centre) or inhibitory (off centre) with a surrounding area of opposite effect. The diagrams on the left show the stimulus in relation to the receptive field. The shaded area represents darkness, the unshaded area light. Arrows indicate stimulus on ( ↑ ) and off ( ↓ ). (After Grinnell, A. D. (1977). In *Animal Physiology: Principles and Adaptations*. (Gordon, M. S., ed.) Macmillan, New York.)

increase in light intensity ('on' cells), while others are exicted by decrease in light intensity ('off' cells). Furthermore, some are excited by light stimulation in the centre of their receptive field and inhibited by light stimulation in the periphery of their field (on centre cells); others show the reverse (off centre cells) (Fig. 9.13). This provides for a complex set of ganglion cell responses for an object moving through the visual field.

**Lateral inhibition**

If more than one ommatidium of a compound eye of *Limulus* is illuminated, the responses in their eccentric cells are less than if they are illuminated individually. This mutual inhibition (known as lateral inhibition) decreases with increase in distance apart of the ommatidia involved. Also the degree to which an eccentric cell is capable of causing lateral inhibition is approximately proportional to its firing frequency, and hence to the level of illumination of the ommatidium.

The purpose of lateral inhibition is to increase contrast. Thus, if part of the eye is illuminated by bright light and the rest by dim light, ommatidia in the former zone will be inhibited, as well as excited,

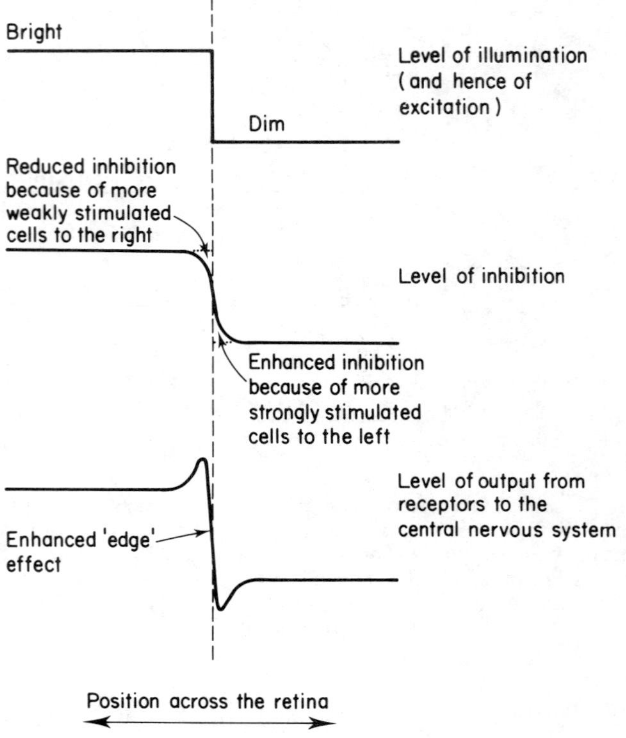


**Fig. 9.14** The effect of lateral inhibition on the output of the sensory cells in the retina of the horseshoe crab *Limulus*. The output is coded in terms of the frequency of action potentials (not shown). The enhanced 'edge effect' is caused by the brightly illuminated cells close to the 'edge' being less strongly inhibited than those further into the brightly illuminated region (because they are close to cells which are only dimly illuminated and hence have a lower inhibitory effect). Conversely, dimly illuminated cells close to the 'edge' are more strongly inhibited than those further into the dimly illuminated region (because they are close to cells which are illuminated by bright light and which hence have a greater inhibitory effect).

more strongly than will those in the latter zone. However, at the interface between the two zones the ommatidia at the bright edge will be inhibited less than those further into the bright area because the former are closer to ommatidia which are only weakly activated and hence have comparatively little inhibitory effect. Conversely, those at the dim edge will be inhibited more than those further into the dim area because they are closer to ommatidia which are producing a marked inhibitory effect (Fig. 9.14).

In most vertebrates, lateral inhibition of the cones occurs via the horizontal cells, while at the level of the bipolar cells there is an even more marked lateral inhibition, affecting information arriving from both the cones and the rods.

## CHEMORECEPTION

Among the lower invertebrates chemoreceptors are found scattered over the surface of the body, generally with a greater density towards the head. In higher invertebrates and in vertebrates they occur in more discrete areas and the chemical sense can be divided into olfaction (smell) and gustation (taste).

### Olfaction

The olfactory receptors are concerned with sampling chemical stimuli brought to the animal by air or water currents. They occur on the appendages of arthropods, notably the antennal flagella, while in vertebrates they are located in the respiratory tract. In addition, snakes transfer odours via their forked tongue to a pair of sensory pits (Jacobsen's organ) in the roof of the mouth. Olfactory receptors are always bipolar primary sensory cells.

Four morphological types of olfactory sensillum have been described on the antennae of insects, although not all occur in any one order: long, thick-walled hairs (sensilla trichodea), thin-walled pegs (sensilla basiconica), pit-pegs (sensilla coeloconica) and placoid organs (sensilla placodea) (Fig. 9.15). The last three types may be exclusively olfactory, but sensilla trichodea are distributed widely over other appendages, where they generally have a tactile function. The olfactory sensilla trichodea differ from the tactile ones in that the cuticle of the hair is perforated with pores, each of which connects with several tubules which pass through the cuticle to the hair lumen. A similar arrangement occurs in the sensilla basiconica. In the sensilla placodea the pores are arranged in radial rows. In the sensilla coeloconica there are no pores and tubules as such; instead radially-oriented, hollow cuticular bars connect the exterior with the hair lumen.

The number of bipolar sensory cells associated with each sensillum is variable, with 1–3 in sensilla trichodea (cf. only one in insect tactile sensilla trichodea, p. 117) and as many as 50 in some sensilla basiconica. The dendrite of each sensory cell contains a basal body, distal to which it bears a ciliary structure with a 9 + 0 axoneme. It is very similar in its fine structure to a mechanoreceptive dendrite (p. 116), except that it does not terminate distally in a tubular body and extends into the hair lumen (Fig. 9.15). In all except the sensilla basiconica the dendrites are unbranched. The dendrites of the sensilla basiconica usually divide into many branches. As in tactile sensilla there are three enveloping cells surrounding the sensory apparatus (p. 117).

The olfactory sensory cells of vertebrates are grouped together to form a respiratory mucosa. Each cell bears a single dendrite from which several cilia arise (Fig. 9.16). These are embedded in mucous and beat with a metachronal rhythm.

Many animals have a very highly developed sense of smell and are extremely sensitive to very low concentrations of certain odours. Two physiological cell types are found in insects at least: odour

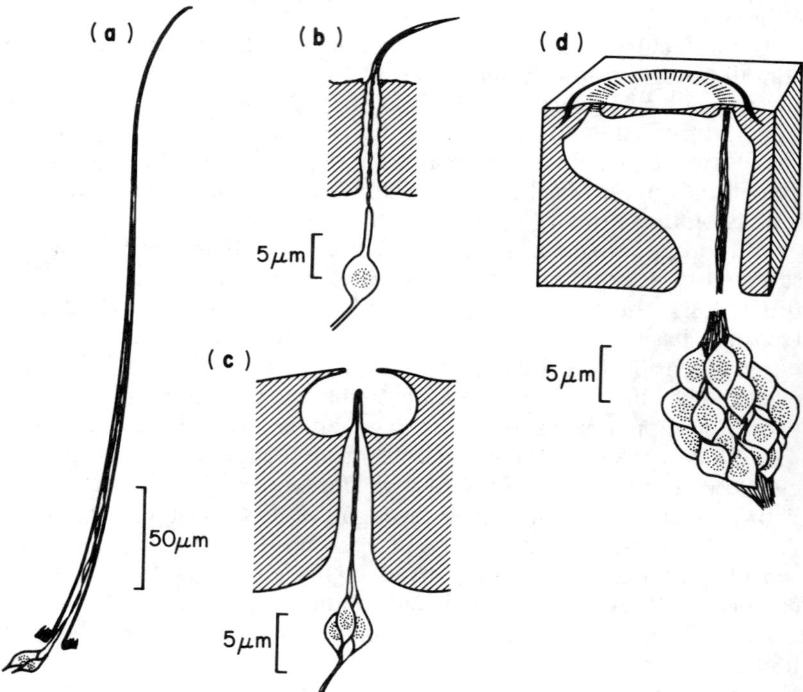


**Fig. 9.15** Diagrams of insect chemosensory sensilla. (**a**) Sensillum trichodeum from the lepidopteran *Antheraea pernyi*; (**b**) sensillum basiconicum from the beetle *Necrophorus vespillio*; (**c**) sensillum coeloconicum from *Locusta migratoria* and (**d**) sensillum placodeum from the bee *Apis mellifica*. Fine detail not drawn to scale. (From Schneider, D. and Steinbrecht, R. A. (1968). In *Symposium of the Zoological Society of London*, **23** (Invertebrate Receptors). (Carthy, J. D. and Newell, G. E. eds.) Academic Press, London.)

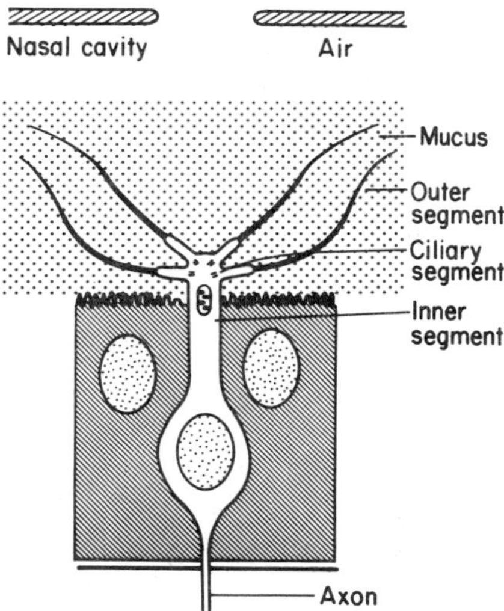


**Fig. 9.16** Diagram of a single receptor from a vertebrate olfactory organ (From Steinbrecht, R. A. (1969). In *Olfaction and Taste. Proceedings of 3rd International Symposium.* (Pfaffman, C. ed.) Rockefeller University Press, New York.)

specialists, each of which responds to a specific chemical such as a pheromone, and odour generalists, which respond to a variety of substances, although any individual cell has a specific set of substances to which it responds. In vertebrates the number of odours which can be recognized is very large, possibly in the region of tens of thousands, and it is thought that a single molecule may be sufficient to activate a receptor. The principal current theory, called the stereochemical theory, is that molecules interact with specific sites on the ciliary membrane, and that the more closely they 'fit' the site the greater the response in the sensory cell. This is similar to the reactions of neurotransmitters with receptor sites on the postsynaptic membrane (Chapter 5). It has been suggested that there is a comparatively small number of types of site and that each type is fitted precisely, and hence activated maximally, by a specific 'primary' odour. Other odours fit and activate one or more types of site to a greater or lesser extent.

**Gustation**

The taste receptors are associated with the physical testing of food. In arthropods they are located on the mouthparts and legs; in vertebrates they are found in the mouth.

The taste receptors of arthropods are called 'contact chemoreceptors'. Some are sensilla trichodea, while others are more robust bristles. They are all innervated by bipolar primary sensory cells, which have the same structure as the olfactory sensory cells, and three enveloping cells surround the sensory apparatus. The dendrites are always unbranched. In insects there are only 2–6 sensory cells associated with each sensillum, but in spiders there are about 20 (Fig. 9.17). They differ from the olfactory receptors in two main ways.

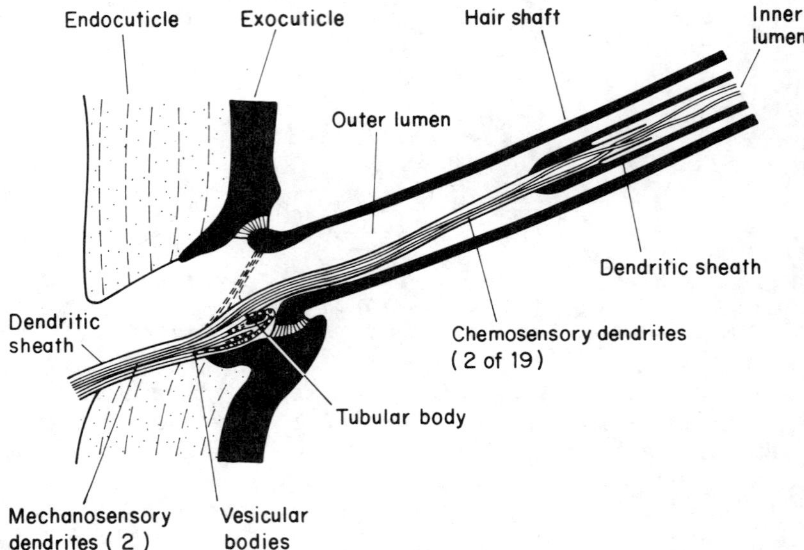


**Fig. 9.17** Diagram of a contact chemoreceptor from the leg of the spider *Ciniflo*. (From Harris, D. J. and Mill, P. J. (1977). *Journal of Comparative Physiology, A*, **119**, 37–54.)

Firstly, there is a single distal pore in the hair, rather than numerous scattered pores. Secondly, one or two of the dendrites possess a tubular body (p. 117) at the base of the hair and so are sensitive to movement of the hair—hence the name 'contact chemoreceptors'.

The vertebrate taste receptors differ from other chemoreceptors in that they are composed of secondary sensory cells, grouped together to form taste buds (Fig. 9.18), and are continuously being replaced. Adjacent receptor cells are joined to each other by tight junctions and the distal border of each cell bears a number of microvilli. They are embedded within the epidermis of the tongue and communicate with the exterior (buccal cavity) via a small pore between the overlying cells. Each taste bud is innervated by a single sensory fibre.

In the blowfly there are four separate receptors, responding to anions, cations, sugars and water respectively. A similar number of primary tastes probably occurs in most or all arthropods and vertebrates, but they are not necessarily the same ones, for example cats do not have a receptor responding to sugars.

There are four taste sensations in man—sweet, sour, salt and bitter. Individual taste buds vary in their degree of specificity, but those which do respond to more than one taste do so preferentially.

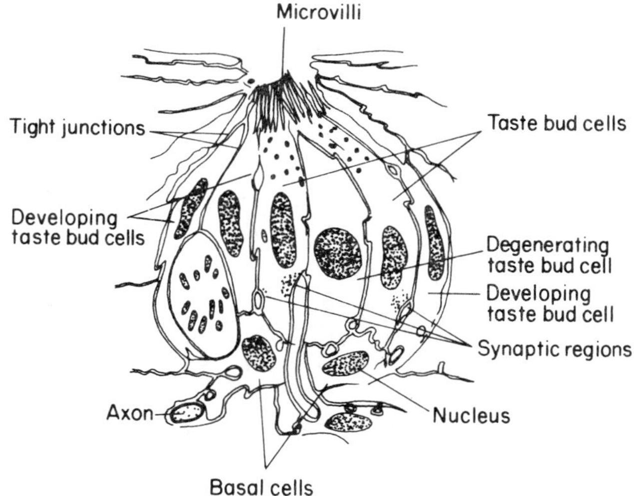


**Fig. 9.18** Diagram of the taste bud of a rabbit. (From Burt, E. T. (1974). *The Senses of Animals*. Wykeham Publications, London.)

Different regions of the tongue vary in their relative sensitivity to the four tastes. Thus the tip of the human tongue is the most sensitive region to sweet stimuli, the back to bitter stimuli. Sensitivity to the other two parameters is more even, although salt sensitivity is slightly greater at the tip, sour at the sides. There are few taste buds in the centre of the tonge or on the under surface.

## THERMORECEPTION

Increase in temperature effects an increase in the firing frequency of most nerve cells, up to a physiological limit. However, some sensory neurons are affected to a greater than average extent ('warm' receptors), while others have a peak firing frequency at a comparatively low temperature ('cold' receptors).

Many invertebrates respond to variations in temperature, but little is known concerning which sensory neurons are thermoreceptors. In arthropods and vertebrates a thermoreceptive function has been ascribed to free nerve endings close to the body surface. In some animals, sense organs which are not primarily thermoreceptors show a marked response to temperature changes. Thus the ampullae of Lorenzini in elasmobranchs (p. 122) and the lateral line system in the aquatic amphibian *Xenopus* (p. 121) act as 'cold' receptors. The latter is sensitive to temperature changes in the region of 1–2°C.

Certain snakes, such as boas and crotalids (pit-vipers), are extremely sensitive to temperature variation and possess 'warm' receptors on their head which respond, in particular, to wavelengths in the infrared ($\lambda$ = 0.5–15 $\mu$m), enabling them to detect warm-blooded prey. Crotalids can detect temperature changes in the order of 0.001°C. In boas the receptors lie in shallow pits between the scales. In crotalids they are found in a single pit on each side of the head, each pit being lined with a membrane containing the peripheral endings of sensory neurons. These neurons give rise to several terminals, each of which is composed of numerous fine branches.

In mammals there are both 'cold' and 'warm' receptors in the skin. The 'cold' receptors are the more numerous and are closer to the surface than the 'warm' receptors.

Thermoreceptors in vertebrates are typically tonic with a large phasic component and this results in the considerable adaptation observed in response to a change in temperature. Warm receptors always show a phasic increase in firing frequency when the temperature is raised and a phasic decrease when the temperature is lowered. 'Cold' receptors show the reverse. Similarly, within an animal's normal physiological range, 'warm' receptors nearly always show an increase in their tonic (adapted) level with increase in temperature. 'Cold' receptors, on the other hand, may show either a lower or a higher adapted level on cooling, depending on the initial and final temperatures. This is because the peak tonic firing level tends to be well above the bottom of the physiological range (Fig. 9.19).

In mammals 'warm' receptors have a maximum tonic firing frequency between 38°C and 43°C, 'cold' receptors between 20°C and 34°C (Fig. 9.19). At about 45°C the firing frequency of the 'warm' receptors is low, and above this temperature the cold receptors start to fire again. This is responsible for the phenomenon of paradoxical cold, experienced when drops of very hot water fall on the skin.

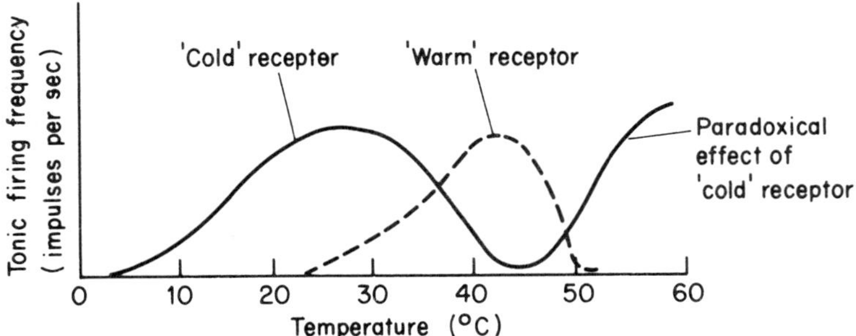


**Fig. 9.19** The relationship between the tonic firing rates of mammalian 'cold' and 'warm' receptors and temperature.

Ultimately some of the more sparsely scattered and deeper 'warm' receptors will also be stimulated and the combined input from both 'cold' and 'warm' receptors produces a sensation of heat.

## ELECTRORECEPTION

Many fish are capable of detecting changes in the electric field surrounding them; this ability may be used for the detection of prey or for orientation. The receptors involved, which are associated with, or derived from, the lateral-line system, are extremely sensitive and are always secondary sensory cells.

In elasmobranchs the receptors are the ampullae of Lorenzini, which also function as mechanoreceptors (p. 122). They are particularly sensitive to low frequency fields (0–20 Hz) and are used by sharks to detect prey. The sensory response is tonic. It has also been suggested that they can be used for orientation with respect to the earth's magnetic field since variations as low as 0.01 $\mu$V $cm^{-1}$ can be detected.

In teleosts the receptors tend to be concentrated in the lateral line, but are also found distributed widely over the surface of the animal. In contrast to those of elasmobranchs they are most sensitive to high frequency fields (60–2000 Hz) and have a phasic response.

Some fish possess an electric organ, comprised of a series of flattened muscle fibres called electroplaques. These electroplaques are only innervated on one face and most of the depolarization occurs on this side. When depolarization does occur an electric field is set up around the animal. In some fish (e.g. the electric ray, *Torpedo*, and the electric eel, *Electrophorus*) the electrical discharges from these organs are strong and are used for defence or offence. However, some teleosts produce a series of very small discharges which are used for orientation purposes. These fish can detect distortions in the field caused by objects within it which have a different conductivity to that of the surrounding water. Conductors cause a decrease in sensory activity, while insulators have the reverse effect. In gymnotids (knife fishes) the basic discharge frequency tends to remain constant for long periods of time, whereas in mormyrids (elephant nose fishes) it varies with the level of activity of the fish.

# 10

# *Central Nervous Systems: Integration*

## INTRODUCTION

In some cnidarians, such as *Velella* and the sea anemone *Calliactis*, there are two networks of nerve cells, called nerve nets. One of these is syncitial, with the individual neurons fused together, and hence conduction is multidirectional and relatively fast. In the other there are synapses between the nerve cells and these impart directionality on the flow of nervous information (see Chapters 1 and 5). In free-swimming medusae there is a subumbrellar nerve net and concentrations of nerve cells into ganglia, which lie around the periphery of the bell and are interconnected by nerve rings. A subepidermal nerve net is present in ctenophores, but is not generally well-developed in platyhelminths, and is not found in phyla above this level of organization. In *Calliactis* there are, in addition to the nerve nets, two slow conducting systems, one involving conduction between the ectodermal cells, the other conduction between the endodermal cells. Such conducting systems which do not comprise neurons are termed 'neuroid' systems. They are not unique to cnidarians; for example the epidermal cells of early larval amphibians are capable of conducting potentials.

In all swimming cnidarians the effector system can be subdivided into one concerned with localized activity and one concerned with locomotion. The trend in higher groups is for sensory information to be integrated centrally and for the periphery to become progressively more subject to central control; this is achieved by an increase in the concentration of nerve cell bodies into plexuses and ganglia, the latter linked together to form a central nervous system. There is also a tendency for the ganglia to become more and more concentrated towards the anterior end of the animal, a process called cephalization.

In most platyhelminths there is a pair of anterior ganglia, each member of which gives rise to a longitudinal nerve cord. These are often connected to each other by transverse nerves (Fig. 10.1). In

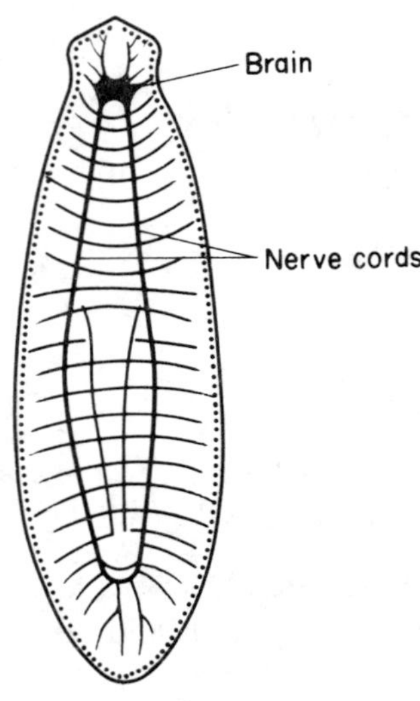


**Fig. 10.1** Diagram of the nervous system of the triclad turbellarian *Procerodes* (Platyhelminthes) to show the paired, longitudinal nerve cords. (From Lang, A. (1881). *Mitteilungen aus der Zoologischen Station zu Neapel*, **3,** 53–76.)

pseudocoelomates there is a cerebral ganglion, or at least a circumoesophageal nerve ring. In annelids and arthropods there is a single cerebral ganglion or brain (formed by the fusion of paired cerebral ganglia) and a double ventral nerve cord. consisting of one ganglion per segment, consecutive ganglia being joined by paired connectives. Each ganglion is formed from the fusion in the mid-line of two primitive ganglia. In higher arthropods there is considerable condensation of the nervous system, the number of posterior ganglia being reduced by incorporation of their nerve cell bodies within one of the more anterior ganglia. In addition, there is often condensation at the posterior end of the abdomen (Fig. 10.2). It is usual for condensation to proceed during the growth of an individual and this is especially dramatic in endopterygote insects, which undergo complete metamorphosis.

In most groups of molluscs there are several pairs of ganglia with

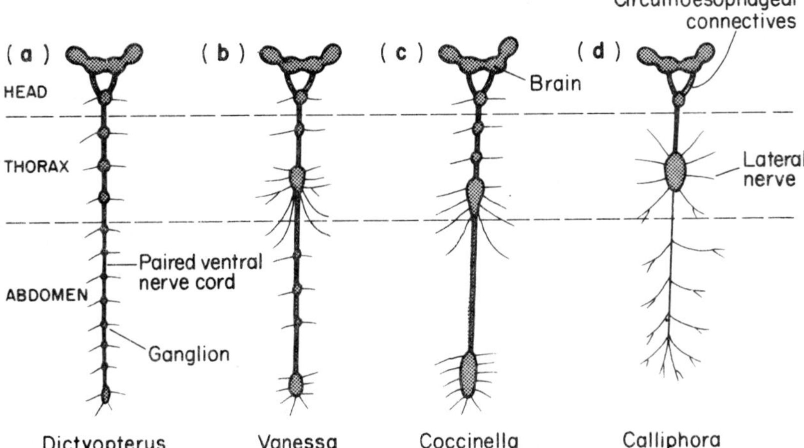


**Fig. 10.2** Diagrams of insect nervous systems illustrating condensation. (**a**) The cockroach *Dictyopterus*; (**b**) the lepidopteran *Vanessa*; (**c**) the beetle *Coccinella* and (**d**) the fly *Calliphora*. (After Brandt, E. (1878–1879). *Horae Societatis Entomologicae Rossicae (Trudӯ Russkago Éntomogicheshago Obshchestva*, **15**.)

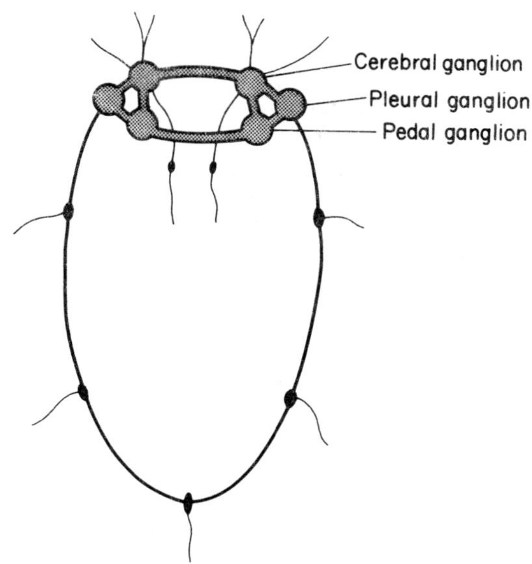


**Fig. 10.3** Diagram of the nervous system of a gastropod mollusc. (After Guiart, J. (1901). *Mémoires de la Société Zoologique de France*, **14,** 5–219.)

interconnecting nerves (Fig. 10.3), but in cephalopods the ganglia are mainly incorporated into a single brain. In echinoderms there are nerve rings, with radial nerves running out into the arms. In vertebrates the degree of cephalization is considerable, but still some local integration and control is carried out in the nerve cord.

**Arthropod central nervous system**

The arthropod central nervous system is composed of a dorsal brain (supraoesophageal ganglion), connected by a pair of circum-oesophageal connectives to a ventral suboesophageal ganglion, from the posterior end of which a paired ventral nerve cord arises interconnecting one of more ventral ganglia. Each of these ganglia bears pairs of lateral nerves, which are mostly mixed (i.e. contain both sensory and motor nerve fibres). In addition there is usually a median nerve associated with each ventral ganglion.

Information from the sense organs enters the central nervous system mainly through the lateral nerves. Axons from mechano-receptors on the body and appendages normally synapse with interneurons in the ganglion which they enter, but also run to ganglia further up the nerve cord, where they synapse with other inter-neurons (Fig. 10.4). Axons entering the brain from some mechano-receptors on the head run posteriorly, at least as far as the suboesophageal ganglion.

Interneurons which receive their input entirely from sensory neurons are called first order (primary) interneurons. Some pass along the nerve cord and synapse with other, higher order, inter-neurons, often collecting sensory information entering other ganglia on the way; others are contained within a single ganglion (amacrine cells of microneurons—see Chapter 1, Fig. 1.1g) and synapse either with other interneurons and/or with motor neurons; in the latter case they are involved in local reflexes.

Probably the best known local reflex in arthropods is the 'resist-ance reflex', so-called because passive movement of an appendage is 'resisted' by an active reflex movement in the opposite direction. It is elicited by stimulation of joint proprioceptors. This reflex is particu-larly well-documented in decapod crustaceans, where the receptors involved are the joint chordotonal organs (p. 140). Stimulation of one of these receptors by passive movement of the appropriate joint elicits excitation of the antagonistic muscle and, where a specific inhibitor is present, inhibition of the synergistic muscle as well. For example, in the crabs (Brachyura) passive opening of the most distal limb segment, the dactylopodite, stimulates sensory cells in the PD organ (p. 143); this produces a reflex response both in the slow closer motor axon (faster movements also produce a response in the fast closer motor axon) and in the opener inhibitor (Fig. 10.5). However, closing of the dactylopodite elicits a response in the opener/stretcher motor axon (a single motor axon innervates both the

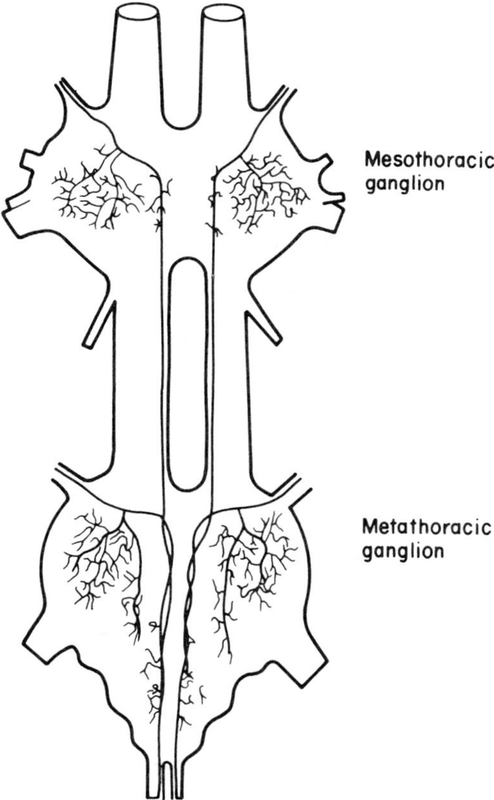


**Fig. 10.4** Diagram showing the central projections of the sensory neurons from the wing stretch receptors in the mesothoracic and metathoracic ganglia of the locust, *Locusta migratoria*. (From Huber, F. (1975). In '*Simple*' *Nervous Systems*. (Usherwood, P. N. R. and Newth, D. R., eds.) Edward Arnold, London. (Preparation by Bentlage and Huber.)

opener muscle of the dactylopodite and the stretcher muscle of the propodite in all decapod crustaceans), but not in the inhibitor to the closer muscle because, in this case, it is a common inhibitor and not specific to the closer muscle (Fig. 10.5).

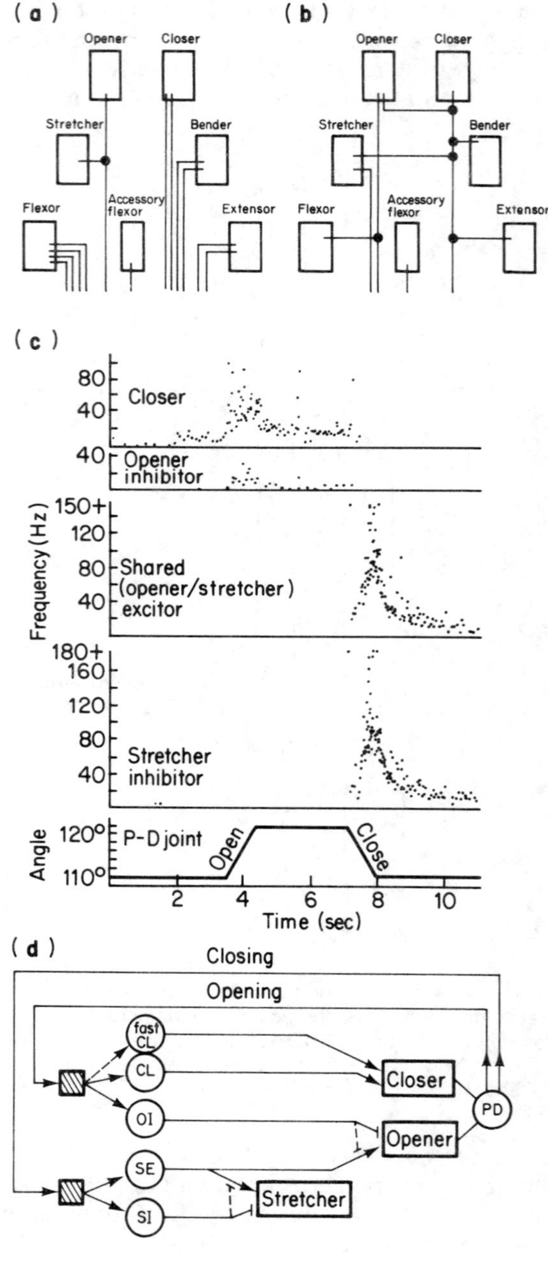
(a)
Opener
Closer
Stretcher
Bender
Flexor
Accessory flexor
Extensor
(b)
Opener
Closer
Stretcher
Bender
Flexor
Accessory flexor
Extensor
(c)
Closer
Opener inhibitor
Frequency (Hz)
Shared (opener/stretcher) excitor
Stretcher inhibitor
Angle
P-D joint
Open
Close
Time (sec)
(d)
Closing
Opening
fast CL
CL
OI
SE
SI
Closer
Opener
Stretcher
PD

Those interneurons which collect sensory information from the same side of the animal on which they lie are referred to as homolateral or ipsilateral interneurons, those which collect sensory information from the opposite side are called heterolateral or contralateral interneurons; while those which receive input from both sides are called bilateral interneurons (Fig. 10.6).

In the abdomen most of the primary and other low-order interneurons convey their information anteriorly (ascending interneurons), but in the circumoesophageal connectives there is quite a high proportion of descending low-order interneurons. The very high-order, pre-motor or command interneurons (Chapter 11) are predominantly descending interneurons which convey commands from the brain or other high level integrating centres and elicit specific behavioural patterns.

Much of the work on the integrative properties of interneurons has been carried out on crayfish. The circumoesophageal connectives in crayfish each contain about 3200 nerve fibres, most of which are interneurons, although there are three bundles of sensory fibres from specific groups of tactile receptors on the head. The size of the sensory field of individual interneurons varies from a small group of hairs to most or all of the proprioceptive input from the whole animal. Of those interneurons which carry tactile and proprioceptive input from various parts of single head appendages (eyes, antennules and antennae) most are homolateral (Fig. 10.7) and only those associated with the statocysts (p. 150) are known to continue

---

**Fig. 10.5** Diagrams showing the patterns of (**a**) excitatory and (**b**) inhibitory motor innervation of the muscles operating the three most distal joints of the limbs of crabs. Note the shared opener/stretcher excitor; also that the opener muscle shares an inhibitor with the flexor muscle and that the stretcher muscle has its own inhibitor, while the only inhibitory innervation of the closer muscle is a branch of the common inhibitor. (**c**) Instantaneous frequency plots of efferent (reflex) activity in various motor axons during imposed movements of the most distal joint (the dactylopodite) of a leg of the crab *Cardisoma guanhumi*. The bottom trace is a monitor record of these movements. (**d**) Model of a control system for resistance reflexes. The shaded squares represent 'control' units in the central nervous system. PD, joint chordotonal organ monitoring movement and position of the dactylopodite; →, excitatory connections; ⊣, inhibitory connections; CL, closer (excitor) motor neuron; fast CL, fast closer (excitor) motor neuron; OI, opener inhibitor motor neuron; SE, shared (opener/stretcher) excitor motor neuron; SI, stretcher inhibitor motor neuron. ((**a**), (**b**) After Wiersma, C. A. G. (1941). *Journal of Comparative Neurology*, **74,** 63–79; Wiersma, C. A. G. and Ripley, S. H. (1952). *Physiologia Comparata et Oecologia*, **2,** 391–405; Cohen, M. J. (1964). *Quarterly Journal of Microscopical Science*, **104,** 551–9 and Dorai Raj, B. S. (1964). *Journal of Cellular and Comparative Physiology*, **64,** 41–54. (**c**), (**d**) From Spirito, C. P. *et al.* (1972). *Zeitschrift für vergleichende Physiologie*, **76,** 1–15.)

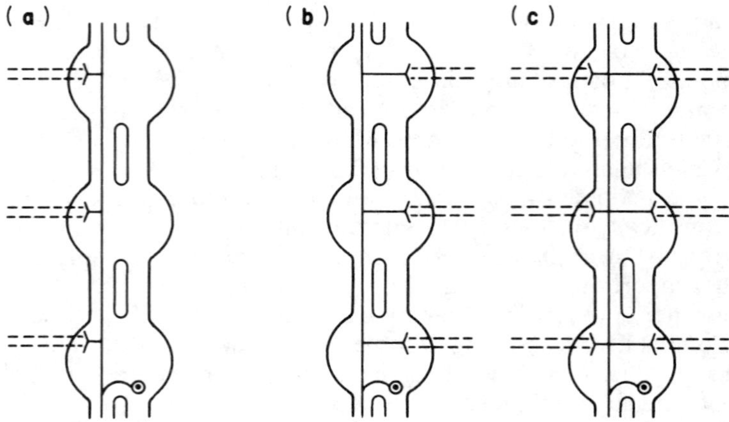


**Fig. 10.6** Diagrams of examples of (**a**) a homolateral or ipsilateral interneuron; (**b**) a heterolateral or contralateral interneuron and (**c**) a bilateral interneuron in the arthropod central nervous system. Note that the interneurons shown collect information from consecutive segments; also that this is not the case with all interneurons. (After Hughes, G. M. and Wiersma, C. A. G. (1960). *Journal of Experimental Biology*, **37,** 291–307.)

posteriorly as far as the abdominal nerve cord. There are numerous interneurons which respond to stimulation of more than one head appendage or of parts of the head or of a combination of both; a greater proportion of these are bilateral and a few extend as far as the abdominal nerve cord. Of the 50 identified interneurons which respond exclusively to stimulation of the head region, all but one integrate either tactile or proprioceptive information, but not both. There are also some descending interneurons which respond to stimulation of posterior regions of the body, either exclusively or together with regions of the head. These tend to have very extensive sensory fields, are mostly bilateral, and many integrate both tactile and proprioceptive inputs. There are a few interneurons in the connectives which respond to visual stimuli, either alone or together with mechanoreceptive information. In some cases the sensory fields of interneurons include inhibitory as well as excitatory zones. Those interneurons with large and/or complex sensory fields (which includes all those containing visual information) are of a very high order and some are probably command interneurons (see Chapter 11). Of the total population of identified descending interneurons in the circumoesophageal connectives, over 80% integrate information from only a single type (modality) of input.

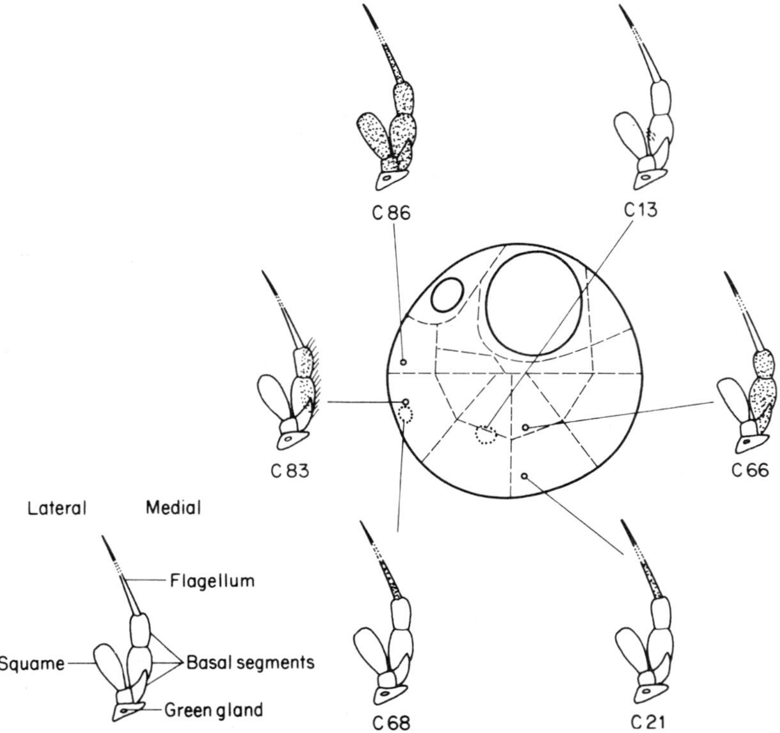


**Fig. 10.7** Diagram of a cross-section through the right circumoesophageal connective of a crayfish (*Procambarus clarkii*) to show the location of the two bundles of sensory axons (C13 and C68) and the four interneurons (C21, C66, C83 and C86) which respond exclusively to stimulation of the ipsilateral antenna; together with ventral views of the right antenna to illustrate the sensory fields (shaded areas). C is the prefix used to indicate that these units have been identified in the circumoesophageal connectives. The insert shows the parts of a right antenna. (From Wiersma, C. A. G. and Mill, P. J. (1965). *Journal of Comparative Neurology*, **125,** 67–94.)

## Vertebrates

In spite of the high degree of cephalization in vertebrates many reflex actions do not involve the brain directly, but occur in the spinal cord, although aspects of the response are affected by information from the brain.

As an example of vertebrate reflexes, those concerned with the knee joint and its involvement in the posture of the animal will be considered. Steady standing requires that the legs should be kept extended with the knee joint (and other joints) stiff. This is brought about by contraction of the appropriate knee extensor muscle, elicited by commands from the brain which pass down the spinothalamic tract and activate the extensor motor neurons. Tension is maintained in the muscle by continuous firing of the motor neurons. The flexor muscle of the joint is also maintained under slight tension.

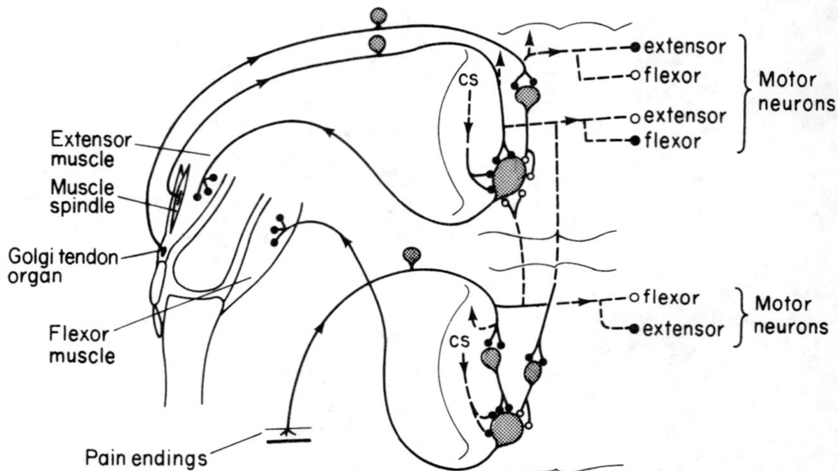


**Fig. 10.8** Diagram showing reflex pathways involving the knee joint of a cat. For simplicity the central neurons are displayed on two sections of the nerve cord. Note that the three sensory systems all send information anteriorly to the brain and have a reciprocal effect on the corresponding contralateral motor neurons. cs, corticospinal tracts from the brain; —● excitatory endings; —○ inhibitory endings. (From Roeder, K. D. (1963). *Nerve Cells and Insect Behaviour.* Harvard University Press, Cambridge, Mass; after Eccles, J. C. (1957). *The Physiology of Nerve Cells.* The Johns Hopkins Press, Baltimore.)

The muscle spindles (p. 135) in both muscles are active and their input to the central nervous system provides a feedback pathway to the motor neurons, which aids in the maintenance of posture. Thus even a slight extension of one of the muscles elicits an increase in its muscle spindle output; this causes an increase in the motor output to the muscle and a concomitant decrease in the motor output to its antagonist. Shortening of the muscle has the reverse effect. Hence the status quo of the posture is maintained. This will now be considered in more detail.

If the animal is loaded (e.g. a man may be given a weight to hold) there is a tendency for each knee extensor muscle to be stretched. This results in an increased discharge from the muscle spindles

(p. 135) and this input to the central nervous system directly excites the ipsilateral extensor motor neurons (Fig. 10.8). The result is an increase in their discharge frequency and a resultant increase in the tension of the ipsilateral knee joint extensor muscle. This is called the stretch or myotatic reflex. The muscle spindle activity also excites interneurons which inhibit the ipsilateral flexor motor neurons, causing a reduction in their activity and hence a reduction in the tension of the ipsilateral knee joint flexor muscle, the antagonist. The input from the muscle spindles also produces a reflex response in the contralateral extensor and flexor motor neurons which is opposite in effect, i.e. it inhibits the extensor motor neurons and excites the flexor motor neurons. However, these are much weaker reflexes than the ipsilateral ones and presumably aid in equilibrating the load between the limbs of the animal. Furthermore, there is a corresponding set of reflexes initiated by the muscle spindles in the flexor muscle.

If the loading on the animal is excessive the Golgi tendon organs (p. 145) in the extensor tendon are activated. The input to the central nervous system from these inhibits the extensor motor neurons, thereby reducing their output and allowing flexon (bending) of the knee joint (Fig. 10.8). This jackknife reflex overrides the stretch reflex and thus acts as an overload protection device for the muscle. As with the stretch reflex there is a weak contralateral effect of opposite sign.

Another protective mechanism comes into action if a foot encounters a sharp object. Pain endings in the skin are stimulated and their discharge has an inhibitory effect on the extensor motor neurons and an excitatory effect (via an interneuron) on the flexor motor neurons (Fig. 10.8), causing rapid flexing of the knee to lift the foot off the ground. The contralateral reflex, which again is of opposite sign, coupled with the stretch reflex at the other knee joint, enables the other limb to support the body. This protective reflex is initiated before one is conscious of pain and can be partly suppressed if the pain is consciously anticipated. In all of these reflexes information is also transmitted to the brain.

Figure 10.9 summarizes the various inputs to a single motor neuron. It should be obvious that such motor neurons do not act as simple relaying stations. The arrival of an action potential at a presynaptic terminal either increases (if it is excitatory) or decreases (if it is inhibitory) the likelihood of a postsynaptic impulse. In other words, the motor neuron output is a function of the sum of all its excitatory and inhibitory inputs. Furthermore, these will not all have the same importance, this being dependant on the number and

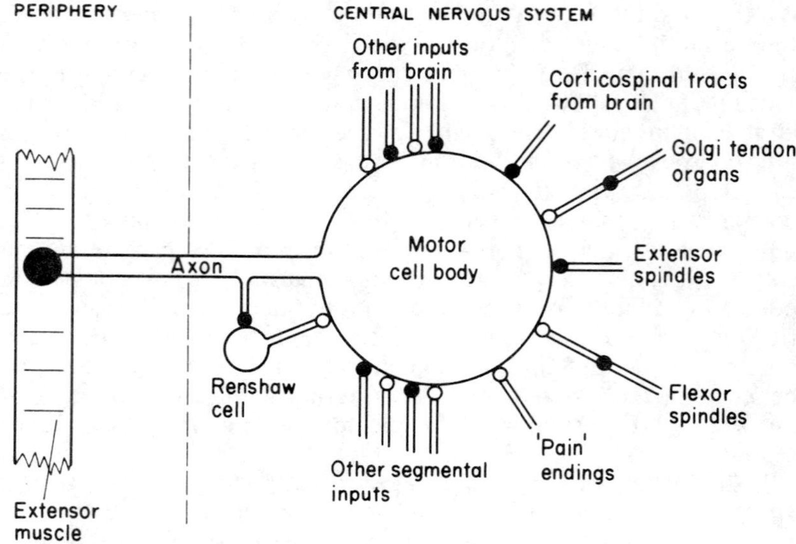


**Fig. 10.9** Diagram showing the inputs to a single knee extensor muscle motor neuron of a cat. Many of the inputs represented as single (e.g. Golgi tendon organs, extensor spindles, flexor spindles and 'pain' endings) are each representative of numerous inputs. —●, excitatory endings; —○, inhibitory endings. (From Roeder, K. D. (1963). *Nerve Cells and Insect Behaviour.* Harvard University Press, Cambridge, Mass.)

position with respect to the spike-initiating zone of the synaptic terminals of each presynaptic input.

As a further complication, the motor axon has a side branch which synapses with an interneuron called a Renshaw cell. Each impulse in the motor neuron causes a rapidly-adapting high frequency impulse train in the Renshaw cell. This has an inhibitory effect on the motor neuron; a good example of a negative feedback device, which presumably serves the function of a governor, protecting the muscle from excessive excitation.

## THE VERTEBRATE BRAIN

The brain appears somewhat different in the various classes of vertebrates (Fig. 10.10). However, it is always divisible into three main regions: hind, mid and fore (Fig. 10.11). In addition there is, in all vertebrates, a pair of olfactory lobes at the anterior end of the brain. These are particularly well-developed in those animals such as elasmobranchs which rely to a considerable extent on their olfactory

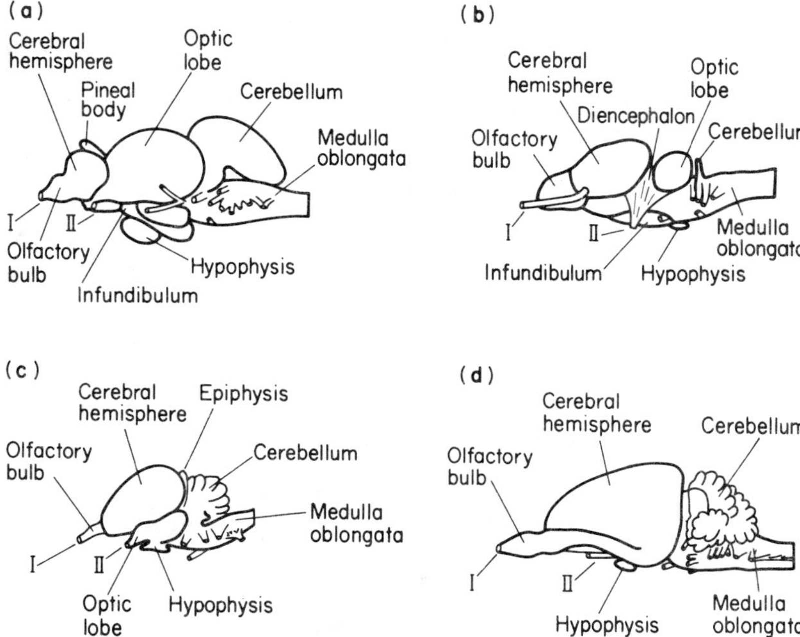


**Fig. 10.10** Diagrams of lateral views of the brains of (**a**) cod, (**b**) a frog, (**c**) a goose and (**d**) a horse. ((**a**), (**d**) After Wiedersheim, *Vertebrata*; (**b**) after Gaupp, E. (1896). *Anatomie des Frosches*, (Ecker, A. and Wiedersheim, R.). Vol. 1, third edition. Friedrich Vieweg und Sohn; (**c**) after Butschli and Ihle.)

sense. Also, on the ventral surface of the forebrain lies the pituitary gland, which secretes a number of hormones.

Within the brain is a series of cavities (ventricles) which are interconnected with each other and with the central canal of the spinal cord (Fig. 10.12). The hind brain contains the fourth ventricle; the midbrain contains the duct which links the third and fourth ventricles (the cerebral aqueduct); the forebrain comprises a posterior diencephalon which contains the third ventricle, and a pair of anterior lobes (the telencephalon) each of which contains a lateral ventricle. The cavities of the brain and spinal cord contain cerebrospinal fluid; materials can be exchanged between this fluid and the blood at two thin-walled, highly vascularized regions called choroid plexuses. The anterior choroid plexus lies in the anterior dorsal wall of the third ventricle; the posterior choroid plexus lies in the posterior dorsal wall of the fourth ventricle (Fig. 10.11). Elsewhere the lining of the ventricles is composed of nervous tissue.

The spinal (nerve) cord has a peripheral zone of myelinated nerve fibres (the white matter) and a central zone which is composed mainly of cell bodies (the grey matter). In transverse sections of the cord the grey matter is 'H' shaped. Within the grey matter there are four main columns on each side which run longitudinally along the

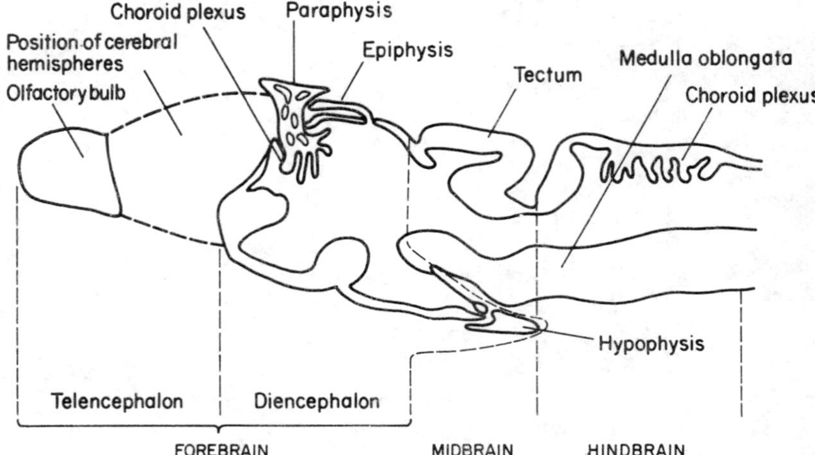


**Fig. 10.11** Diagram of a median section of the vertebrate brain to show the principal divisions. (After Gaupp, E. (1896). *Anatomie des Frosches*, (Ecker, A. and Wiedersheim, R.). Vol. 1, third edition. Friedrich Vieweg und Sohn.)

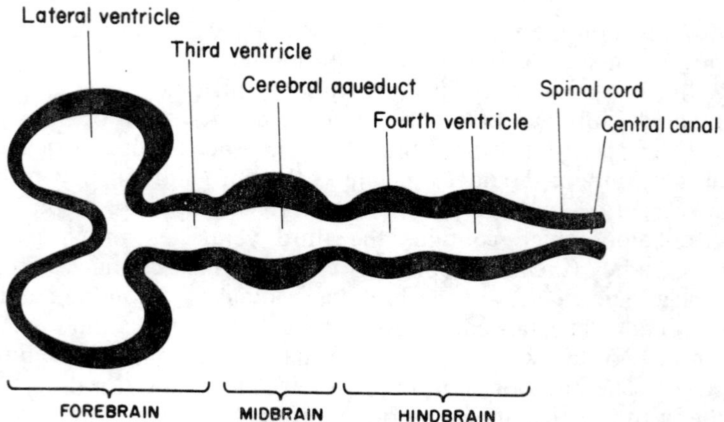


**Fig. 10.12** Diagram to show the positions of the ventricles of the vertebrate brain. (From Gardner, E. (1952). *Fundamentals of Neurology*, 2nd edition. W. B. Saunders.)

nerve cord. The somatic and visceral sensory columns lie dorsally, while the somatic and visceral motor columns lie ventrally (Fig. 10.13). This basic pattern is maintained through the hindbrain (Fig. 10.14) and into the posterior region of the midbrain.

**Hindbrain**

The floor and sides of the hindbrain are collectively called the medulla oblongata or brain stem, and in higher vertebrates the anterior region of this is referred to as the pons. The pons is the origin of cranial nerves IV to VII, the medulla of cranial nerves IX to XII. As mentioned above, the basic pattern of the sensory and motor columns of the nerve cord is also found in the hind brain. From

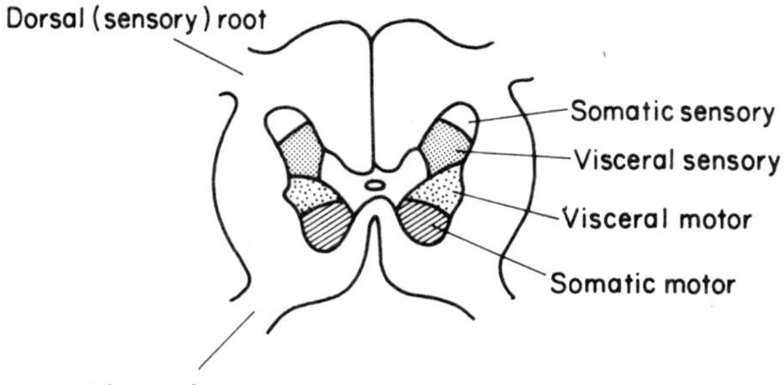


**Fig. 10.13** Diagram showing the distribution of the sensory and motor regions in a transverse section of the spinal cord of a vertebrate. (After Minckler, J. (1972). In *Introduction to Neuroscience*. (Minckler, J. ed.) C. V. Mosby, Saint Louis.)

ventral to dorsal on each side these columns are somatic motor, visceral motor (divisible into branchial and autonomic), visceral sensory and somatic sensory columns. However, in higher vertebrates the columns in the brain are more or less separated into discrete groups of cells called nuclei. The relationship between these nuclei and the cranial nerves is shown in Fig. 10.14. In addition to the main columns a special respiratory centre has developed in the motor region and there is a special sensory area for the acoustico-lateralis system above the somatic sensory column. In land vertebrates the acoustic part persists; in mammals there are distinct centres for hearing and balance. A notable feature of the medulla in fishes and in amphibians which possess tails is the presence of a pair of giant Mauthner cells, the axons of which extend along the whole nerve cord. These cells, which are closely associated with the acoustico-lateralis centre, are command neurons (see Chapter 11) for the locomotory system.

Also in the medulla is the reticular formation, which extends posteriorly into the anterior part of the nerve cord and anteriorly through the midbrain. It receives sensory input from all over the body, although it is not in the direct route of sensory input to the higher centres. The hindbrain and nerve cord portions of this

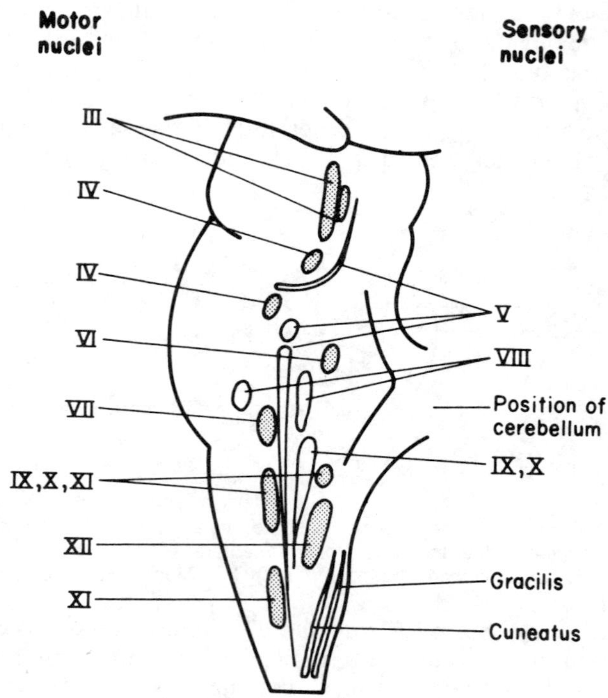


**Fig. 10.14** Diagram of a longitudinal section through the mid and hind brain and spinal cord of a mammal to show the arrangement of the sensory and motor nuclei. (After Minckler, J. (1972). In *Introduction to Neuroscience*. (Minckler, J., ed.) C. V. Mosby, Saint Louis.)

structure serve as a motor coordinating and relaying system. However, in higher vertebrates the major pathways to the motor nuclei bypass the reticular formation. In birds the motor pathways from the corpus striatum run first to the tegmentum and thence to the motor nuclei; in mammals the motor pathways from the cerebral cortex run direct to the motor nuclei (see below).

Two other regions, which will be discussed in more detail when dealing with the midbrain portion of the reticular formation (p. 210), are the nuclei of raphe and the locus coeruleus. The nuclei of raphe lie in the midline and extend from the anterior region of the medulla through the pons to the posterior region of the midbrain. The locus coeruleus consists of a pair of nuclei lying in the dorsal region of the pons.

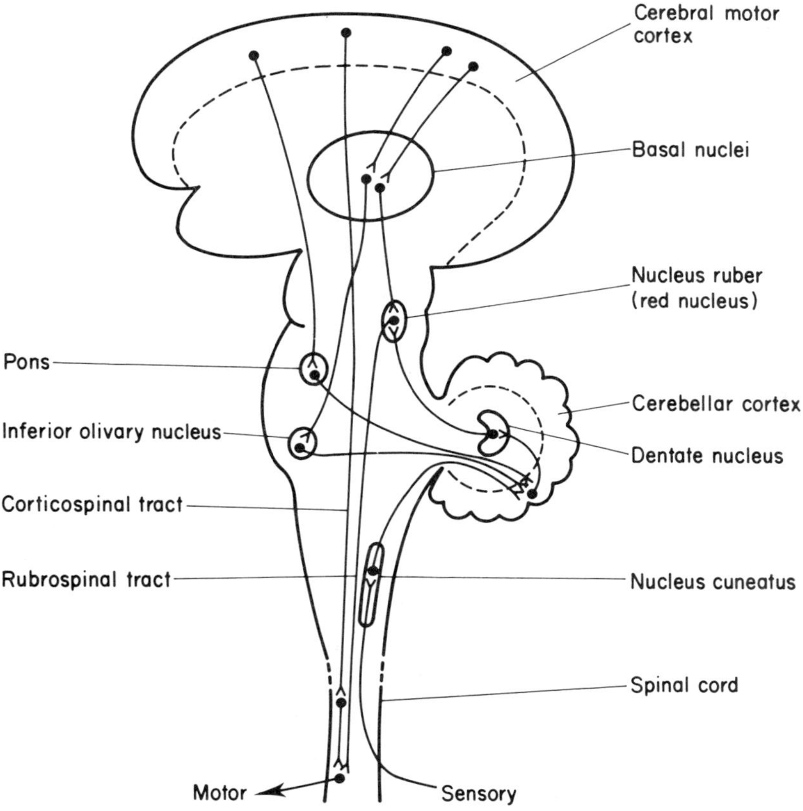

**Fig. 10.15** Diagram to show the main interconnections between the cerebellum and the other regions of the brain of a mammal. (After Minckler, J. (1972). In *Introduction to Neuroscience.* (Minckler, J., ed.) C. V. Mosby, Saint Louis.)

A structure called the cerebellum lies on the dorsal surface at the anterior end of the hindbrain. Its primitive role is the maintenance of equilibrium, using information from the receptors of the inner ear. However, in most, if not all, classes of vertebrate this input is integrated with that from the muscle spindles, which ascends into the cerebellum via a pair of posterior peduncles (tracts) (Fig. 10.15).

There is, in addition, some input to the cerebellum from the various skin receptors, from the visual system and, in lower vertebrates, from the olfactory system. The cerebellum is small in amphibians and most reptiles, but is well-developed in fish, birds and mammals.

The cerebellum also receives information from the higher centres which elicit muscular movements. In mammals the motor cortex of the cerebral hemispheres is primarily responsible for this control, and the information runs first to the pons and thence to the cerebellum

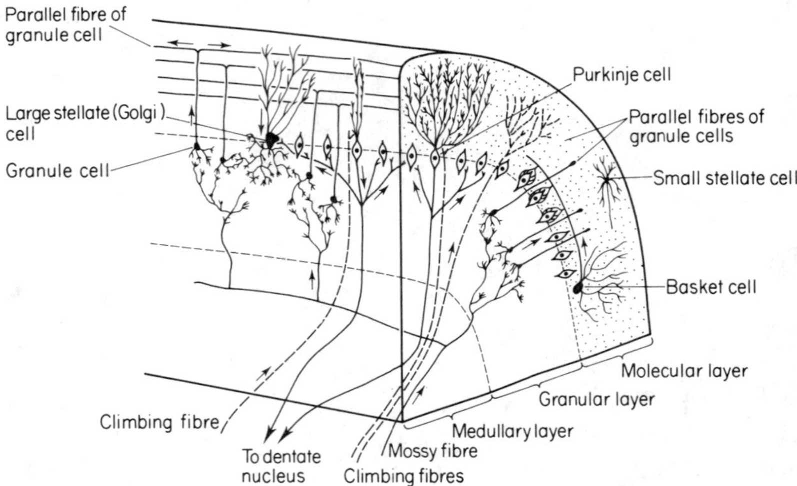


**Fig. 10.16** Diagram to show the arrangement of the principal cellular components and their interconnections in the mammalian cerebellum. The arrows indicate the direction of information transmission. (After Crosby, E. C., Humphrey, T. and Laver, E. W. (1962). *Correlative Anatomy of the Nervous System*. The Macmillan Co., New York.)

via a pair of lateral peduncles. Indeed, in mammals the cerebellum has an important role in the control of motor functions and, commensurate with this, a convoluted pair of cerebellar hemispheres has evolved. In these hemispheres there is a peripheral cellular cortex (grey matter) surrounding the internal white (fibrous) matter. The cortex is organized into layers and contains a number of different cell types (Fig. 10.16). The large Purkinje cells, which have highly branched dendritic trees, receive both excitatory inputs (from the granule cells and the climbing fibres) and inhibitory inputs; their axons convey information to the central nucleus of the cerebellum.

The output from the cerebellum is via paired anterior peduncles to, in most vertebrates, the tegmentum of the midbrain, from where it passes to the various motor nuclei of the midbrain, hindbrain and nerve cord. However, in mammals the output runs direct to the thalamus of the midbrain and then to the cerebral cortex.

**Midbrain**

The roof of the midbrain forms the tectum, the cells of which lie peripheral to the white matter, as in the cerebellar cortex and the cerebral cortex. In lower vertebrates the tectum is primarily concerned with vision and is termed the optic tectum. However, the tectum also receives input from the acoustico-lateralis and olfactory systems and from the somatosensory nuclei, and is interconnected to the cerebellum. In fishes and amphibians it is the main association and motor control centre of the central nervous system. While it is still extremely important in this respect in reptiles, in birds it is partly subservient to the corpus striatum of the cerebral hemispheres. In mammals the cerebral cortex is the major region of association and motor control, and the tectum is relatively unimportant, with most sensory information (including visual) being relayed via the thalamus (in the diencephalon) to the cerebral cortex. Indeed, in mammals the tectum is reduced to two pairs of nuclei, the corpora quadrigemina. The anterior pair (representing the optic lobes of lower vertebrates) are responsible for visual reflexes; the posterior pair relay auditory information to the cerebral cortex via the thalamus.

The side walls of the midbrain constitute the tegmentum, which is an anterior continuation of the motor areas of the medulla oblongata, and acts as a coordinating and relaying station for information directed to the motor nuclei from the diencephalon, tectum and cerebellum.

The reticular formation has already been mentioned when dealing with the hindbrain (p. 207). The very considerable sensory input which it receives is associated with the importance of the midbrain portion in arousing the cerebral cortex and keeping it alert. Consequently the midbrain portion is termed the reticular activating system (RAS). When changing from wakefulness to sleep the activity of the RAS is suppressed. In mammals two states of sleep occur. Light sleep is almost always the first stage in adults and is typified by the maintenance of tension in the neck muscles. This is followed by deep sleep (alternatively called REM (rapid eye movement) sleep or paradoxical sleep), which is characterized by rapid eye movements and fast cortical waves, similar to those of wakefulness, coupled with lack of tension in the neck muscles. (The presence of the fast cortical waves has given rise to the term 'paradoxical sleep'.) It is during this deep sleep that dreaming occurs. Light sleep is apparently induced by suppression of the RAS by the nuclei of raphe (p. 207), the cells of which contain the neurotransmitter 5-HT (p. 63); while deep sleep results from suppression of the RAS by the locus coeruleus (p. 207), the cells of which contain the neurotransmitter noradrenaline (p. 63). In the adult cat about 35% of its time is spent in wakefulness, 50% in light sleep and 15% in deep sleep. The time spent in deep sleep as a proportion of the time spent in light sleep is thus 30%. This proportion is also quite high (about 20%) in other carnivores, such as the dog, and in man, but in ruminants is only 5–10%.

**Forebrain (Diencephalon)**

The side walls of the diencephalon contain a number of sensory and motor nuclei, comprising the dorsal thalamus and the ventral thalamus respectively. The dorso-lateral region of the diencephalon forms the epithalamus; the floor forms the hypothalamus. In some animals one or a pair of pineal organs arise from the roof.

The epithalamus is of comparatively little importance. In contrast, the hypothalamus is the primary site of integration for the internal (visceral) activities of the body and hence is interconnected with the autonomic nervous system. Apart from its visceral sensory input, it also receives information from olfactory and gustatory (taste) receptors. It exercises control over the pituitary gland, with some nuclei secreting hormones which travel to the neurohypophysis of the pituitary, and it regulates body temperature in homoiotherms. In mammals it also regulates, for example, heart rate, blood pressure and respiratory rate.

In lower vertebrates some sensory information is relayed to the cerebral hemispheres via the dorsal thalamus for synthesis with olfactory information. The importance of the dorsal thalamus as a sensory relaying centre increases with the development of the cerebral hemispheres as the major association centre of the brain and indeed, in mammals, most (if not all) somatic sensory information, except olfactory, is routed this way to the cerebral cortex. The three main pairs of nuclei of the dorsal thalamus are the ventrobasal complex or ventral nuclei (somatosensory information, p. 216), the medial geniculate nuclei (auditory information, p. 218) and the lateral geniculate nuclei (visual information, p. 219). The ventral thalamus is a motor coordinating centre and also relays information from the cerebral hemispheres to the motor nuclei.

**Forebrain (Telencephalon)**

The telencephalon consists of a pair of cerebral hemispheres, each with an olfactory bulb connected to its anterior end, and indeed, the hemispheres originated as centres for the coordination of olfactory stimuli. This is still the case in cyclostomes, where the coordinated information is relayed posteriorly to the hypothalamus or via the epithalamus to the tectum, in which centres most of the correlation with other sensory input occurs. However, during the course of evolution the cerebral hemispheres have come to contain the primary association and command centres of the brain.

The original olfactory nucleus is called the paleopallium (Fig. 10.17a). At an early stage in evolution two other cellular areas

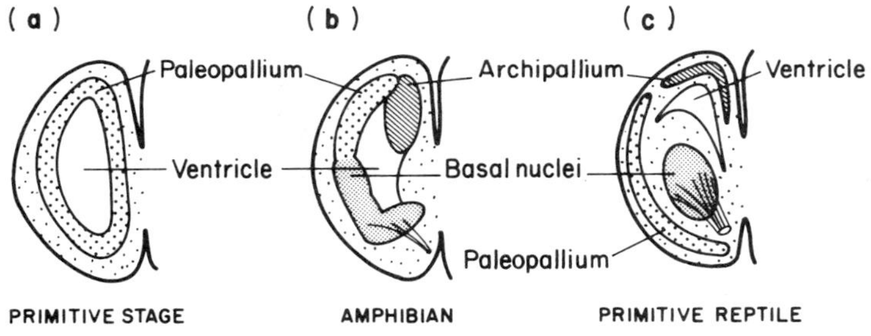


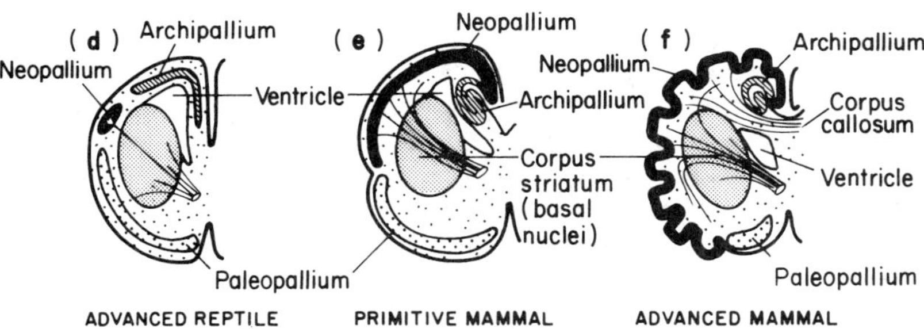


**Fig. 10.17** Diagrams of transverse sections through the left cerebral hemisphere of various vertebrates. (From Romer, A. S. and Parsons, T. S. (1977). *The Vertebrate Body*, 5th edition. Copyright © 1977 by W. B. Saunders Company. Copyright 1970, 1962, 1955, and 1949 by W. B. Saunders Company. Adapted by permission of Holt, Rinehart and Winston.

developed in the cerebral hemispheres, a ventral basal nucleus and a dorso-medial archipallium, with the resultant restriction of the paleopallium to the lateral region. This is the stage obtaining in modern amphibians (Fig. 10.17b). In successive stages leading to the reptiles and mammals, the basal nucleus has remained internal in each cerebral hemisphere (and is called the corpus striatum in mammals because of the number of tracts traversing it), while the paleopallium and the archipallium have moved peripherally to form the cerebral cortex (Fig. 10.17c). In higher reptiles a small neopallium has developed in the cortex between the paleopallium and the archipallium (Fig. 10.17d). This has become progressively more extensive during mammalian evolution (Fig. 10.17e), with the resultant displacement of the paleopallium ventrally to form the pyriform (olfactory) lobe, and the archipallium medially and internally to form the hippocampus (Fig. 10.17f). The hippocampus is concerned with 'emotional' behaviour and is connected to the hypothalamus via a tract called the fornix.

In teleosts and birds, both of which groups rely little on olfaction, the cellular regions of the cerebral hemispheres are arranged somewhat differently. In teleosts the basal nucleus of each hemisphere is internal, but so also is the rest of the grey matter, the epistratum; a cerebral cortex as such has not developed. In birds there is a poorly-developed cerebral cortex which consists largely of the archipallium, there being no neopallium in birds. However, the basal nucleus (called the corpus striatum, as in mammals) is very large.

The corpus striatum becomes progressively more important as a correlation centre during the course of evolution, integrating olfaction with the other sensory inputs, which are relayed to it via the dorsal thalamus. It reaches its maximum state of development in birds, where it is probably the seat of the multitudinous innate behaviour patterns of the members of this class. Its dorsal region, the hyperstriatum, is the centre responsible for memory and learning. The output of the corpus striatum is via the ventral thalamus to the midbrain tegmental region.

However, in mammals it is the neopallium which is the seat of memory and learning. Throughout mammalian evolution the neopallium has become more and more extensive and elaborate, reaching its peak of development in the highly folded cerebral cortex of man. In placental mammals the neopallia of the two cerebral hemispheres are interconnected by a large fibre tract, the corpus callosum. Commensurate with its development, the neopallial cerebral cortex has progressively taken over the higher correlative and associative functions of other centres such as the corpus striatum and the tectum. The corpus striatum, however, has remained concerned with the regulation of muscle tone. As mentioned above (p. 211) all of the sensory input to the neopallium, except olfaction, is relayed via the dorsal thalamus. In reptiles the output is via the ventral thalamus to the motor nuclei, but in mammals there is a direct tract (the pyramidal tract) to the motor nuclei. There is also output to the cerebellum via the pons.

In primitive mammals the basic pattern of the brain can still be seen, but in most mammals the elaboration of the cerebral cortex has involved a posterior and ventral extension of the cerebral hemispheres, thereby covering the midbrain and part of the cerebellum (Figs. 10.18, 10.19). The folds in the cortex are called convolutions, while the gaps between them are termed fissures. The two hemispheres are separated on the dorsal aspect by the ***median***

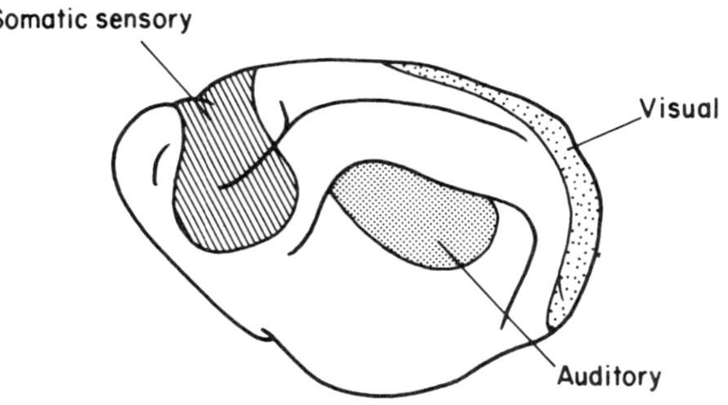


**Fig. 10.18** Diagram showing a lateral view of the cerebral cortex of the cat to illustrate the sensory projection areas. (After Best, L. G. (1972). In *Introduction to Neuroscience* (Minckler, J. ed.). C. V. Mosby, Saint Louis.)

***longitudinal fissure***. Each hemisphere has two main fissures at right angles to the longitudinal axis—the ***central fissure*** on the dorsolateral surface and the ***sylvian fissure*** on the ventro-lateral surface (Fig. 10.19a). These delimit four regions in each hemisphere—the frontal, parietal, occipital and temporal lobes.

Functionally, the cortex can be divided into three zones—sensory, motor and association (Fig. 10.19b). The sensory cortex comprises a somatosensory cortex in the parietal lobe, an auditory cortex in the temporal lobe and a visual cortex in the occipital lobe. The motor cortex, which is primarily concerned with the coordination of voluntary actions, is located in the frontal lobe anterior to the central fissure. The remainder of the frontal lobe is concerned with 'higher' brain functions, such as thought, and is referred to as the association cortex. Most sensory information ultimately ends up on the opposite side of the brain to that on which it enters the animal. Similarly, motor centres in the cortex control the opposite side of the animal.

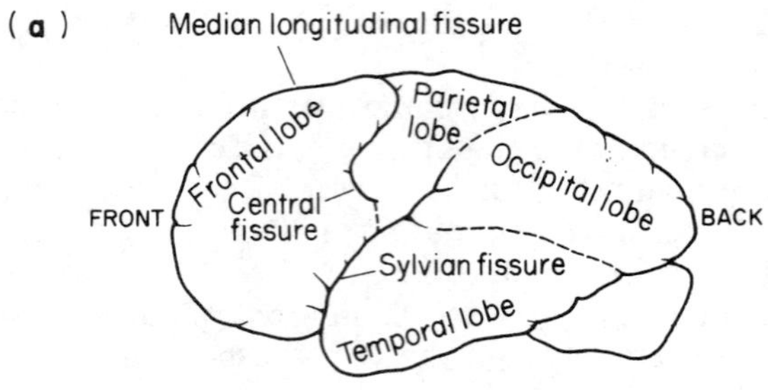


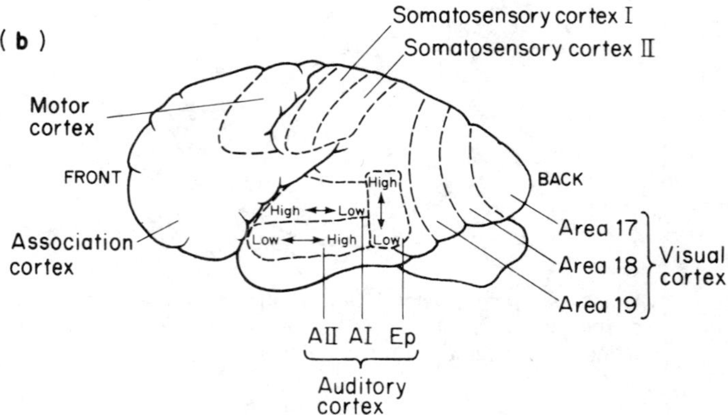


**Fig. 10.19** Diagrams of lateral views of the cerebral cortex of man showing (**a**) the principal fissures and anatomical areas and (**b**) the physiological areas. (After Ludel, J. (1978). *Introduction to Sensory Processes*. W. H. Freeman and Co., San Francisco. Copyright © 1978.)

## Synopsis of brain structure and function

The cerebellum arose as an integrating centre for the acousticolateralis system, the tectum for the visual system and the paleopallium of the cerebral hemispheres for the olfactory system. Each region, as it developed, came to receive input from other sensory modalities for comparison and integration, and exercised some measure of control over the motor nuclei. Furthermore, these are the only areas of the brain in which the cellular layer has become peripheral, forming a cortex. Functionally, a corresponding centre for the visceral system has developed in the hypothalamus.

During evolution the cerebral hemispheres assumed increasing dominance over the other two somatic centres. This has been so marked in the case of the visual system that, in mammals, most visual input is relayed to the neopallium via the dorsal thalamus, without passing to the tectum. However, the cerebellum has retained an important correlative function and, in mammals, strong interconnections occur between it and the cerebral hemispheres. Nevertheless, it is subservient to the cerebral hemispheres in higher vertebrates. In reptiles and, more particularly, in birds the corpus striatum has gained dominance, whereas in mammals it is the neopallium which has increased in importance to become the primary centre for correlation, association and learning. Indeed, the mammalian neopallium has a direct output to the motor nuclei, in contrast to that of the corpus striatum of birds, which is relayed via the ventral thalamus.

We are now in a position to consider what happens to different modalities of sensory information once they enter the central nervous system. As an example the mammalian system will be described.

**Somatosensory information**

Somatosensory information is that from the skin receptors—touch, pressure, temperature and pain. There are two pathways or systems for somatosensory information—the lemniscal and the extralemniscal (spinothalamic). Information from all of the categories of skin receptors probably enters each system, but there appears to be a predominance of touch sensitivity in the lemniscal system and of temperature sensitivity and pain in the extralemniscal system.

The lemniscal system is a relatively fast pathway involving only three orders of neurons before the sensory cortex is reached (Fig. 10.20a). The first order (sensory) neurons enter the nerve cord and run anteriorly in the dorsal tract, on the same side as they enter the nerve cord, to the dorsal tract nuclei of the medulla, where they synapse with second order neurons (first order interneurons, cp. p. 196). The second order neurons convey the information along ribbon-like tracts, the medial lemnisci, which cross over to the ventrobasal complex on the contralateral side of the thalamus. Third order interneurons then relay the information, without any further crossing over, to an area of the somatosensory cortex called somatosensory cortex I (Fig. 10.19b). Thus the right side of the body is represented on the left side of the thalamus and cortex, and vice versa.

Both the ventrobasal complex and somatosensory cortex I contain a very precise topographic projection (map) of the surface of the body. Thus adjacent areas of the body are represented in adjacent

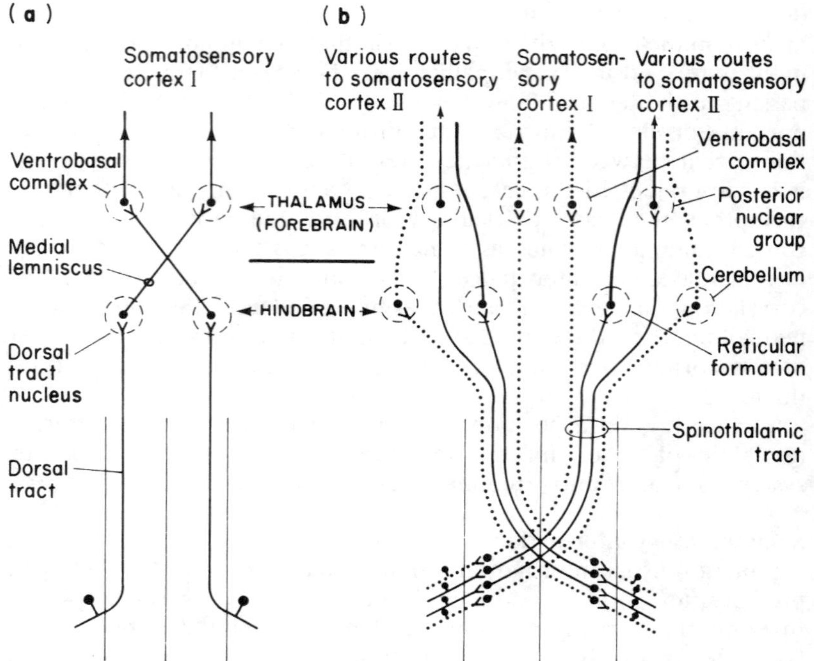


**Fig. 10.20** Diagram showing the central pathways of somatosensory information. (**a**) The lemniscal system and (**b**) the extralemniscal system. ——, major pathways; ·······, minor pathways.

areas of these parts of the brain (i.e. stimulation of adjacent areas of the body activates neurons in adjacent areas in both the ventrobasal complex and somatosensory cortex I). Furthermore, within each location the neurons responding to each stimulus modality are grouped together. In somatosensory cortex I the cells responsive to a single stimulus modality (for each region of the body) are arranged in a column at right angles to the surface of the cortex, and different stimulus modalities are represented by adjacent columns of cells. It follows that each neuron at both of these levels has its own receptive field. This field is unique for each neuron, although the receptive fields of adjacent neurons may overlap. In the ventrobasal complex the size of the receptive field is indicative of the sensitivity of the part of the body concerned. Thus sensitive areas (e.g. fingers and lips) contain more receptors than other, less sensitive regions, and the size of the receptive fields of the central neurons is correspondingly small. This is also the case in somatosensory cortex I, although here all of the receptive fields are fairly small and, in most cases, are surrounded by an inhibitory region, which presumably serves to enhance localization of a stimulus.

The extralemniscal system provides a much slower pathway to the cortex, with up to seven neurons between the periphery and the cortex (Fig. 10.20b). The first order (sensory) neurons enter the nerve cord and immediately synapse ipsilaterally with second order neurons. These cross over to the opposite side of the cord and run anteriorly in the spinothalamic tracts, most going to the reticular formation in the brain stem or to the posterior nuclear group in the thalamus, but with some running to the ventrobasal complex or the cerebellum. Most of the information in the extralemniscal system ultimately reaches somatosensory cortex II, the area of cortex adjacent and posterior to somatosensory cortex I (Fig. 10.19b). In complete contrast to the ventrobasal complex, there is no topographical relationship between the periphery and the neurons in the posterior nuclear group of the thalamus, either in terms of area or stimulus modality. There is some anatomical relationship in somatosensory cortex II, but it is not nearly as precise as in somatosensory cortex I. Furthermore, many of the neurons in both the posterior nuclear group and somatosensory cortex II are multimodal, i.e. they respond to more than one stimulus modality, and their receptive fields are very large.

Information from the head region enters the medulla directly, from where most is sent to the ventrobasal complex of the thalamus and thence to somatosensory cortex I.

**Auditory information**

Sensory information from each ear enters the brain via the VIIIth (auditory) cranial nerve, and the first order (sensory) neurons synapse in the brain stem in the dorsal or ventral cochlear nuclei or in the superior olivary nuclei (Fig. 10.21). The second order neurons connect these nuclei to the inferior colliculi in the midbrain. Third order neurons then relay the information to the medial geniculate nuclei of the thalamus, from where fourth order neurons transmit it to the auditory cortex. There is some crossing-over of information, notably at the lower levels, and so, unlike in the somatosensory system, information from each ear arrives on both sides of the cortex.

Each neuron of the auditory cortex responds maximally to a particular, small range of frequency of sound. The auditory cortex can be subdivided into three regions, AI, AII and Ep (Fig. 10.19b), in all of which there is a gradation of response with respect to the frequency of sound, with neurons at one end of each region responding to high frequencies, those at the other end to low frequencies, and intermediate frequencies represented by neurons between the two ends; i.e. there is a tonotopic map in each region.

To detect the direction of a sound, the time of arrival, relative intensity and phase difference between the ears are utilized. Thus a sound occurring to one side of an animal will arrive at the ear on that side first, where it will also sound louder than, and be out of phase

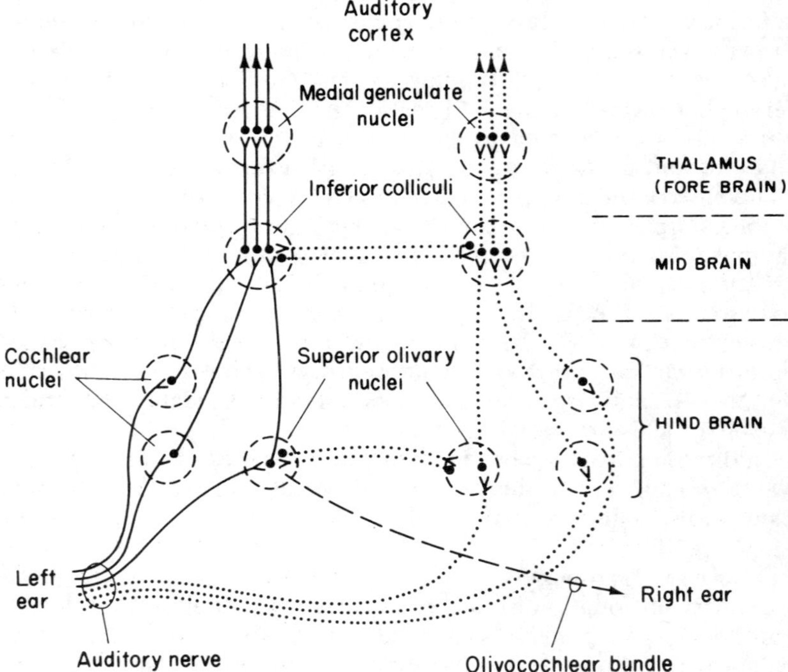


**Fig. 10.21** Diagram showing the central pathways of auditory information from the left ear. ——, major pathways; ·······, minor pathways; ––––, olivocochlear bundle. (After Ludel, J. (1978). *Introduction to Sensory Processes*. W. H. Freeman and Co., San Francisco. Copyright © 1978.)

with, the sound arriving at the opposite ear, because the sound waves have to travel around the head. It is difficult to locate sounds whose source is equidistant from each ear, i.e. to distinguish a sound from directly in front from one directly behind, since the time of arrival, the intensities and the phase will be the same at both ears.

In the superior olivary nuclei some neurons have a greater response to sounds arriving at the left ear before the right ear, and to sounds which are louder at the left ear than at the right ear; others respond in the reverse manner. Thus the time of arrival of a sound and its intensity are directly correlated in these neurons. Furthermore, there is a central mechanism which enhances the localization of sound. Some neurons run from each superior olivary nucleus to the contralateral ear (in the olivocochlear bundle), where they have an inhibitory effect on the cochlear afferents. Since each superior olivary nucleus receives most of its information from the ipsilateral ear, sounds which occur first and are louder at one ear cause greater inhibition of the contralateral input.

**Visual information**

The information from the eyes travels in the optic nerves to the optic chiasma, where the nerves apparently cross each other. What really happens here, however, is that the axons from the lateral region of each retina remain on the ipsilateral side, while the axons from the medial region of each retina cross over to the contralateral side of the brain (Fig. 10.22). Central to the optic chiasma, the axons run in the optic tracts. Much of the visual information travels direct to the lateral geniculate nuclei of the thalamus, from where it is carried by second-order neurons to the visual cortex. However, some axons run to the pregeniculate nuclei and others to the superior colliculi. These are motor centres which control, respectively, the muscles of the iris and the extraocular (eye movement) muscles.

The ganglion cells of the retina, whose axons constitute the optic nerves and tracts, exhibit four types of receptive field, all of which are circular (p. 182, see Fig. 9.13). This basic shape of the receptive fields is preserved by the cells of the lateral geniculate nuclei, where details of colour are analysed, but at this level they are all of the centre-surround type. Some have an on-centre and an off-surround, or vice versa, irrespective of the wavelength of the light. Most, however, have a central zone excited by one wavelength and a surround inhibited by a different wavelength. Four types of cell are colour-coded in this way with respect to red and green lights; four more with respect to yellow and blue lights (Fig. 10.23). These colour-coded neurons receive their input from the three types of cones. Thus the red-green cells integrate information from the 530 nm and 565 nm cones, while the yellow-blue cells integrate information from the 440 nm and 565 nm cones (p. 179).

Other aspects of vision are analysed in the visual cortex, where the receptive fields of individual cells are more complicated. The dendrites and somas of the second order neurons in the lateral geniculate nuclei are organized into layers and the information from

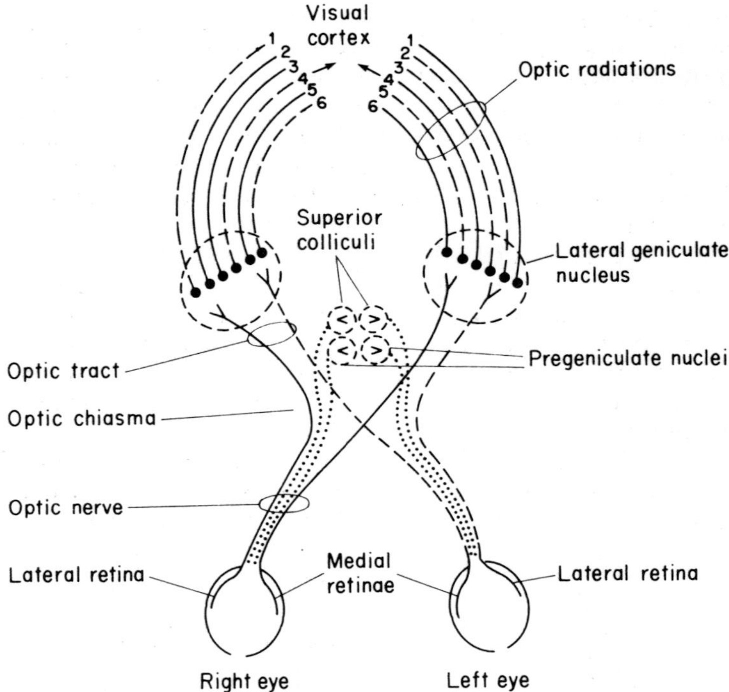


**Fig. 10.22** Diagram showing the central pathways of visual information. ——, major pathways from the right eye; ----, major pathways from the left eye; ········, minor pathways. (After Ludel, J. (1978). *Introduction to Sensory Processes*. W. H. Freeman and Co., San Francisco. Copyright © 1978.)

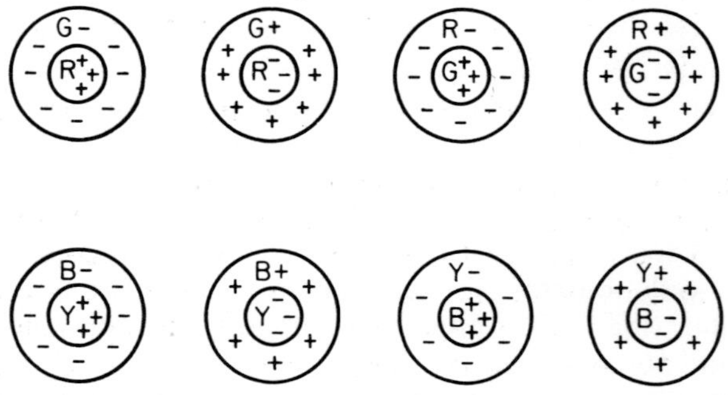


**Fig. 10.23** Diagrams to show the receptive fields of colour-coded neurons in the lateral geniculate nuclei of the thalamus. B, blue; G, green; R, red; Y, yellow; +, excitatory; −, inhibitory. (After Ludel, J. (1978). *Introduction to Sensory Processes*. W. H. Freeman and Co., San Francisco. Copyright © 1978.)

the two eyes is kept separate at this level. On each side, information from the ipsilateral eye is processed by layers 2, 3 and 5, and information from the contralateral eye by layers 1, 4 and 6 (Fig. 10.22). These second order neurons run to area 17 (the most posterior area) of the visual cortex (see Fig. 10.19b) in the optic radiations. Third order neurons then carry the information to area 18 and fourth order neurons to area 19. The information from the two eyes is combined in the visual cortex and each of the three areas contains a precise map of the retina (a retinotopic map). For example, in area 17 the fovea is represented at the posterior end of the area, while the periphery of the retina is represented by the anterior border of the area. Furthermore, cells with a similar type and orientation of receptive field (see below) from a given region of the retina occur in a column; adjacent columns containing cells with different orientations of the receptive field.

Areas 17, 18 and 19 all contain simple and complex cells. The simple cells have ellipsoidal receptive fields with both on and off zones (Fig. 10.24). Maximal excitation of these cells is achieved when

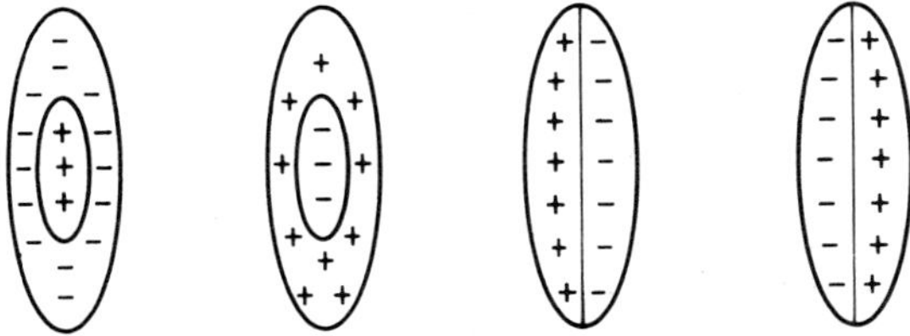

**Fig. 10.24** Diagrams to show the receptive fields of simple cells in the visual cortex. Note that, in addition to the different types of receptive field, the orientation of the visual field is variable for different cells (not shown). +, excitatory; −, inhibitory. (After Ludel, J. (1978). *Introduction to Sensory Processes*. W. H. Freeman and Co., San Francisco. Copyright © 1978.)

the on zone is completely covered by light, without any of the off zone (which is inhibitory) being covered. This is achieved experimentally by using a bar of light of appropriate length, width and orientation (different cells have differently oriented receptive fields). If the bar is moved away from its optimum position there will be a reduction in the firing frequency of the cell due, in the simple cells, to stimulation of the off zone. The complex cells, however, do not have an off zone. Nevertheless, the optimal form of stimulus is the same as for simple cells (a light bar), except that the length of the bar of light in the receptive field is unimportant. Areas 18 and 19 contain, in addition, lower order and higher order hypercomplex cells. The lower order hypercomplex cells are similar to complex cells, except that the length of the bar of light in the receptive field is important. Higher order hypercomplex cells are similar to lower order ones, in that the width and the length of the light bar are important, but the orientation of the bar is not critical.

### Olfactory information

The axons in the olfactory nerve end in the olfactory nucleus within the olfactory bulb. From here the information passes along the olfactory tract to the cerebral hemispheres. In cyclostomes the cellular layer, the paleopallium, is solely concerned with olfaction and this information is subsequently relayed to more posterior centres (p. 211). The olfactory input also runs to the archipallium and the basal nuclei when theses develop. However, in mammals, with the development and extension of the neopallium (p. 212) the olfactory lobe (paleopallium) has become restricted to the ventrally-situated pyriform lobe.

## THE STOMATOGASTRIC AND AUTONOMIC NERVOUS SYSTEMS

In the higher invertebrates and in the vertebrates there is some separation of the innervation of the internal organs from that of the peripheral sense organs and skeletal muscles. In invertebrates, the visceral system is called the ***stomatogastric (or stomodeal) nervous system*** and it is involved with the innervation of only the anterior regions of the alimentary canal. In vertebrates it is a far more comprehensive system, innervating the viscera, heart and glands, and is called the ***autonomic nervous system***.

### The stomatogastric nervous system

The stomatogastric nervous system is found in annelids, arthropods and molluscs and reaches its peak of development in certain insects, decapod crustaceans and cephalopod molluscs. In polychaetes, the group of annelids in which this part of the nervous system is best developed, it consists of two pairs of stomatogastric nerves, one pair arising from the brain, the other from the circumoesophageal connectives. Where the latter pair leave the connectives there is sometimes a discrete stomatogastric ganglion. The nerves contain both sensory and motor neurons, and branch to form a 'nerve ring' around the gut. From this, branches innervate the pharynx and oesophagus.

In insects there is typically a ***frontal ganglion*** which is connected to the brain and to the circumoesphageal connectives (Fig. 10.25). Anteriorly, nerves arise from it to innervate the mouth and upper lip;

posteriorly it is linked to the ***hypocerebral ganglion***, from which a ***recurrent nerve*** passes backwards to the ***ventricular ganglion***. The foregut is innervated by branches of the recurrent nerve and by nerves arising from the ventricular ganglion. The recurrent nerve contains both sensory and motor axons. In addition there is a neurohaemal organ, called the ***corpus cardiacum***, which is linked by one or two nerves to the brain and is also connected to the hypocerebral ganglion. It innervates a pair of endocrine organs, the ***corpora allata***. In decapod crustaceans a pair of commissural ganglia are linked to a median ***oesophageal ganglion*** and a more posterior, median ***stomatogastric ganglion***. Nerves containing both sensory and

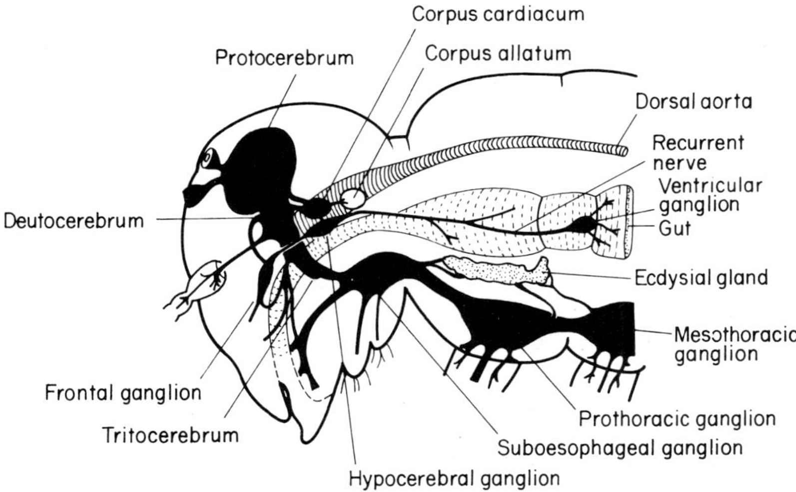


**Fig. 10.25** Diagram of a lateral view of the insect stomatogastric nervous system and its relationship with the central nervous system. (From Weber, H. (1952). *Fortschritteder Zoologie*, **9,** 18–231.)

motor axons leave the oesophageal and stomatogastric ganglia to innervate the foregut.

In arthropods the hind gut is innervated direct from the central nervous system, but there is some indication that in insects the midgut is innervated by the stomatogastric system. The heart is regulated via the central nervous system but, again in insects, the stomatogastric system may exercise some degree of control.

In cephalopod molluscs the stomatogastric system consists of a pair of nerves which run from the buccal ganglia to a ***gastric ganglion***, which innervates the gut. In gastropods there is a gut plexus which has connections with both the buccal and the visceral ganglia. As in arthropods, the stomatogastric system contains both sensory and motor elements.

### The autonomic nervous system

In vertebrates, the smooth muscles of the viscera and the cardiac muscles possess the intrinsic capability of contraction, but their

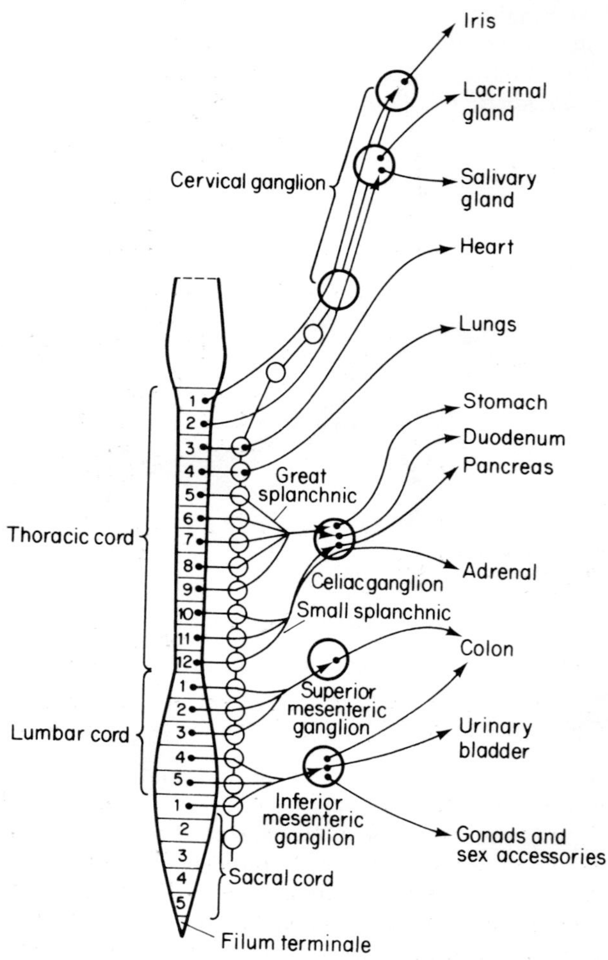


**Fig. 10.26** Diagram of the mammalian sympathetic nervous system on one side of the animal. (After Turner, C. D. and Bagnard, J. T. (1976). *General Endocrinology*, 6th edition. Copyright © 1976 by W. B. Saunders Company. Copyright 1948, 1955, 1960, 1966, and 1971 by W. B. Saunders Company. Reprinted by permission of Holt, Rinehart and Winston.)

activity, and that of the glands, is regulated by the autonomic nervous system in conjunction with the endocrine system. The autonomic nervous system is divisible into the ***sympathetic*** and ***parasympathetic nervous systems***. Anatomically the sympathetic system consists of a chain of interconnected ganglia lying on each side of the nerve cord with connections to the thoracic and lumbar spinal nerves. Short 'pre-ganglionic' fibres originate in the central nervous system and

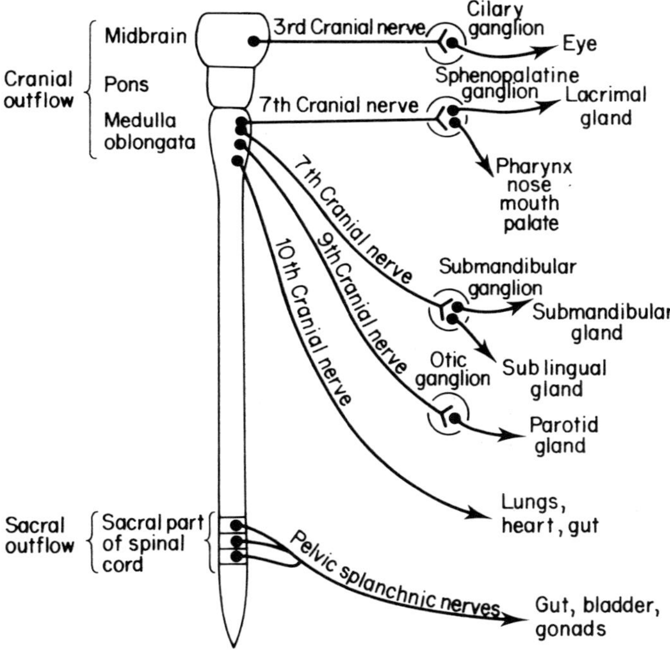


**Fig. 10.27** Diagram of the mammalian parasympathetic nervous system on one side of the animal. (From Basmajian, J. V. (1964). *Primary Anatomy*. Williams and Wilkins, Baltimore.)

pass out to the sympathetic ganglia where they synapse with 'post-ganglionic' neurons which innervate the internal organs. Some cranial nerves also contain sympathetic axons (Fig. 10.26).

In contrast, the 'pre-ganglionic' neurons of the parasympathetic system lie in the brain stem and in the sacral region of the nerve cord, and their axons are considerably longer than those of the sympathetic system, synapsing with 'post-ganglionic' neurons lying either in the parasympathetic ganglia (which are situated some distance from the nerve cord) or else directly in the walls of the end organs (Fig. 10.27).

The 10th cranial nerve carries both sympathetic and parasympathetic axons.

The two parts of the autonomic nervous system are generally antagonistic in function, and the parasympathetic system can be considered as being concerned with the basic control of the internal organs, while the sympathetic system is capable of excercising a dominant effect under conditions of stress. For example, activity in the parasympathetic system slows down the rate of heart beat, while activity in the sympathetic system speeds it up. An exception to this concerns the salivary glands, where activity in both systems is excitatory, although each controls different constituents of the saliva. Furthermore, the adrenal medulla, sweat glands, skin and the capillaries in the muscles only receive innervation from the sympathetic system. The neurotransmitters concerned with the sympathetic and parasympathetic systems have been discussed in Chapter 5.

# 11

# *Neuroethology: The Control of Behaviour*

The neural mechanisms underlying patterns of behaviour are primarily intrinsic properties of the central nervous system. The way in which central neurons interact determines the specific sequence of the motor output governing a particular piece of behaviour. The initiation of such a pattern and its subsequent modulation are determined to varying extents (depending on the behaviour pattern concerned) by sensory input.

In the previous chapter some examples of reflexes were considered. Thus input from the pain receptors of the skin of the foot in a vertebrate can produce reflex flexion of the knee joint to remove the foot from the source of pain. Also, passive displacement of one of the leg joints of a decapod crustacean elicits a resistance reflex which attempts to restore the leg joint to its original position. Such reflexes are very simple behavioural patterns.

A reflex may be defined as a rapid, specific behavioural response, normally resulting from a brief sensory stimulus, which involves either the initiation or the modification of motor output. Many reflexes involve movement of only a single joint, as in the above examples (although in both of these cases other joints may be involved in similar reflexes as a result of the same stimulus). Others involve a response in many different muscles, such as the prey-capturing strike of mantids, or even involve most of the motor mechanisms of the animal as in the reflex escape behaviour of certain animals such as crayfish (tail flip), earthworm (withdrawal into its burrow) and dragonfly larva (jet-propulsive swimming). Taxes, which are orientation movements of the animal (normally responses to a sustained stimulus such as light intensity or the gravitational field), are also reflex behaviours which involve the whole animal.

The threshold for a reflex is generally low because reflexes tend to be safety mechanisms, often of survival value to the animal. Furthermore, increase in the strength of the stimulus usually reduces the latency (time between stimulus and response) and also tends to increase the duration of the response; the flexion reflex illustrates

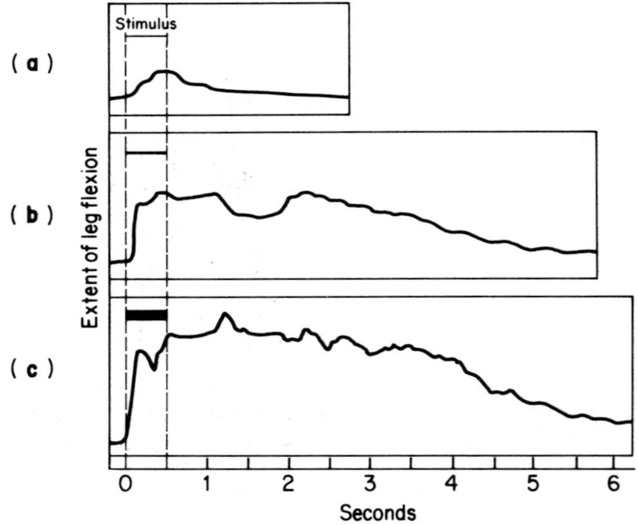


**Fig. 11.1** The effects of increasing the strength of the stimulus (**a–c**) on the flexion reflex of the dog. Note the increase in persistence and decrease in latency (time between stimulus and response) with increase in stimulus strength. (From Manning, A. (1979). *An Introduction to Animal Behaviour*, 3rd edition. Edward Arnold, London; after Sherrington, C. S. (1906). *The Integrative Action of the Nervous System*. Scribner's, New York.)

these two phenomena (Fig. 11.1). In some cases, if the stimulus is below threshold, repetitive stimulation will elicit a response (temporal summation); alternatively, simultaneous below-threshold stimulation of two adjacent (or close) parts of the sensory field may prove effective (spatial summation). This is shown in Fig. 11.2 for the scratch reflex in the dog.

Repetitive, low frequency stimulation can also be used to maintain a reflex, as in the case of the crayfish defence reflex, where the animal assumes an antagonistic posture with outstretched claws in response to a visual stimulus. Some reflexes can be elicited by more than one stimulus modality. Thus many escape responses can be caused by both visual and tactile stimuli. Certain reflexes require a maintained stimulus before they achieve maximum strength and this, presumably, involves a progressive increase in the number of motor neurons activated (motor recruitment). Repetitive or continuous stimulation of a reflex causes habituation or fatigue of the response; shown in Fig. 11.3a for the withdrawal reflex of the tubicolous

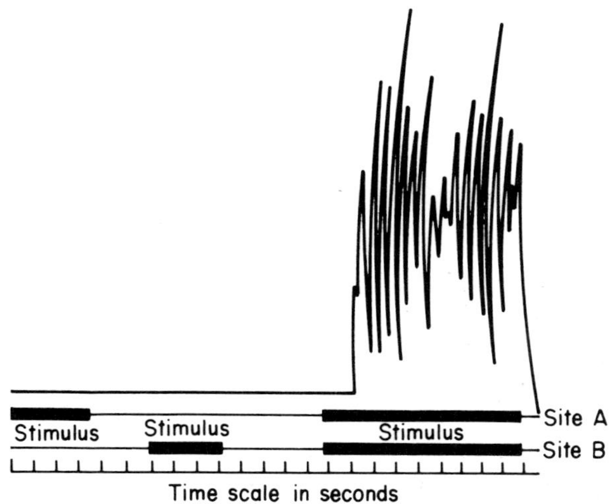


**Fig. 11.2** The effect of spatial summation on the scratch reflex of the dog. Movements of the top trace indicate movements of the dog's leg. A and B are two points on the shoulder skin. Note that no response is evoked if the two areas are stimulated separately. (From Manning, A. (1979). *An Introduction to Animal Behaviour*, 3rd edition. Edward Arnold, London; after Sherrington, C. S. (1906). *The Integrative Action of the Nervous System.* Scribner's, New York.)

polychaete *Branchiomma*. In this example the stimulus is a sudden decrease in illumination. Furthermore if, after habituation is complete, the stimulus is changed to a moving shadow (Fig. 11.3b), there is complete recovery of the withdrawal reflex followed by habituation to the new stimulus; but the habituation is slower than before.

The reflex contraction of another polychaete, *Nereis*, provides a similar example, but, in this case, recovery of the reflex after habituation is only partial. Note that in these examples both stimuli are visual, i.e. they belong to the same stimulus modality. However, the reflex contraction of *Nereis* habituates rapidly to either visual or mechanical stimulation and, if habituation to either of these modalities is followed by stimulation with the other, there is again recovery of the response and subsequent habituation, but habituation to the new stimulus is normal in this case.

The scratch reflex of the dog is another type of example. The reflex starts to decrease in intensity after about 20 seconds of continuous stimulation. However, if the site of stimulation is changed, the scratch reflex recovers. Also, following habituation of the scratch reflex, the flexion reflex (which uses largely the same complement of muscles) can be elicited. There is evidence that habituation is

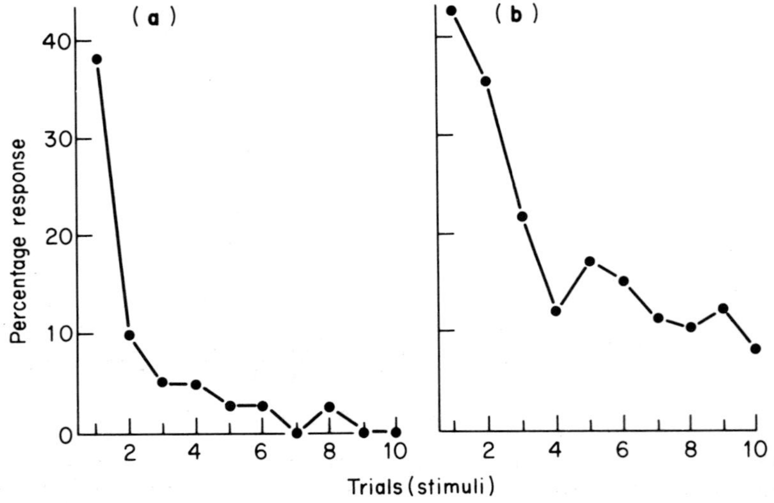


**Fig. 11.3** Habituation of the rapid withdrawal (escape) response in the polychaete annelid *Branchiomma* to visual stimulation. (**a**) Sudden decreases in illumination are immediately followed by (**b**) moving shadow stimuli. (From Nicol, J. A. C. (1950). *Journal of the Marine Biological Association*, **29,** 303–20.)

primarily a property of synapses within the central nervous system, and the last observation lends support to this. Indeed, interneurons can show habituation to repetitive sensory stimulation, with recovery of their response followed by further habituation if the site of sensory stimulation is changed (Fig. 11.4). After a period of rest from stimulation, reflexes can be initiated again with their former strengths.

In many instances a reflex may be suppressed by the central nervous system. Thus suppression of the flexion reflex in man requires a 'conscious' effort. Suppression of the decapod limb joint resistance reflex is 'automatic' when the animal is walking normally, and only becomes manifest when a leg joint is prevented from assuming its 'correct' position (i.e. as determined by the normal motor output) in the locomotory cycle. The latter can be explained if the sensory input resulting from leg movements is being compared continuously with the motor programme. If the two form the 'expected' match then no corrective (reflex) activity ensues, whereas if there is a difference the subsequent motor output is affected in an attempt to restore the leg to its correct position in the movement cycle.

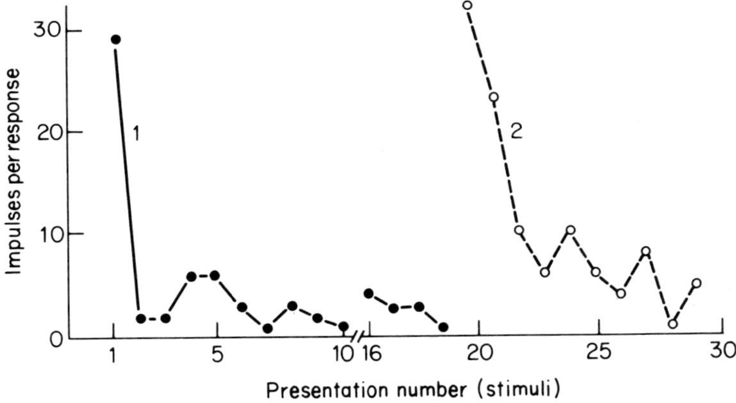


**Fig. 11.4** Habituation of the response of a visual interneuron in the locust *Schistocerca gregaria* to repetitive stimulation of one region of the visual field (1). Moving the site of stimulation by 12° results in recovery, followed by habituation again (2). (From Horne, G. and Rowell, C. H. F. (1968). *Journal of Experimental Biology*, **49**, 143–69.)

Indeed, central inhibition is an important aspect of behavioural control and there is evidence that different reflexes which utilize the same motor pathways inhibit each other and hence compete for dominance. Thus the scratch reflex can be inhibited by the flexion reflex and is resumed after stimulation of the latter ceases (Fig. 11.5). Another example of mutually exclusive reflexes is the escape and defence reflexes of the crayfish. In this case the same type of visual stimulus may elicit either of the reflexes, but not both. In young animals it is almost exclusively the escape reflex which is elicited; in old animals the defence reflex more often than not dominates. Often when a reflex is released from inhibition a reflex rebound occurs, in that the reflex is stronger than before it was inhibited; this is illustrated for the scratch reflex of the dog in Fig. 11.5.

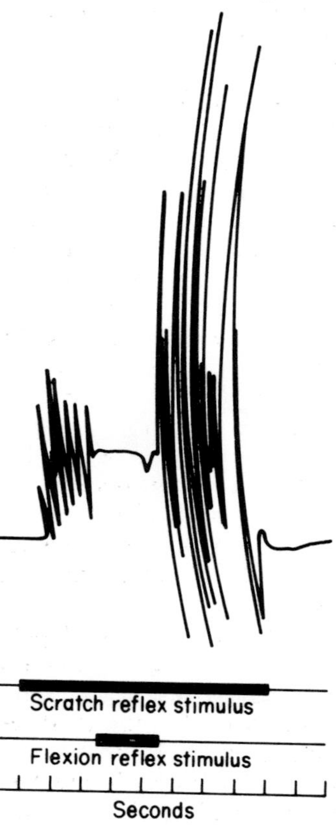


**Fig. 11.5** Inhibition of the scratch reflex by the flexion reflex in the dog. Movements of the top trace indicate movements of the dogs leg. The heavy lines on the stimulus traces indicate the periods of stimulation. Note the reflex rebound of the scratch reflex when the flexion reflex stimulus is removed. (From Manning, A. (1979). *An Introduction to Animal Behaviour*, 3rd edition. Edward Arnold, London; after Sherrington, C. S. (1906). *The Integrative Action of the Nervous System.* Scribner's, New York.)

Reflex behavioural patterns are not always as 'simple' as the above examples, with a single stimulus often eliciting one response. Thus a single, initial stimulus may result in a sequence of stimulus-response reflexes, as in the feeding reflex of the crayfish. In this sequence, if an object is presented to a claw, the tactile stimulus to the inner surface of the chela results in closure of the dactylopodite against the propodite (the two most distal limb segments). This is followed by flexion of the limb joints to bring the object close to the mouth. If the chemoreceptors then indicate that the object is food, the mandibles start working to break it down into small particles for ingestion; otherwise it is rejected.

There are many forms of behaviour which are much more complex than reflexes. Rhythmic, maintained behavioural patterns such as swimming, terrestrial locomotion, flight and ventilation may persist for long periods; throughout life in the case of mammalian ventilation. These have been termed homogeneous sequences, the same pattern being repeated at either regular or irregular intervals. They almost invariably include reflexes imposed on a basic endogenous (central) pattern; for example, the resistance reflex of decapod crustaceans and reflexes involving the organs of balance (see Chapter 8) in both invertebrates and vertebrates are integral parts of the locomotory system. However, the extent of sensory (peripheral) influence varies from one behaviour to another. Some headway has been made towards understanding these homogeneous sequences in neurological terms, notably in arthropods.

There are, however, many complex behaviour patterns which have not yet attracted the attention of neurobiologists to the same extent. These include, for example, threat and courtship displays, displacement activities and feeding. They are mostly heterogeneous sequences, in that a sequence of different patterns is generated in a predictable order. Like homogeneous sequences they are primarily endogenous patterns but often include one or more reflex responses, such as the swallowing reflex following food-seeking. Many heterogeneous sequences contain a homogeneous sequence. This is particularly obvious where locomotion is involved, as in the escape response of the nudibranch mollusc *Tritonia*. It should be noted that this response can also be classified as a reflex (although a complex one; see p. 251) and illustrates how behaviour patterns form a more or less continuous spectrum of types. However, as an aid to discussion, it is convenient to attempt to classify them.

Many complex behaviour patterns, like reflexes, are triggered by a specific external stimulus (or stimuli), which may itself be quite complex. Thus ventilation may be initiated by a particular level of environmental carbon dioxide concentration; flying in orthopterans (locusts, crickets and grasshoppers) can be triggered by a current of air deflecting a group of sensory hairs on the head, provided that the animal does not have any tarsal contact with the substrate; the swimming escape response of *Tritonia* can be started by contact with a starfish, and the complex courtship sequence of the male cricket

*Gryllus* is normally triggered by the sight of a conspecific female, but can also be elicted by the song of a conspecific female. The first two of the above examples are homogeneous sequences; the last two are heterogeneous sequences. In some other cases, however, the reason for a particular behaviour starting is less obvious, although the internal physiological state of the animal is undoubtedly important, as well as the environmental stimuli which it is receiving. The extent to which subsequent sensory input is important varies from one behaviour to another and this is discussed below (p. 250).

The role of inhibition is well-established in complex behavioural patterns. During walking, excitation of one muscle is accompanied by inhibition of the motor neurons innervating its antagonist; also excitation of, say, the flexors of one limb is accompanied by inhibition of those of the contralateral limb. This is called reciprocal inhibition. One of the roles of the brain, in insects at least, appears to be to provide inhibition of various motor activities. Removal of the head in insects often results, for example, in increased locomotor activity.

Many of the characteristics ascribed to reflexes are also found in complex behavioural patterns, but are obviously the result of the interaction of many mechanisms, and in many cases the relationships are somewhat obscure. The latency between stimulus and response is very variable. It may be brief, measured in milliseconds, or it may be measured in minutes, and, although there may be a tendency for increase in stimulus strength to shorten the latency, this is generally masked by other variables such as the physiological state of the animal. Also the behavioural response may take some time to attain its maximum intensity. Thus chaffinches take about 2½ minutes to reach their maximum alarm call frequency when presented with an owl, after which the response habituates. Furthermore, removal of the stimulus (the owl) does not result in immediate cessation of the response. Chaffinches habituated to the presence of an owl only show a partial recovery of the alarm response when the owl is replaced by a stoat (i.e. both visual stimuli). In the case of young passerine birds begging for food, the response can be habituated using visual stimulation, but reappears when jolting of the nest is used subsequently as a stimulus (i.e. the use of a different stimulus modality). After a period of rest, renewed stimulation with the same stimulus modality often elicits the full strength of the behavioural pattern once more, but in some cases recovery is incomplete. There are cases where summation can occur to stimuli of different modalities, and there are instances which are analogous to the reflex rebound described above.

We will now look at some of the neurological information available. Since some examples of reflexes have already been dealt with above and in the previous chapter, and since little information is available concerning many of the more complex behavioural patterns, the following account will concentrate largely on the rhythmic behaviour patterns of homogeneous sequences.

## HOMOGENEOUS SEQUENCES

### Motor bursts

Homogeneous sequences have been investigated in a number of systems, notably among arthropods. In general, the motor output from the central nervous system consists of rhythmic bursts of activity, alternating in two groups of antagonistic motor neurons (Fig. 11.6).

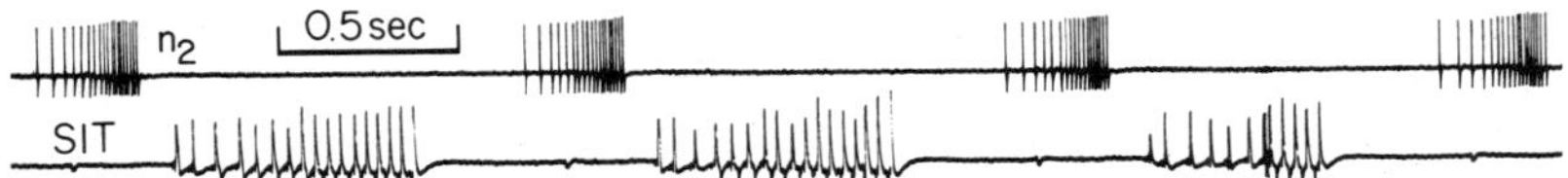


**Fig. 11.6** Recordings from a dragonfly larva showing the alternation of expiratory bursts (comprising action potentials in a single expiratory motor neuron) in a lateral segmental nerve ($n_2$) with inspiratory bursts in an inspiratory muscle (SIT). Note the build up in frequency of the action potentials in the former and the fairly steady firing frequency in the latter. (From Mill, P. J. (1970). *Journal of Experimental Biology*, **52**, 167–75.)

In most large insects ventilation is effected by raising and lowering the floor of the abdomen (sterna)—expiration and inspiration respectively. Raising the sterna produces an increase in abdominal pressure, which causes the air in the tracheae to be forced out of any spiracles which are open or, in the somewhat unusual respiratory system of dragonfly larvae, causes water to be expelled from the branchial chamber (a modified part of the hind gut) through the anus. Lowering the sterna effects movement of air or water respectively in the reverse direction. This rhythmic activity may be continuous for long periods or be periodic (i.e. groups of cycles separated by periods of quiescence), depending both on the species and on the physiological condition of the individual.

Expiration always involves the active contraction of segmental muscles. However, inspiration in some insects is a purely passive movement effected by the elasticity of the abdominal sclerites (e.g. the cockroach *Periplaneta*), in some cases aided by resilin (e.g. the beetles *Orcytes* and *Melolontha*). Hence the motor output in each abdominal segment consists solely of a series of expiratory bursts. In other insects there are inspiratory as well as expiratory muscles (Fig. 11.6). Typically the expiratory muscles are innervated by motor neurons in the lateral nerves in each segment; the inspiratory muscles by motor neurons in the median nerves. The significance of this is that the motor neurons in the median nerves send a branch to each side and so the corresponding muscles on each side receive identical motor output. There is one main pair of dorsoventral expiratory muscles in each abdominal segment involved in ventilation, and each is innervated by a very small number of motor neurons. In dragonfly larvae only one of these is an expiratory motor neuron, but in locusts, cockroaches and mantids there is more than one. Additional muscles are involved in expiration and some of these may be particularly important when ventilation is vigorous. Commonly included are other dorsoventral muscles, and longitudinal muscles may also be activated during expiration. In dragonfly larvae the latter probably serve simply to prevent increase in abdominal length as the internal pressure during expiration rises (otherwise this pressure rise would be negated). However, in some insects (e.g. mantids) longitudinal contraction is part of the normal expiratory movement and enhances the internal pressure during expiration.

In the dragonfly larva there are only two inspiratory muscles in the whole abdomen, but in other insects where they occur they are segmentally arranged and there is sometimes more than one pair per segment (e.g. *Schistocerca*). In the absence of a ventilatory pattern, both expiratory and inspiratory motor neurons remain inactive. In strong ventilation additional pumping mechanisms may be employed, synchronized with the principal abdominal movements. These include longitudinal contractions of the abdomen as well as head and prothoracic pumping movements. All three are utilized in *Schistocerca*.

A second aspect of the ventilatory system is the operation of the spiracles which, in large air-breathing insects, are opened and/or closed in synchrony with ventilatory movements (see below). In adult dragonflies the spiracles have only a closer muscle, opening being effected by the elasticity of the cuticle. This also applies to the second pair of spiracles in cockroaches and *Schistocerca*, but the other spiracles of these animals have both closer and opener muscles. Innervation of the closer muscles is via the median nerves; that of the opener muscles is variable (median or lateral nerves or both). The innervation of the spiracular muscles of *Schistocerca* is shown in Fig. 11.7.

Unlike the motor neurons to the ventilatory muscles, those to the spiracular closer muscles tend to fire at a low frequency when the animal is not ventilating. This 'free-running' is commonly seen in cockroaches, but the superimposed ventilatory pattern tends to obscure it in *Schistocerca*, although it can be observed in the latter under certain experimental conditions (Fig. 11.8). The effect of this

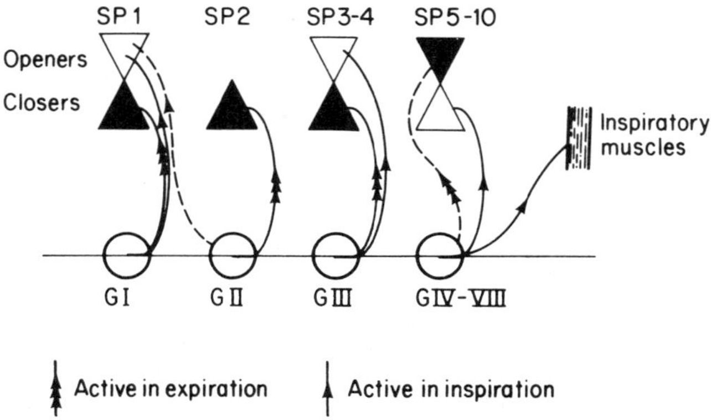


**Fig. 11.7** Diagrammatic representation of the innervation of the spiracle muscles of the locust *Schistocerca gregaria*. ▲, muscles active during expiration; △, muscles active during inspiration. ——, median nerves, ----, lateral nerves. G, thoracic (I–III) and abdominal (IV–VIII) ganglia; SP, spiracles (1–3 thoracic, 4–10 abdominal). (From Miller, P. L. (1974). In *The Physiology of Insecta*, 2nd edition, Vol. 6. (Rockstein, M., ed.) Academic Press, New York.)

free-running is to keep the spiracles closed for most of the time when the animal is not ventilating, thereby conserving water.

During abdominal ventilation, the closer and, when present, the opener muscles receive rhythmic bursts of impulses via their motor neurons. The bursts are fairly complex in structure. For example, during low ventilatory rates in *Schistocerca*, the closer motor neurons of the first and second spiracles fire at a high frequency at the start of

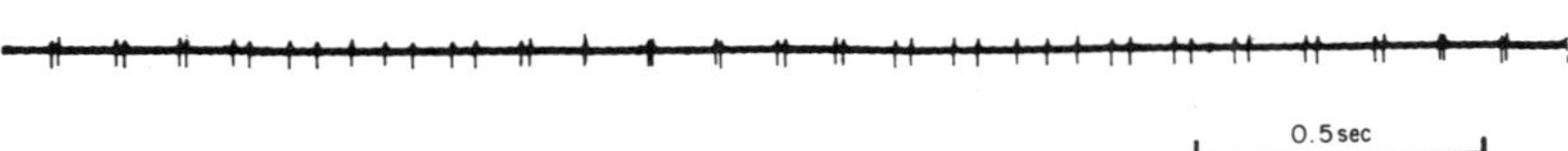


**Fig. 11.8** 'Free-running' activity in the two motor axons innervating the closer muscle of a second spiracle of a locust from which the metathoracic ganglion has been removed. Note that the innervation is via a median nerve, in which each motor axon bifurcates, one branch going to each side. Hence there is an identical pattern on the two sides (not shown). (From Miller, P. L. (1965). In *The Physiology of the Insect Central Nervous System* (Treherne, J. E. and Beament J., eds.). Academic Press, London.)

the burst, slow down ('pause'), then increase in frequency again at the end of the burst. The opener bursts to the first spiracles of *Schistocerca* are even more complex. Reference to Fig. 11.7 shows that this muscle is innervated by two motor neurons from the prothoracic ganglion and one from the mesothoracic ganglion. During weak ventilation they are all inactive or fire at low frequencies. With increase in strength of ventilation the two prothoracic motor neurons start to fire with a burst towards the end of the closer burst. (They do, however, have an opening effect on the spiracle, since the conduction time to the periphery is slower in the opener than in the closer motor neurons; also the opener muscle relaxes more slowly than does the closer muscle.) The mesothoracic motor neuron fires during opening. With further increase in strength of ventilation the prothoracic motor neurons extend their firing into the opening period. There is thus a progressive increase in the effectiveness of the opener motor neurons with increase in strength of ventilation. It should be noted that the two rhythms do not strictly alternate since two of the opener motor neurons fire mainly during the closer burst.

Most leg joints in arthropods move predominantly in one plane and each is operated primarily by a pair of antagonistic muscles; although many joints have one or more additional muscles. During walking, a rhythm of alternating motor bursts occurs in the motor neurons innervating each pair of antagonistic muscles. This rhythm is shown in Fig. 11.9 for the levator and depressor muscles of the coxa of *Periplaneta*.

The flight system in dragonflies possesses direct wing muscles, three for elevation and two for depression of each wing; in other insects (e.g. *Schistocerca*) these movements are effected by the dorso-ventral and dorsal longitudinal muscles respectively of the pterothoracic segments. The elevator muscles are each innervated by 3–5 motor neurons in dragonflies and 6–8 motor neurons in *Schistocerca*: while the depressor muscles are each innervated by 4–15 motor neurons in dragonflies and about five in *Schistocerca*. The rhythm consists of alternating bursts of action potentials in the motor neurons innervating these two sets of muscles. There are, in addition, a number of accessory muscles, controlling, for example, the attitude of the wing during each flight cycle.

In crayfish and lobsters the biramous abdominal appendages are called swimmerets, although they are only used for locomotion in the younger stages. However, they still beat regularly in adults, providing a current of water which is concerned with respiration. In the lobster *Homarus*, each swimmeret is controlled by twelve muscles, three of which retract the appendage (power stroke muscles) and two of which protract it (return stroke muscles); the others are concerned with, for example, opening the rami during the powerstroke. There is a rhythmic alternation of motor bursts in the powerstroke and returnstroke motor neurons, with the motor neurons innervating the remaining muscles contributing to one or other of the bursts.

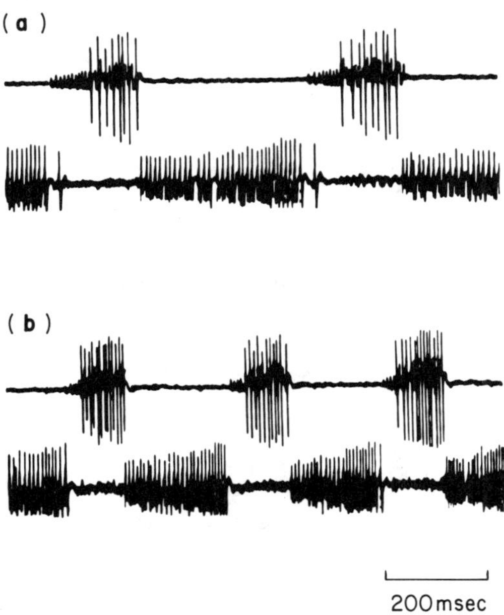


**Fig. 11.9** Recordings from the cockroach *Periplaneta americana* to show alternating activity in coxal levator and depressor muscles during walking at two different speeds ((**b**) faster than (**a**)). In both recordings the levator activity is at the top, the depressor activity at the bottom. Note the increase in firing frequency with increase in walking speed. (From Pearson, K. G. (1972). *Journal of Experimental Biology*, **56,** 173–93.)

Certain features of the above rhythms are common to more than one behaviour, while others are unique to a specific behaviour pattern. In some rhythms alteration in frequency of the cycle is brought about mainly by changes in the duration of one of the pairs of antagonistic motor bursts. Thus, in locust ventilation the duration of the inspiratory bursts remains fairly constant while the expiratory bursts decrease in duration with increase in ventilatory frequency (Fig. 11.10a). Similarly, in walking in *Periplaneta* the duration of the coxal depressor bursts remains fairly constant over most of the range of stepping frequency (albeit with some decrease at high stepping frequencies) while that of the coxal depressor bursts decreases with increase in stepping frequency (Fig. 11.10b). Levation of the coxal joint coincides approximately with protraction of the limb, and it has been shown from studies on the gait (walking pattern) of the stick insect *Carausius* that protraction time remains almost constant, while retraction time decreases with increase in walking speed, which is in

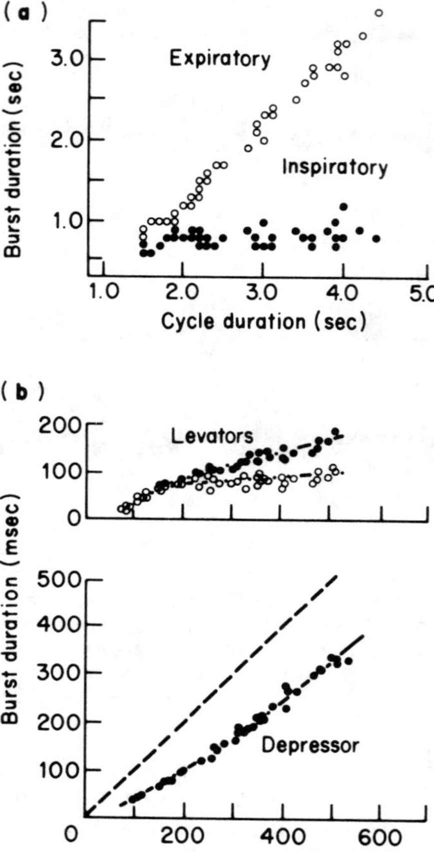


**Fig. 11.10** Variation in the burst duration with cycle duration of (**a**) expiratory and inspiratory motor bursts in the locust *Schistocerca gregaria* and (**b**) two levator and one depressor motor axons innervating the coxal muscles of the cockroach *Periplaneta americana*. ((**a**) From Lewis, G. M., Miller, P. L. and Mills, P. S. (1973). *Journal of Experimental Biology*, **59,** 149–68; (**b**) from Pearson, K. G. (1972). *Journal of Experimental Biology*, **56,** 173–93.)

accord with the above. There are also other rhythms in which at least one of the bursts is similarly affected. Thus the bursts to the swimmeret powerstroke muscles in *Homarus* decrease in duration with increase in frequency of beating; in *Schistocerca* the bursts to the closer muscles of the first and second pairs of spiracles decrease in duration with increase in ventilatory frequency, the expiratory 'pause' becoming shorter and eventually disappearing. Conversely, in the locust flight system, where each unit only fires once or twice per cycle, the burst length increases with increase in flight frequency (Fig. 11.11).

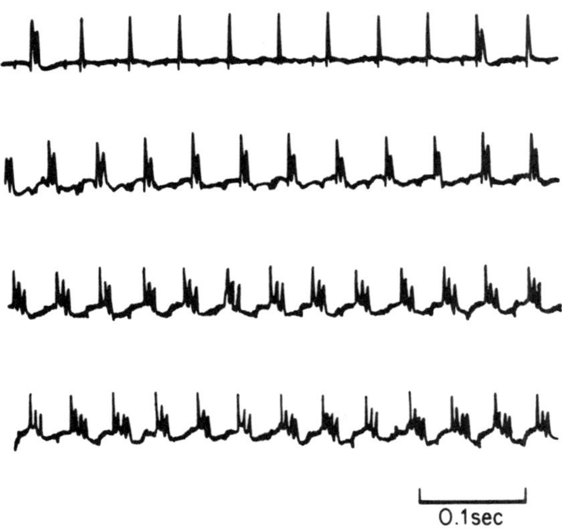


**Fig. 11.11** Recordings showing the increase in burst duration in a flight muscle with increase in wing-beat frequency in the locust *Schistocerca gregaria*. (From Wilson, D. M. (1968). *Advances in Insect Physiology*, **5,** 289–338.)

In some rhythms there is an obvious starting point because the rest position is nearly always the same. This is the case in ventilation, where an insect usually rests in the fully inspired state. The consequence of this is that a sequence of ventilatory movements starts with expiration, and this is followed by inspiration after a short and fairly constant delay.

In some instances the bursts of the antagonistic rhythms appear never to overlap. This is so in dragonfly larval ventilation (Fig. 11.5) and in locust flight. However, overlap of the antagonistic bursts occurs under certain circumstances in the swimmeret beating system of astacurans and in insect walking. For example, at high frequencies of swimmeret beating in *Homarus* each powerstroke burst starts during the preceding return stroke, thereby acting as a brake on the latter (Fig. 11.12).

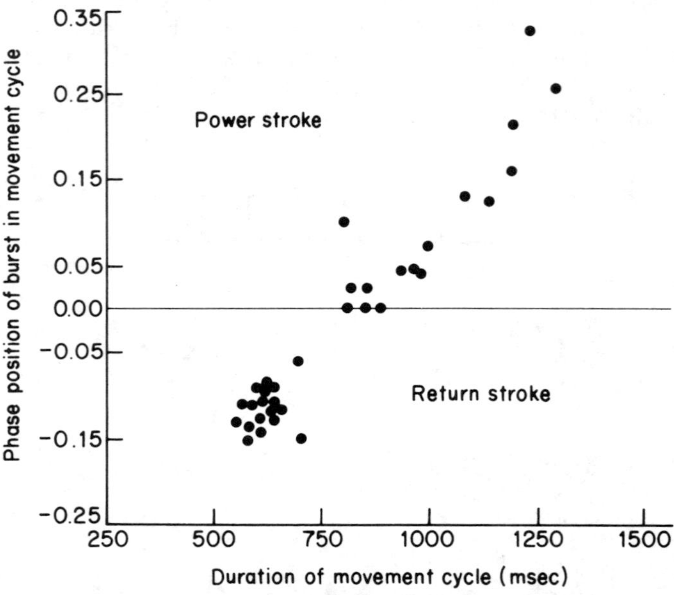


**Fig. 11.12** The phase position in the swimmeret movement cycle of the lobster at which a powerstroke muscle began to fire, plotted against cycle duration. Note that at cycle durations less than about 800 ms this powerstroke muscle is active towards the end of the return stroke. (From Davis, W. J. (1969). *Journal of Experimental Biology*, **50**, 99–118.)

*Firing patterns of individual motor neurons within bursts*

The number of motor neurons innervating each muscle is always small in arthropods (see Chapter 1). The pattern of firing of many motor neurons in these rhythmic bursts involves an initial high frequency followed by some adaptation during the burst (and sometimes a further slight increase in frequency towards the end of the burst). At high cycle frequencies there is less adaptation. This is the pattern in, for example, the expiratory motor neurons of *Schistocerca* (Fig. 11.13a). There are, however, other motor neurons which differ from this. Thus the expiratory motor neuron innervating the main expiratory muscle in dragonfly larvae fires initially with a low frequency which increases to a maximum at or near the end of the burst (see Fig. 11.6); the muscle potentials show facilitation as the firing frequency increases. However, at higher ventilatory frequencies this motor neuron fires at a fairly high and more constant frequency throughout the burst. The inspiratory motor neurons of insects also differ in their firing pattern. They tend to fire at a fairly constant frequency throughout the burst (e.g. dragonfly larvae (Fig. 11.6) and locust (Fig. 11.13b). Furthermore, each motor neuron innervating the elevator and depressor muscles of the wings of the locust rarely fires more than twice in each burst.

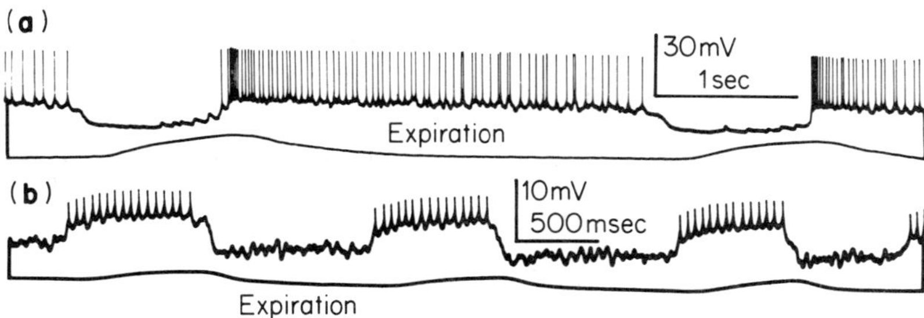


**Fig. 11.13** Intracellular recordings from (**a**) an expiratory motor neuron and (**b**) an inspiratory motor neuron of the locust *Schistocerca*. Lower traces show dorsoventral movements of the floor of the abdomen – down indicates expiration; up indicates inspiration. (From Burrows, M. (1974). *Philosophical Transactions of the Royal Society, B,* **269,** 29–48.)

The decrease in duration of the bursts to the swimmeret powerstroke muscles with increase in frequency of beating, mentioned above, is accompanied by an increase in the number of active motor neurons (motor recruitment) and in the frequency of firing of individual motor neurons. However, the duration of firing of any one powerstroke motor neuron is independent of the beating frequency. Increase in the latter therefore results in decreasing delays between the onset of firing of individual motor neurons in a burst. Motor recruitment is also seen in walking in *Periplaneta*. The coxal levator and depressor muscles are each innervated by slow and fast motor neurons (Chapter 1). At low walking speeds only the slow motor neurons are active and their firing frequency increases with increase in walking speed (Fig. 11.9). At faster speeds the fast motor neurons are recruited. This also occurs in the tibial flexor and extensor muscles. Furthermore, peripheral inhibition (Chapter 1) plays an important part, at least at this joint. Thus, the extensor muscle is also innervated by an inhibitory motor neuron. This is silent at low walking speeds, but at fast walking speeds it fires with a burst just before the excitatory flexor motor neurons start to fire. It reduces tension in the extensor muscle and hence has a braking effect. Another example of motor recruitment is seen in the expiratory muscles of the dragonfly larva when longitudinal abdominal contractions are coupled with rapid dorsoventral expiratory movements to produce jet-propulsive swimming (Fig. 11.14).

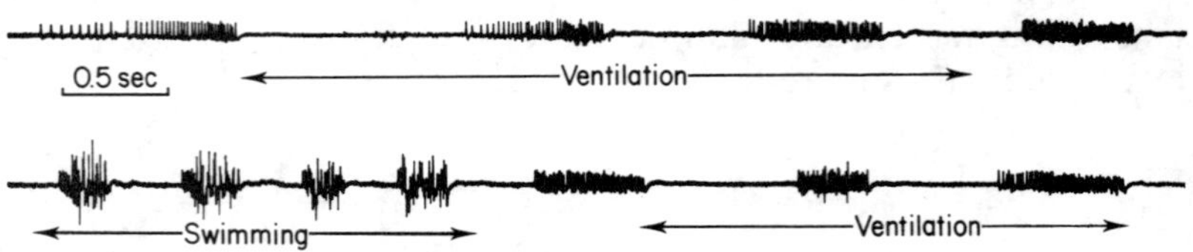


**Fig. 11.14** Extracellular recordings from a respiratory (expiratory) dorsoventral muscle in an unrestrained dragonfly larva to show motor recruitment during the change from ventilation to swimming. (From Mill, P. J. and Pickard, R. S. (1975). *Journal of Comparative Physiology*, **97**, 324–38.)

*Intrasegmental relationships*

The rhythmic motor output in a single segment is relatively simple in, for example, ventilation, where the muscles in the segment tend to be synchronized both in expiration and in inspiration. However, if we add to this the rhythmic output to the spiracular muscles, the system assumes an added degree of complexity. For example, in a resting animal the spiracular movements of any one segment are linked in a specific way with the ventilatory cycle; i.e. the spiracles open during expiration or during inspiration, or remain open or closed throughout the whole cycle. Temporary changes, however, may occur in which there is a reversal. This has been demonstrated in the first spiracles of the praying mantid *Sphodromantis*, which are normally closed during expiration and open during inspiration (Fig. 11.15). Furthermore, changes in the state of activity of the animal often result in a change in the synchronization between spiracular and ventilatory movements. For example, in a resting locust the second pair of spiracles open only during inspiration, whereas in the initial stages of flight they remain open throughout the whole ventilatory cycle.

Another type of complexity concerns such activities as walking, where several joints must move in a particular sequence. Here the timing of the outputs to the different joints requires considerable precision. In flight and in swimmeret beating other subsidiary movements, such as pronation of the wings and closing of the rami respectively, occur at specific points in the cycle, and so again there has to be precise timing of the sequence of motor outputs emanating from a single ganglion (Fig. 11.16).

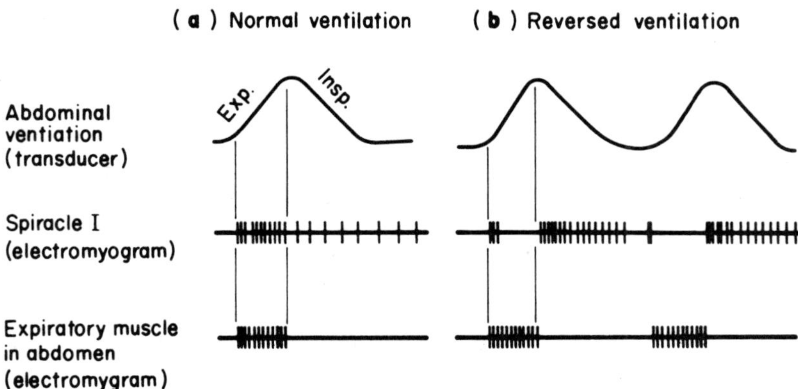


**Fig. 11.15** Activity in the closer muscle of the first spiracle of the praying mantid *Sphodromantis* during (**a**) normal ventilation (spiracle closed during expiration) and (**b**) reversed ventilation (spiracle open during expiration). (From Miller, P. L. (1974). In *The Physiology of Insecta*, 2nd edition, Vol. 6. (Rockstein, M., ed.) Academic Press, New York.)

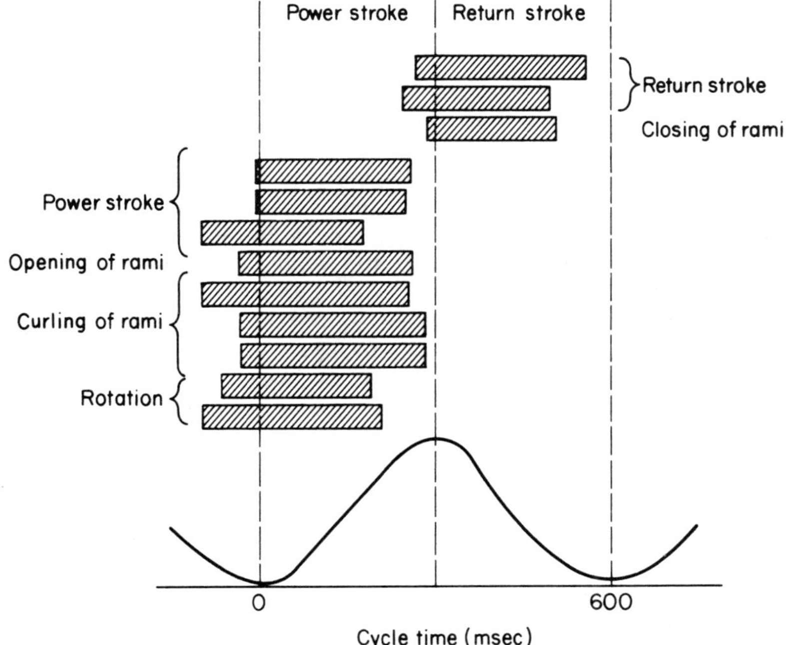


**Fig. 11.16** Diagram showing the sequence of muscle activity in the twelve muscles controlling a single swimmeret in the lobster *Homarus*. (From Davis, W. J. (1968). *Journal of Experimental Zoology*, **168,** 363–78.)

*Intersegmental relationships*

Another aspect of the motor output which has received some attention is the relative timing of the motor output in different segments. The ventilatory rhythm of *Schistocerca*, cockroaches, mantids and adult dragonflies appears to emanate synchronously from each segmental set of motor neurons and only a statistical analysis (in *Schistocerca*) of the timing of the onset of the bursts in successive segments has revealed that there is a tendency for there to be an anterior–posterior sequence. Ventilation in larval dragonflies differs in that there is a marked posterior–anterior sequence with an intersegmental delay in the order of 100–150 milliseconds per segment (Fig. 11.17). A similar posterior–anterior sequence is seen in

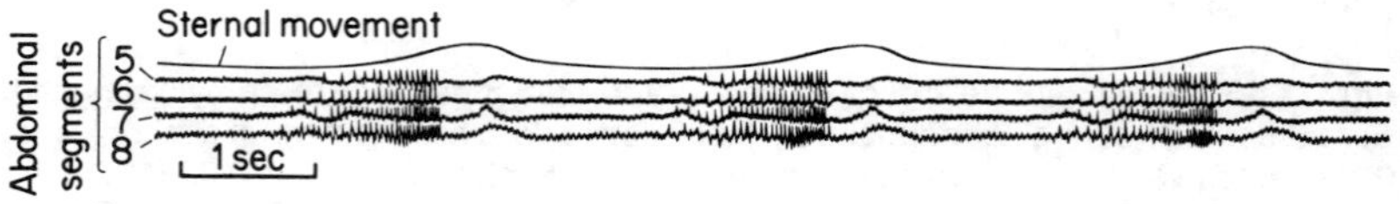


**Fig. 11.17** Extracellular recordings of expiratory bursts in the respiratory (expiratory) dorsoventral muscles of four consecutive abdominal segments (5–8) of a dragonfly larva. The top trace shows dorsoventral movements of the floor of the abdomen (sternal movements) – up indicates expiration. (From Pickard, R. S. and Mill, P. J. (1972). *Journal of Experimental Biology*, **56**, 527–36.)

the swimmeret beating of astacurans; here the intersegmental delay is about 150 milliseconds. In insect walking there is also a posterior–anterior sequence. Figure 11.18 illustrates a model of the gait (stepping pattern) of insects, in which protraction time remains constant (see above), as do the delays between protraction of the hind and middle legs and between the middle and front legs on each side. Alteration of frequency is brought about by change in the delay between protraction of the front and hind legs (which includes retraction), i.e. between the end of one cycle of movement and the start of the next. Furthermore, legs on opposite sides of the same segment are directly out of phase (i.e. alternate) with one another. (It

---

**Fig. 11.18** Diagram illustrating a model of insect walking. The horizontal axis indicates time. Solid bars show protraction (leg off the ground). $L_1$, $L_2$, $L_3$, first, second and third left legs; $R_1$, $R_2$, $R_3$, first, second and third right legs. Solid enclosures show the fixed patterns on each side; dashed enclosures indicate legs moving at (or nearly at) the same time. (**a**) – (**d**) Show increases in stepping frequency. Note that frequency changes involve only the interval between protraction in a first leg (end of one cycle) and protraction in the third leg of the same side (start of the next cycle). The legs on opposite sides of the same segment are exactly in opposite phase to each other (i.e. a phase value of 0.5). (From Wilson, D. M. (1966). *Annual Reviews of Entomology*, **11**, 103–22.)

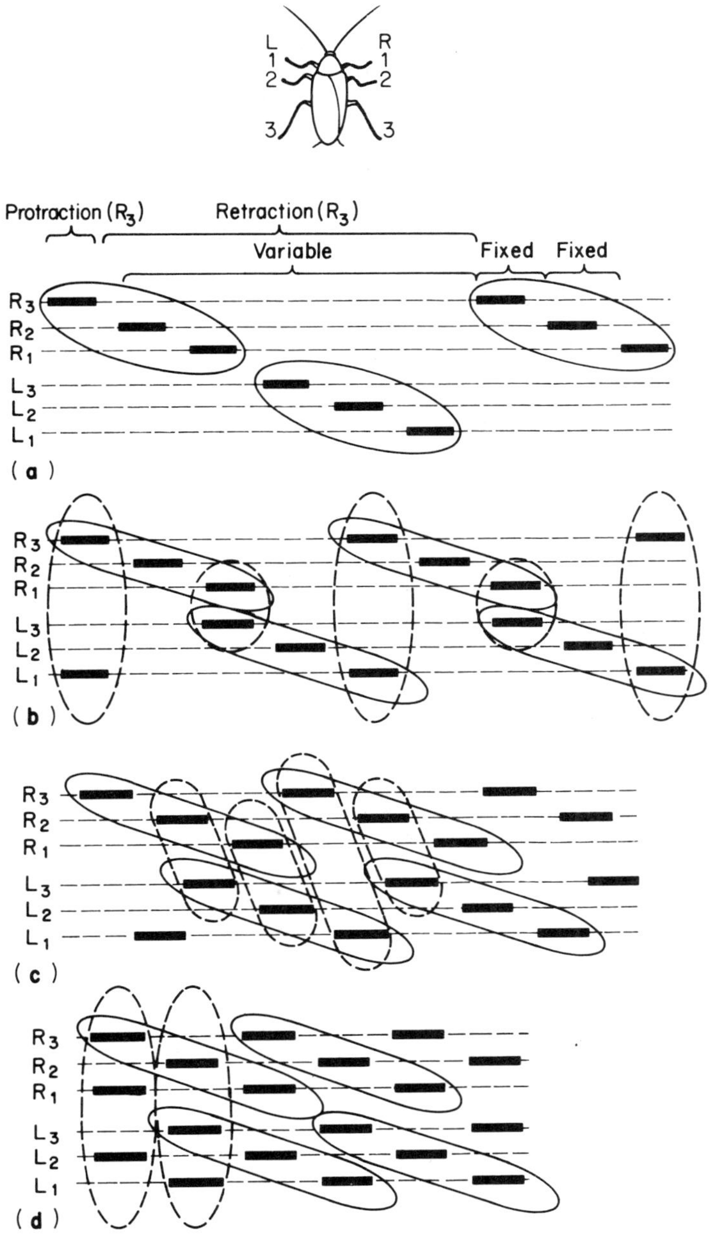

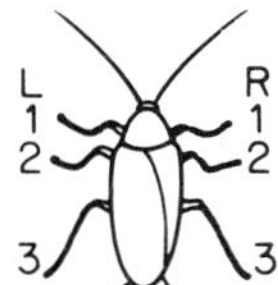


Protraction ($R_3$) Retraction ($R_3$)

Variable Fixed Fixed

$R_3$
$R_2$
$R_1$
$L_3$
$L_2$
$L_1$

(a)

$R_3$
$R_2$
$R_1$
$L_3$
$L_2$
$L_1$

(b)

$R_3$
$R_2$
$R_1$
$L_3$
$L_2$
$L_1$

(c)

$R_3$
$R_2$
$R_1$
$L_3$
$L_2$
$L_1$

(d)

is interesting to observe here that the legs on opposite sides of the same segment move synchronously when an animal swims.) A similar stepping pattern to the above seems to hold for forward-walking decapod crustaceans such as lobsters and crayfish, but crabs may have a basic alternating tetrapod gait.

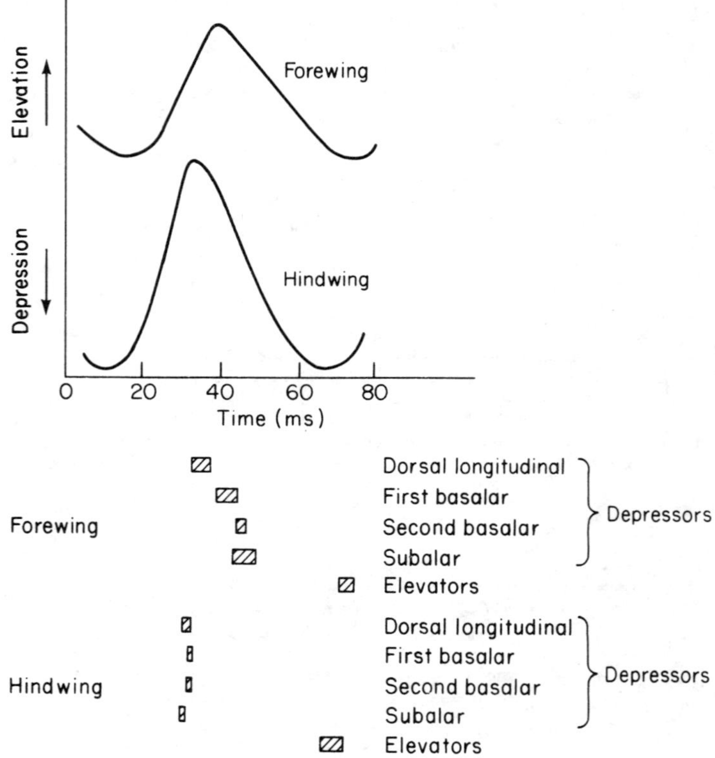


**Fig. 11.19** Sequence of wing movements in the locust *Schistocerca* and the duration of activity in the depressor and elevator wing muscles. (After Wilson, D. M. and Weis-Fogh, T. (1962). *Journal of Experimental Biology*, **39**, 643–67.)

In locust flight the hind wings lead the fore wings, but the amount by which they lead varies throughout the cycle. Thus, at maximum elevation they lead by 6–7 msec, while at maximum depression their lead is only about half this. The relative timing of some of the motor units involved is shown in Fig. 11.19.

**The central control system**

It is now pertinent to consider how the above patterns may be produced. The following account illustrates the direction in which the evidence and current thoughts are leading. It is apparent from recordings obtained intracellularly from motor neurons (see Fig. 11.13) that their activity is the result of activity in presynaptic neurons, which may involve excitation, the removal of inhibition or a mixture of both. It is generally accepted that there is a local control centre (oscillator) in each half of each ganglion involved in the rhythm, and that this may consist of one or more interneurons. Its function is to control the timing of motor neuron firing in the corresponding half segment, both within and between the members of the two antagonistic groups. Each local control centre is almost certainly coupled via interneuron(s) with its contralateral counterpart, as well as with the local control centres on the ipsilateral side of adjacent ganglia. Such interneurons have been termed ***coordinating interneurons*** and their role is to regulate the phase relationships between adjacent local control centres. They may be excitatory, ensuring that adjacent centres remain in phase with each other (as in ventilation) or inhibitory, so that adjacent centres are out of phase (as in walking). The local control centres and their coordinating interneurons may be considered together as the ***pattern generator***, the components of which are activated by information from 'higher' centres of the central nervous system via ***command interneurons***.

One of the local control centres, often referred to as the ***pacemaker***, normally leads the wave of activity. If the ganglion containing it is removed, another local control centre may take over this role in some systems. Thus, in the crayfish swimmeret pattern generator the pacemaker resides in the 5th abdominal ganglion, but the control centre in either the 4th or 3rd abdominal ganglion can assume its function. It seems likely that the command interneurons activate all of the local control centres and that either the one which receives the information first (e.g. as in locust ventilation) or the one with the lowest threshold (e.g. as in walking, swimmeret beating and ventilation in larval dragonflies) assumes the role of pacemaker. In the first case the direction of the wave of activity is determined primarily by the direction of the information flow in the command interneurons, and the role of the coordinating interneurons is, presumably, to enhance the excitation of successive local control centres. In the second case there always appears to be a considerable delay between the excitation of successive local control centres, and the role of the coordinating interneurons could be to control this delay. This could either be because activity in the command interneurons must be combined with activity in the coordinating interneurons for excitation of other local control centres to occur, or because the coordinating interneurons actively inhibit adjacent local control centres when they are active.

Activity in the command interneurons serves to initiate and maintain the rhythmic behaviour pattern, and there is evidence that several command interneurons are concerned with each behaviour. Triggering of the command interneurons may be the result of an external stimulus and/or result from the physiological state of the animal (see p. 233).

**Sensory modulation**

Homogeneous sequences are basically endogenous and indeed can often continue in the absence of any sensory input, although the latter may be important in initiating the sequence. However, sensory input often modulates (and corrects) the endogenous motor output and appears to be of particular importance in activities such as locomotion, where environmental perturbations can have a marked effect on the behavioural pattern (e.g. one of the legs may meet an obstruction while it is being protracted).

As far as ventilation is concerned the concentration of carbon dioxide is especially important and acts on the command system via carbon dioxide receptors in the anterior ganglia. Where proprioceptive input is important it generally acts on the local control centres (or in some cases directly on the motor neurons), where it may alter the intensity (amplitude) and/or the timing (phase) of the motor output. Proprioceptive input is probably of comparatively little importance in ventilation, although the rhythm is monitored by abdominal receptors. In *Schistocerca* there is a stretch receptor at the base of each wing which is activated on the upstroke. Their input appears to be averaged and to have a tonic effect on the wing beat frequency, removal resulting in both decreased frequency and amplitude of the wing beat. The importance of the resistance reflexes initiated by the limb chordotonal organs in crustacean walking has already been discussed (Chapter 10), but other limb sense organs also modify locomotion in arthropods. For example, in some insects, hair plates at the bases of the legs are important in controlling the length of the stride, their removal resulting in over-stepping. Also, ablation of the femoral chordotonal organ in a locust leg results in a decrease in activity of the slow excitatory motor neuron innervating the tibial extensor muscle and a consequent reduction in the speed of walking. There are many other examples of proprioceptive modulation of behaviour and it should also be noted that sensory input as a whole is probably important in maintaining the general excitatory level of the central nervous system.

## HETEROGENEOUS SEQUENCES

Studies of some heterogeneous sequences have shown that many of the parameters discussed above for homogeneous sequences also apply to them. There is evidence for command interneurons, local control centres, coordinating interneurons, sensory triggering and sensory modulation. Furthermore, as was mentioned earlier (p. 233) many heterogeneous sequences include one or more homogeneous sequences. Two examples of heterogeneous sequences will be examined briefly.

A comparatively simple example (simple in behavioural terms at least) is that of the escape response of the nudibranch mollusc

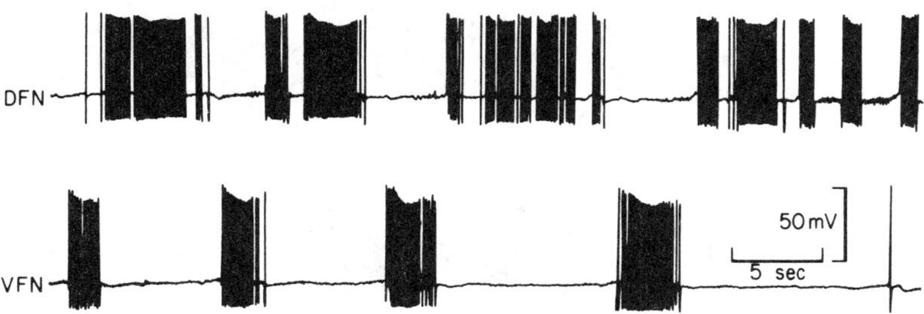


**Fig. 11.20** Intracellular recordings of alternating bursts in a dorsal flexor neuron (DFN) and a ventral flexor neuron (VFN) during the swimming sequence of the escape response of the nudibranch mollusc *Tritonia diomedia*. Note that the subgroups in the DFN bursts are particularly prominent towards the end of the sequence and each elicits a distinct dorsal flexion. (From Willows, A. O. D., Dorsett, D. A. and Hoyle, G. (1973). *Journal of Neurobiology*, **4**, 255–85.)

*Tritonia*. However, it contains four sequences—reflex withdrawal at the site of stimulation, preparation for swimming, swimming, and cessation of activity. The first stage appears to be a reflex of the peripheral neuromuscular system, but the others are elicited by activity in motor neurons in the pedal ganglia. Swimming consists of 3–7 rhythmic dorsal and ventral flexions of the animal, produced by the appropriate longitudinal muscles, and examples of the motor bursts from an antagonistic pair of motor neurons are shown in Fig. 11.20. The bursts of the dorsal flexion motor neurons tend to be longer than those of the ventral flexion motor neurons, and the former also tend to be comprised of groups of pulses. There is a close correlation in the bursts among the cells of each type and there is evidence that the swimming sequence is initiated by a burst of activity in several 'trigger' interneurons.

Perhaps one of the most complex heterogeneous behaviours studied so far is that of courtship in orthopterans. This involves a

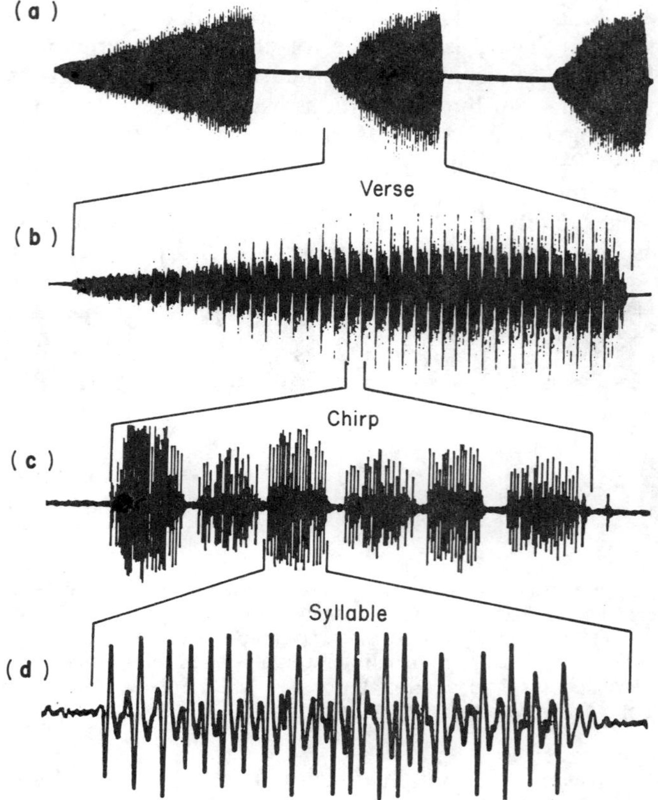


**Fig. 11.21** Recordings of the song of the grasshopper *Chorthippus biguttulus* to illustrate the terminology. (**a**) Three verses; (**b**) one verse (duration about 2.8 sec); (**c**) one chirp (duration about 65 msec) and (**d**) one syllable (duration about 8.5 msec) consisting of a number of oscillations. (From Elsner, N. (1974). *Journal of Comparative Physiology*, **88,** 67–102.)

number of sequences, including locomotion and various types of song pattern. In crickets, sounds are produced by closing movements of the wings, when a file under each tegmen is rubbed against a scraper on the other wing. In grasshoppers, sounds are elicited by upward and downward movements of the hind legs, each movement causing a group of small pegs on each hind leg to hit one of the anterior wing veins. Each closing movement of the wings in crickets, and both the upward and downward leg movements in grasshoppers, produces a vibration, referred to as a 'syllable', and several syllables occur in close succession to form a 'chirp' (Fig. 11.21). A sequence of chirps is

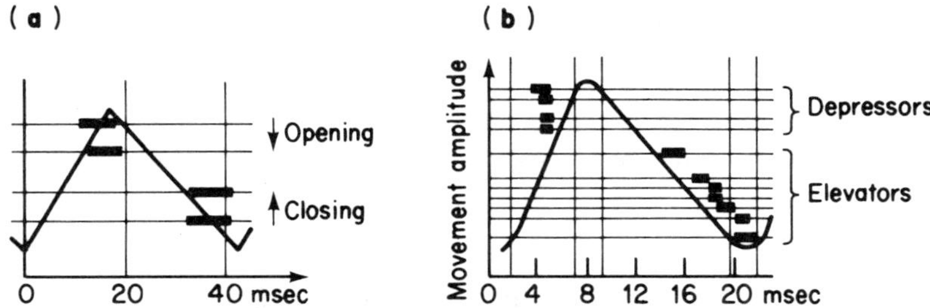


**Fig. 11.22** Sequences of stridulatory movements and the duration of activity (bars) in the muscles involved. (**a**) In the cricket *Gryllus campestris* note the close synchromy of the synergists. (**b**) In the grasshopper *Gomphocerippus rufus* there is close synchrony of the depressors, but the elevators show progressive recruitment. ((**a**) From Huber, F. (1975). In '*Simple*' *Nervous Systems*. (Usherwood, P. N. R. and Newth, D. R., eds.) Edward Arnold, London; after Kutsch, W. (1969). *Zeitschrift für vergleichenae Physiologie*, **63,** 335–78; (**b**) after Elsner, N. (1968). *Zeitschrift für vergleichende Physiologie*, **60,** 308–50.)

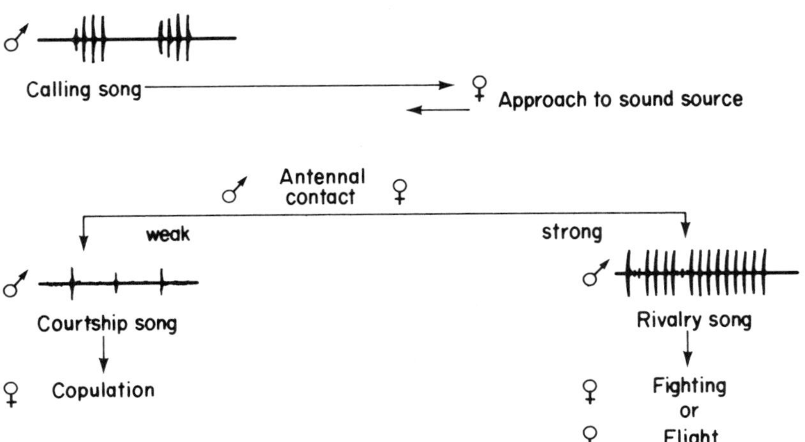


**Fig. 11.23** Song patterns of the cricket *Gryllus campestris*. (From Huber, F. (1977). *Rheinisch–Westfälische Akademie der Wissenschaften*, Vorträge N **205**.)

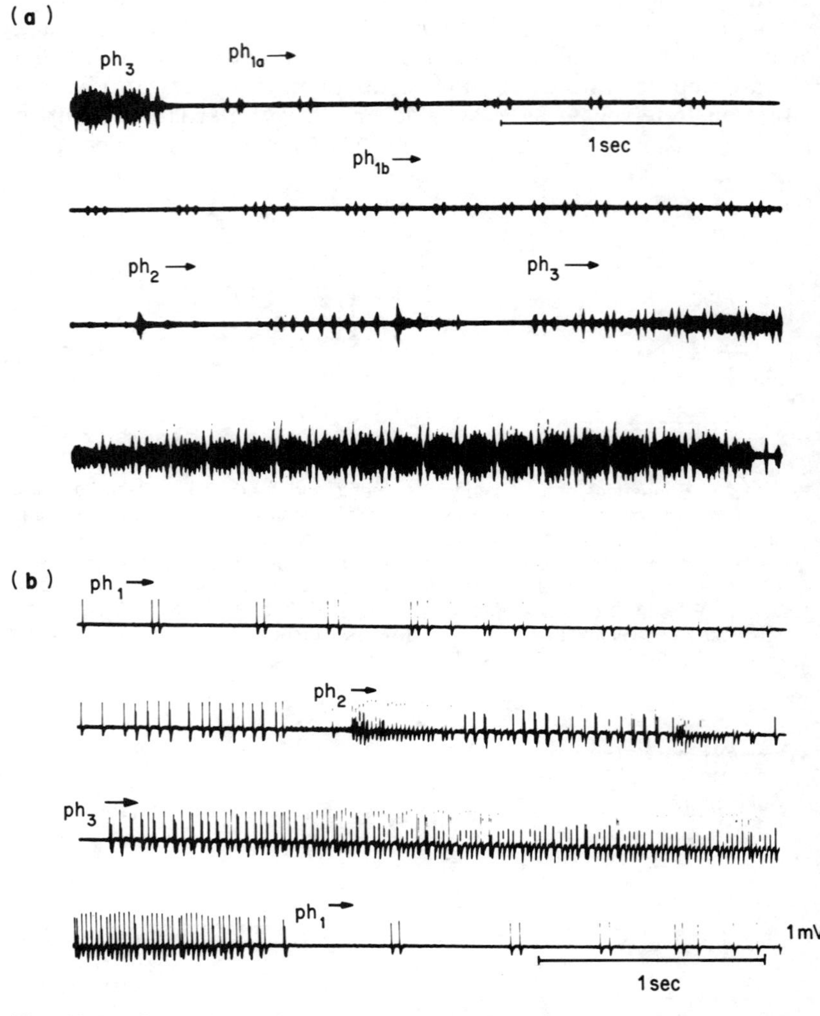


**Fig. 11.24** Courtship display in the male grasshopper *Gomphocerippus rufus*. (**a**) Song sequence (sounds caused by stridulation). (**b**) Recording of activity in a fast motor neuron innervating a leg depressor muscle. $ph_1$, phase 1 with head-shaking and stridulation (low frequency at first, higher later); $ph_2$, phase 2 with hind-leg jerking and stridulation; $ph_3$, stridulation with the syllables grouped into chirps, etc. ((**a**) From Loher, W. and Huber, F. (1966). *Symposia of the Society for Experimental Biology*, **20,** 381–400; (**b**) from Huber, F. (1975). In '*Simple*' *Nervous Systems*. (Usherwood, P. N. R. and Newth, D. R., eds) Edward Arnold, London. (By Elsner, N.))

known as a 'verse'. In the cricket *Gryllus campestris* the bursts of motor output to both the opener and closer muscles of the wings are closely synchronized (Fig. 11.22a); but in the grasshopper *Gomphocerippus rufus* this close synchronization only occurs between the motor bursts to the downstroke muscles, the upstroke muscles being activated sequentially (Fig. 11.22b).

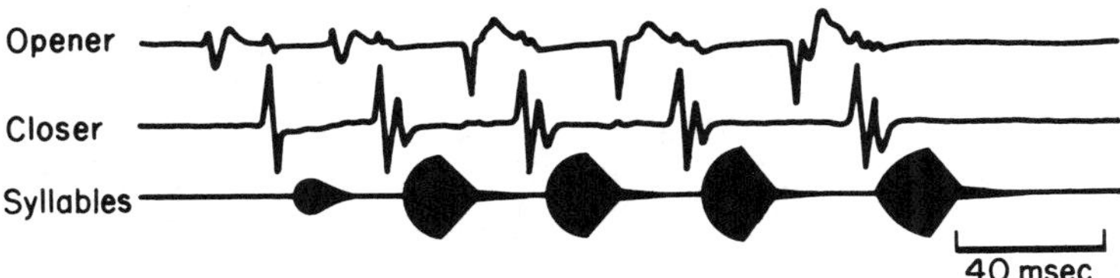


**Fig. 11.25** Recording of alternating activity in an opener and in a closer muscle, together with the syllables resulting from wing closure (bottom trace) in a single calling chirp of the cricket *Gryllus campestris*. (After Kutsch, W. (1969). *Zeitschrift für vergleichende Physiologie*, **63,** 335–78.)

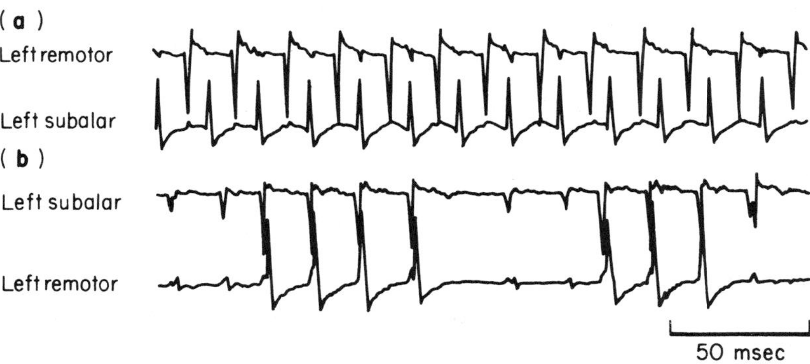


**Fig. 11.26** Recordings of activity in two muscles (remoter and subalar) in the grasshopper *Gomphocerippus rufus*. (**a**) Alternation during flight and (**b**) synchronization during stridulation. (From Elsner, N. (1968). *Zeitschrift für vergleichende Physiologie*, **60,** 308–50.)

The male of *Gryllus* has a repertoire of three songs. The calling song is emitted to attract a conspecific female. This is followed, after antennal contact between the two animals, either by the courtship song together with other mating behaviour, or by the aggressive rivalry song which leads to either fighting or flight (Fig. 11.23). The calling song consists of a group of chirps repeated at regular intervals, the courtship song of sporadic chirps and the rivalry song of almost continuous chirping with occasional pauses. The male of *Gom-*

*phocerippus* has a calling song and a courtship song. The latter is part of a courtship display which can be separated into three phases—head shaking, hind leg jerking and stridulation (Fig. 11.24), and is repeated several times.

In these songs there are at least two superimposed rhythms—there is the rhythmic movement of the wings or legs to produce the syllables of a chirp, and also the rhythm of the chirps. Current evidence indicates that these two rhythms are independent processes. The local control centres are located in the mesothoracic ganglion in crickets, but in the metathoracic ganglion in grasshoppers. In addition, in the calling song of *Gryllus* the verses are repeated rhythmically, and a slow rhythm can also be seen in the third phase of the courtship sequence of *Gomphocerippus* (Fig. 11.24).

Each motor neuron (both slow and fast) only fires once or twice during a burst (Figs 11.24 and 11.25). Figure 11.25 illustrates the alternating activity in an opener and in a closer muscle in *Gryllus* and the resulting syllables in a single chirp. In *Gomphocerippus* these same muscles alternate during flight (Fig. 11.26a) but are synchronized during stridulation (Fig. 11.26b). Also, within the innervation to any one muscle, slow motor neurons are activated before fast motor neurons and, if there is more than one fast motor neuron, they are always activated in the same sequence.

## CONCLUSION

There are thus many aspects of complex behavioural patterns which can be described in terms of their neural components. We are, however, at a very early stage in our attempt to unravel and understand behaviour in terms of the underlying neural control mechanisms. The problems are immense, particularly as different patterns of behaviour are continually interacting and competing with one another for dominance. However, there is much promise for the future. There is now a detailed knowledge of a number of simple reflexes and we are progressing in our understanding of rhythmic behaviour patterns and of more complex heterogeneous sequences. Significantly, there are signs that neurobiologists and ethologists are coming to appreciate the implications of each others work more and more, so that the field of neuroethology is one of the most exciting and rapidly expanding fields of biological research.

# *Bibliography*

A number of references are given in the legends to the figures; these have been chosen as far as possible to give a wide representation of the literature and, while some are from review articles or books, many are from original papers. The intention of the following list is primarily to provide details of introductory texts to specialized areas and books containing review articles for the student who wishes to read more about particular aspects of the subject. So much has been written that it is only possible to give a selection of the titles available and most of those listed are post-1970.


BARLOW, H. B. and FATT, P. (eds) (1978). *Vertebrate Photoreception.* Academic Press, London and New York.

BARONDES, S. H. (ed.) (1976). *Neuronal Recognition.* Chapman & Hall, London.

BENCH, R. J., PYE, A. and PYE, J. D. (eds) (1975). *Sound Reception in Mammals. Symposia of the Zoological Society of London*, 37. Academic Press, London and New York.

BENNETT M. R. (1972). *Autonomic Neuromuscular Transmission. Monographs of the Physiological Society*, 30. Cambridge University Press, Cambridge.

BOURNE, G. H. (ed.) (1972, 1973). *The Structure and Function of Muscle,* second edition. Vols 1–3. Academic Press, London and New York.

BOUDREAU, J. C. and TSUCHITANI, C. (1973). *Sensory Neurophysiology.* Van Nostrand Reinhold Co. Ltd., New York.

BROWN, A. G. (1981). *Organization in the Spinal Cord: The Anatomy and Physiology of Identified Neurones.* Springer-Verlag, Berlin.

BÜLBRING, E. and SHUBA, M. T. (eds) (1976). *Physiology of Smooth Muscle.* Raven Press.

BULLOCK, T. H. and HORRIDGE, G. A. (1965). *Structure and Function in the Nervous Systems of Invertebrates.* 2 vols. W. H. Freeman & Co. Ltd, San Francisco.

BUTCHER, L. L. (ed.) (1978). *Cholinergic-Monaminergic Interactions in the Brain.* Academic Press, London and New York.

CARTHY, J. D. and NEWELL, G. E. (eds) (1968). *Invertebrate Receptors. Symposia of the Zoological Society of London*, 23. Academic Press, London and New York.

COTTRELL, G. A. and USHERWOOD, P. N. R. (eds) (1977). *Synapses.* Blackie & Son, Glasgow.

CROSBY, E. C., HUMPHREY, T. and LAUER, E. W. (1962). *Correlative Anatomy of the Nervous System.* Macmillan, London.

DAVSON, H. (1972). *The Physiology of the Eye*, 3rd edition. Academic Press, London and New York.

DAVSON, H. (ed.) (1969–1977). *The Eye*, 2nd edition. Vols 1, 2A, 2B and 3. Academic Press, London and New York.

DAVSON, H. and GRAHAM, L. T. (eds) (1975). *The Eye*, 2nd edition. Vols 5 and 6. Academic Press, London and New York.

ECCLES, J. C. (1957). *The Physiology of Nerve Cells.* The Johns Hopkins Press, Baltimore.

ECCLES, J. C. (1969). *The Inhibitory Pathways of the Central Nervous System. The Sherrington Lectures, IX.* Liverpool University Press.

FREEMAN, R. D. (ed.) (1979) *Developmental Neurobiology of Vision. NATO Advanced Study Institutes Series. Series A: Life Sciences*, 27. Plenum Press, New York.

FRISCH, L. (ed.) (1965). *Sensory Receptors. Cold Spring Harbor Symposia on Quantitative Biology, 30.* Cold Spring Harbor Laboratory of Quantitative Biology.

GARROD, D. R. and FELDMAN, J. D. (eds) (1981). *Development in the Nervous System.* Cambridge University Press, Cambridge.

GOLDSPINK, D. F. (ed.) (1981). *The Development and Specialization of Skeletal Muscle. Society for Experimental Biology Seminar Series*, 7. Cambridge University Press, Cambridge.

GORDON, S. A. and COHEN, M. J. (eds) (1971). *Gravity and the Organism.* University of Chicago Press, Chicago.

GRANIT, R. (1970). *The Basis of Motor Control: Integrating the Activity of Muscles, Alpha and Gamma Motoneurons and their Leading Control Systems.* Academic Press, London and New York.

GRANIT, R. (1977). *The Purposive Brain.* M.I.T. Press.

GRINNELL, A. D. and BRAZIER, M. A. B. (eds) (1981). *The Regulation of Muscle Contraction. UCLA Forum in Medical Sciences Series, 22.* Academic Press, London and New York.

GUTHRIE, D. M. (1980). *Neuroethology: An Introduction.* Blackwell Scientific Publications, Oxford.

HAINSWORTH, R., KIDD, C. and LINDEN, R. J. (eds) (1979). *Cardiac Receptors.* Cambridge University Press, Cambridge.

*Handbook of Physiology. Section I. The Nervous System* (1977). (Section editors BROOKHART, J. M. and MOUNTCASTLE, V. B.) American Physiological Society.

HEYM, C. and FORSSMANN, W. G. (eds) (1981). *Techniques in Neuroanatomical Research.* Springer-Verlag, Berlin.

HORN, A. S., KORK, J and WESTERINK, B. H. C. (eds) (1979). *The Neurobiology of Dopamine.* Academic Press, London and New York.

HORRIDGE, G. A. (1968). *Interneurons.* W. H. Freeman & Co. Ltd, San Francisco.

HOYLE, G. (ed.) (1977). *Identified Neurons and Behaviour of Arthropods.* Plenum Press, New York.

HUBBARD, J. I. (1974). *The Peripheral Nervous System.* Plenum Press, New York.

*International Review of Neurobiology* (22 vols to 1981). Academic Press, London and New York.

KANDEL, E. R. (1977). *Cellular Basis of Behaviour: An Introduction to Behavioural Neurobiology*. W. H. Freeman & Co. Ltd, San Francisco.

KANDEL E. R. (1979). *Behavioural Biology of Aplysia: A Contribution to the Comparative Study of Opisthobranch Molluscs*. W. H. Freeman & Co. Ltd, San Francisco.

KARLIN, A., TENNYSON, V. M. and VOGEL, H. J. (eds) (1978). *Neuronal Information Transfer*. Academic Press, London and New York.

KATZ, B. (1966). *Nerve, Muscle and Synapse*. McGraw-Hill, Maidenhead and New York.

KRAVITZ, E. A. and TREHERNE, J. E. (eds) (1981). *Neurotransmission, Neurotransmitters and Neuromodulation*. (Special Issue of *Journal of Experimental Biology*.) Cambridge University Press, Cambridge.

LAMING, P. R. (ed.) (1981). *Brain Mechanisms of Behaviour in Lower Vertebrates. Society for Experimental Biology Seminar Series, 9*. Cambridge University Press, Cambridge.

LAVERACK, M. S. and COSENS, D. J. (eds) (1981). *Sense Organs*. Blackie and Son, Glasgow.

LISSMANN, H. W. (1950). Proprioceptors. In *Symposia of the Society for Experimental Biology*, **4**, 34–59. Cambridge University Press, Cambridge.

LUDEL, J. (1978). *Introduction to Sensory Processes*. W. H. Freeman & Co. Ltd, San Francisco.

LUND, R. D. (1978). *Development and Plasticity of the Brain: An Introduction*, 3rd edition. Oxford University Press, Oxford.

MANNING, A. (1979). *An Introduction to Animal Behaviour*, 3rd edition. Edward Arnold, London.

MARKS, L. E. (1978). *The Unity of the Senses: Interrelations among the Modalities*. Academic Press, London and New York.

MATTHEWS, P. B. C. (1972). *Mammalian Muscle Receptors and their Central Actions*. Edward Arnold, London and New York.

MCGEER, P. L., ECCLES, J. C. and MCGEER, E. G. (1978). *Molecular Neurobiology of the Mammalian Brain*. Plenum Press, New York.

MATZKE, H. A. (1979). *Synopsis of Neuroanatomy*, 3rd edition. Oxford University Press, Oxford.

MILL, P. J. (ed.) (1976). *Structure and Function of Proprioceptors in the Invertebrates*. Chapman & Hall, London.

MILL, P. J. (ed.) (1978). *Physiology of Annelids*. Academic Press, London and New York.

NAUNTON, R. F. and FERNÁNDEZ, C. (eds) (1978). *Evoked Electrical Activity in the Auditory Nervous System*. Academic Press, London and New York.

NEWMAN, P. P. (1974). *Visceral Afferent Functions of the Nervous System*. Edward Arnold, London.

PEARSON, R. and PEARSON, L. (1976). *The Vertebrate Brain*. Academic Press, London and New York.

POPPER, A. N. and FAY, R. R. (1980). *Comparative Studies of Hearing in Vertebrates*. Springer-Verlag, Berlin.

PORTER, R. (ed.) (1978). *Studies in Neurophysiology*. Cambridge University Press, Cambridge.

PRASAD, K. N. (1980). *Regulation of Differentiation in Mammalian Nerve Cells*. Plenum Press, New York.

PYCOCK, C. J. and TABERNER, P. V. (1980). *Central Neurotransmitter Turnover*. Croom Helm, London.

ROBERTS, A. and BUSH, B. M. H. (eds) (1981). *Neurones without Impulses: Their Significance for Vertebrate and Invertebrate Nervous Systems. Society for Experimental Biology Seminar Series, 6*. Cambridge University Press, Cambridge.

ROCKSTEIN, M. (ed.) (1974). *Physiology of Insecta,* 2nd edition. Academic Press, London and New York.

RODIECK, R. W. (1974). *The Vertebrate Retina: Principles of Structure and Function.* W. H. Freeman & Co. Ltd, San Francisco.

SALÁNKI, J. (ed.) (1981). *Neurobiology of Invertebrates.* Pergamon Press, Oxford.

*Scientific American Reprints. The Brain.* (1979). W. H. Freeman & Co. Ltd, San Francisco.

SHEPHERD, G. M. (1979). *The Synaptic Organization of the Brain,* 2nd edition. Oxford University Press, Oxford.

SPEARMAN, R. I. C. and RILEY, P. A. (1980). *The Skin of Vertebrates. Linnean Society Symposium*, 9. Academic Press, London.

S-RÓZZA, K. (ed.) (1981). *Neurotransmitters in Invertebrates.* Pergamon Press, Oxford.

STEIN, D. G., ROSEN, J. J. and BUTTERS, N. (eds) (1974). *Plasticity and Recovery in the Central Nervous System.* Academic Press, London and New York.

STEIN, R. B., PEARSON, K. G., SMITH, R. S. and REDFORD, J. B. (eds) (1977). *The Control of Posture and Locomotion. Advances in Behavioural Biology*, 7. Plenum Press, New York.

STILES, W. S. (1978). *Mechanisms of Colour Vision.* Academic Press, London and New York.

STODDART, D. M. (ed.) (1980). *Olfaction in Mammals. Symposia of the Zoological Society of London*, 45. Academic Press, London and New York.

SZABÓ, T. and CZEH, C. (eds) (1981). *Sensory Physiology of Aquatic Lower Vertebrates.* Pergamon Press, Oxford.

TAVOLGA, W. N. (ed.) (1976). *Sound Reception in Fishes.* Academic Press, London and New York.

TREGEAR, R. T. (ed.) (1977). *Insect Flight Muscle.* Elsevier North-Holland, Netherlands.

TREHERNE, J. E. and BEAMENT, J. W. L. (eds) (1965). *The Physiology of the Insect Central Nervous System.* Academic Press, London and New York.

TRIGGLE, D. J. (1971). *Neurotransmitter-Receptor Interactions.* Academic Press, London and New York.

TRIGGLE, D. J. and TRIGGLE, C. R. (eds) (1976). *Chemical Pharmacology of the Synapse.* Academic Press, London and New York.

UEHARA, Y., CAMPBELL, G. R. and BURNSTOCK, G. (1976). *Muscle and its Innervation: An Atlas of Fine Structure.* Edward Arnold, London.

USHERWOOD, P. N. R. (ed.) (1975). *Insect Muscle.* Academic Press, London and New York.

USHERWOOD, P. N. R. and NEWTH, D. R. (eds) (1975). *'Simple' Nervous Systems.* Edward Arnold, London.

UTTLEY, A. M. (1979). *Information Transmission in the Nervous System.* Academic Press, London and New York.

VRBOVÁ, G., GORDAN, T. and JONES, R. (1978). *Nerve-Muscle Interaction.* Chapman & Hall, London.

WIERSMA, C. A. G. (ed.) (1967). *Invertebrate Nervous Systems: Their Significance for Mammalian Neurophysiology.* University of Chicago Press, Chicago.

WILLIS, W. D. (1979). *Sensory Mechanisms of the Spinal Cord.* John Wiley and Sons, New York.

WOLKEN, J. J. (1975). *Photoprocesses, Photoreceptors, and Evolution.* Academic Press, London and New York.

WOOLDRIDGE, D. E. (1979). *Sensory Processing in the Brain: An Exercise in Neuroconnective Modeling.* John Wiley and Sons, New York.

YOST, W. A. and NIELSON, D. W. (1977). *Fundamentals of Hearing.* Holt-Saunders, Sussex.

# Index